TARGET

UPSC - CMS

Concise and Illustrated Solutions to Combined Medical Services Question Bank (2018-2016)

Kamal KV MBBS, MS (Orthopedics)
Ex-Senior Resident: Safdarjung, ESI: Okhla, Fortis: Noida
Ponseti and Ilizarov Techniques Fellow (Akola)
Madhya Pradesh – Indian Orthopedic Association
Hand Surgery Fellow (Pune), Maharashtra, India

PEEPEE PUBLISHERS AND DISTRIBUTORS (P) LTD.®

Target UPSC - CMS

Published by
Pawaninder P. Vij and Anupam Vij

Peepee Publishers and Distributors (P) Ltd.
Head Office: 160, Shakti Vihar, Pitam Pura
Delhi-110034 (India)

Correspondence Address:
7/31, First Floor, Ansari Road, Daryaganj
New Delhi-110002 (India)
Ph: 41512412, 23246245, 9811156083
e-mail: peepee160@yahoo.co.in
e-mail: peepee160@gmail.com
www.peepeepub.com

First Edition: 2019

ISBN : 978-81-8445-261-7

Dedication

This title is dedicated to all the (past and present) students of **drkamalkv's classes for FMGE and DNB**.

It's their faith and support, which is helping me in surviving this competitive world of coaching.

I started my classes in December 2011, and by God's grace and students support, I am still going on, singly.

I teach all the subjects singly (students call it **1-Man Army**) and theoretically it seems very difficult to teach all subjects singly, but the unconditional support and faith of my dear students had made it practically possible.

Hope this title will serve its purpose.

drkamalkv

Contact:
Cell and WhatsApp: 84 7000 4333
Website: www.**drkamalkvgroup**.co.in
E-mail & Skype-id: **drkamalkvgroup**@gmail.com
Facebook, WeChat, Youtube, Twitter and Instagram: **drkamalkvgroup**

Remembering Our Brave Martyrs

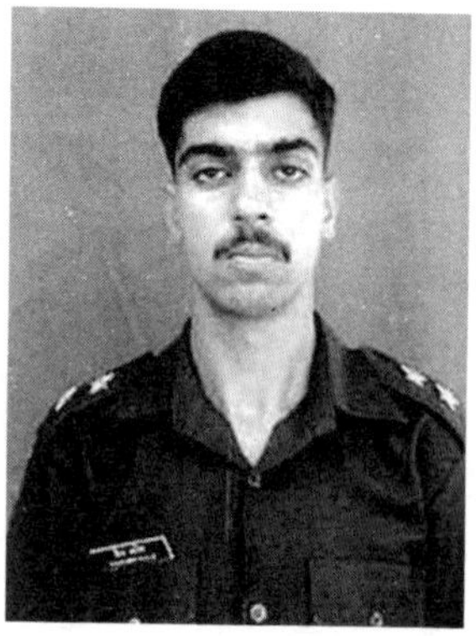

Lt Saurabh Kalia was selected for the Indian Military Academy, in August 1997 through Combined Defence Services and was commissioned on 12 December, 1998. His first posting was in the 4th battalion Jat Regiment (4 Jat) in the Kargil Sector. Saurabh arrived there in mid-January 1999 after reporting at the Jat Regimental Centre, Bareilly on 31 December, 1998.

In the first two weeks of May 1999, several patrols were conducted in the Kaksar Langpa area of Kargil district to check whether the snow had retreated enough for the summer positions to be re-occupied. Lt Saurabh Kalia was the first Indian army officer to observe and report large-scale intrusion of Pakistani army and foreign mercenaries on the Indian side of the Line of Control (LoC) in Kargil. He assumed guard of "Bajrang Post" at 13,000–14,000 feet to check infiltration in the Kaksar area.

On 15 May, 1999 Lt Saurabh Kalia and five other soldiers – Sepoys Arjun Ram, Bhanwar Lal Bagaria, Bhika Ram, Moola Ram and Naresh Singh of the 4 Jat Regiment had gone for a routine patrol of the Bajrang Post in the Kaksar sector in the rugged, treeless Ladakh mountains. After a continuous cross-fire with Pakistani armed forces from across the LOC, he and his troops ran out of ammunition. They were finally encircled by a platoon of Pakistani rangers and captured alive before Indian reinforcements could reach them. No trace of the patrol was left, meanwhile Radio Skardu of Pakistan announced that Captain Saurabh Kalia had been captured by Pakistani troops. It was after this that India discovered hundreds of guerillas had established fortified positions on the peaks of the hills deep inside the Indian side of the Line of Control, with sophisticated equipment and supply lines back to Pakistan Controlled Kashmir.

Lt Saurabh Kalia and his men were in captivity from 15 May, 1999 – 7 June, 1999 (over twenty-two days), and subjected to torture as evident from injuries to their bodies when they were handed over by the Pakistani army on 9 June, 1999. Post mortem examinations revealed that the Pakistanis had tortured their prisoners by burning their bodies with cigarettes, piercing the ear-drums with hot rods, puncturing eyes before removing them, breaking most of their teeth and bones, fracturing their skulls, cutting the lips, chipping of nose, chopping off limbs and private organs of the soldiers, and finally shooting them dead, as evidenced by bullet wounds to the temple. The post mortem also confirmed the injuries were inflicted antemortem (before death).

On 9 June, 1999, Dr N. K. Kalia received the body of his son, Lt Saurabh Kalia, handed over by the Pakistani army to Indian army commanders at the Kargil sector, with evidence of torture.

I am a son of an ex-army man (my father was in Army Education Corps) and I feel, it's my duty to highlight the supreme sacrifices made by our Indian soldiers. One can make donations to army welfare fund by logging onto **www.pmindia.gov.in.**

Preface

The need of a concise and illustrated title for UPSC – CMS exam was felt since long. Most of the available titles in the market are explanatory only and that too detailed, which students find difficult to revise in the end. I have tried to keep the explanation to a minimum but had tried to put plenty of illustrations and tables to simplify the presentation.

Correlation of images with theory helps in understanding the text and also aids in remembering the concept for long. So I can summarize my title as "**Target UPSC–CMS Concise and Illustrated Solutions to Combined Medical Services Question Bank (2018–2016)**".

For the first edition, I am restricting myself to only 3 years of question papers (2016, 2017 and 2018–both sessions).

As I always say, students are the best judge of an author's work. And I personally feel, there is always some room left for further improvement. So, I expect my dear students to share their valuable feedbacks regarding betterment of this text in subsequent editions.

Despite my best efforts, some errors must have crept in. I request dear readers to please forward the same to me.

Hope this title will serve its purpose.

drkamalkv

Contact:
Cell and WhatsApp: 84 7000 4333
Website: www.**drkamalkvgroup**.co.in
E-mail and Skype-id: **drkamalkvgroup**@gmail.com
Facebook, WeChat, Youtube, Twitter and Instagram: **drkamalkvgroup**

Acknowledgements

All thanks to Almighty (for imparting me with this passion of writing books and teaching), to my parents (for imparting qualities of a good human being), my brothers and sister (for giving me some wonderful memories of childhood), my wife (for supporting me in all my endeavours), my daughters (for allowing me to use their share of time with my students) and my dear students (for accepting my all titles with equal enthusiasm and also, who made me academically strong, to an extent).

Thanks are due for everyone behind this project, from the publication house.

drkamalkv

Contact:
Cell and WhatsApp: 84 7000 4333
Website: www.**drkamalkvgroup**.co.in
E-mail and Skype-id: **drkamalkvgroup**@gmail.com
Facebook, WeChat, Youtube, Twitter and Instagram: **drkamalkvgroup**

Contents

CHAPTER

1 CMS EXAMINATION 2018

PAPER - 2

1. **What are the characteristics of ideal health indicators?**
   (a) They should be valid, reliable, sensitive, specific, feasible and relevant
   (b) They should be mainly valid, reliable and sensitive but need not be specific
   (c) They should be mainly valid, reliable and feasible but need not be sensitive
   (d) They should be mainly valid, reliable and relevant but need not be feasible

EXPLANATION

An **ideal health indicator** should be valid, reliable, sensitive, specific, feasible and relevant.

- Valid: it must measure what it is supposed to measure.
- Reliable: the answer should be the same if measured by different people.
- Sensitive: they should show variations in different situations.

Ans. (A) i.e., They should be valid, reliable, sensitive, specific, feasible and relevant.

2. **Which one of the following statements regarding predictive value of a positive test is true?**
   (a) It does not tell about diagnostic power of test
   (b) The more prevalent the disease, the less accurate the test is
   (c) It tells the probability that a patient with positive test has the disease in question
   (d) It tells the probability that a patient with positive test does not have the disease in question

EXPLANATION

Predictive value

- Positive predictive value is the probability that subjects with a positive screening test truly have the disease.
- Negative predictive value is the probability that subjects with a negative screening test truly don't have the disease.

Ans. (C) i.e., It tells the probability that a patient with positive test has the disease in question.

3. **The yield of a screening test CAN NOT be increased by which of the following?**

(a) Including entire population
(b) Including high risk population
(c) Improved sensitivity
(d) Improved specificity

EXPLANATION

Yield of a screening test can be improved by including the entire population rather than limiting to high risk population.

Ans. (B) i.e., Including high risk population

4. **Which one of the following statements regarding the growth chart is NOT true?**

(a) It is used as a tool for growth monitoring and diagnosis

(b) It is used for planning and policy making

(c) It is used as tool for action against the Anganwadi worker

(d) It is used as tool for teaching and evaluation of effectiveness of programme

EXPLANATION

The assessment of growth by objective anthropometric methods of weight, length/height, and body mass index (BMI) is crucial in child care to assess the nutritional status and for the identification of growth failure. Reference data are central to growth monitoring and they help doctors, health care workers, and policymakers to diagnose under nutrition, overweight and obesity, and other growth related and endocrine conditions. Thus the growth chart is a "passport' to child health care.

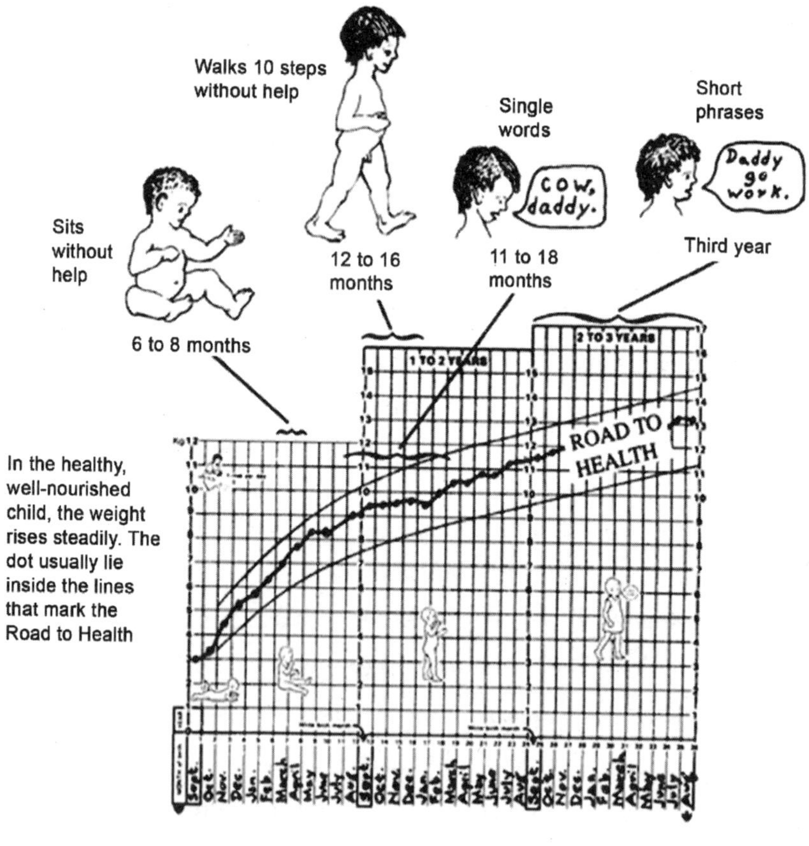

Ans. (C) i.e., It is used as tool for action against the Anganwadi worker

5. **Flattening of the growth curve in the growth chart signifies:**

(a) Child is on a healthy path

(b) Child is severely malnourished

(c) Child is showing signs of growth failure

(d) Child does not need special care

EXPLANATION

Abnormal flattening or falling of child weight's curve signals growth failure which is an early indicator of PEM (protein energy malnutrition).

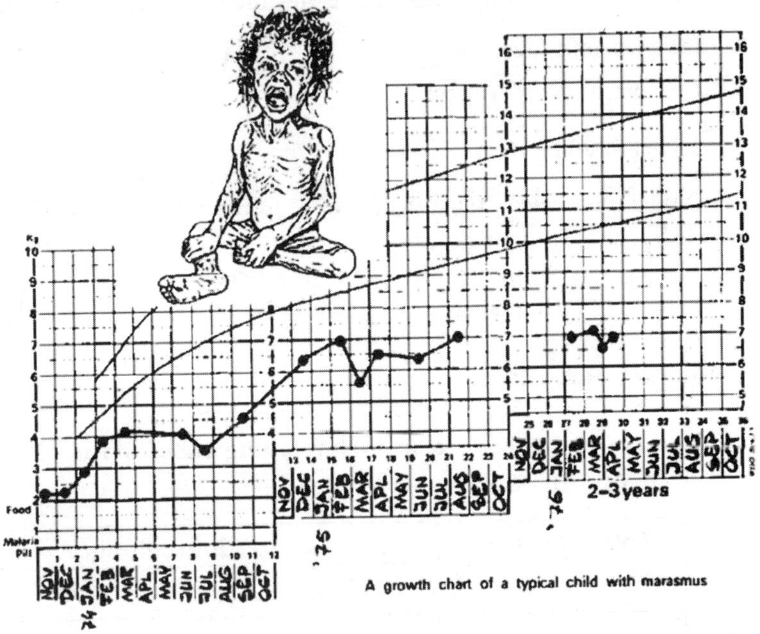

A growth chart of a typical child with marasmus

Ans. (C) i.e., Child is showing signs of growth failure

6. A well of contaminated water resulted in an outbreak of diarrhoea in a community. Which type of epidemic will this exposure present with?

1. Propagated epidemic
2. Common source – continuous exposure
3. Common source – point exposure

Select the correct answer using the codes given below:

(a) 1 and 2 only (b) 3 only (c) 1, 2 and 3 (d) 2 only

EXPLANATION

Continuing common Source outbreak

- As with the point source outbreak, a group of people are exposed to a single noxious influence. But here the exposure continues over a longer time (e.g., a contaminated water supply that doesn't get fixed), so the outbreak persists for longer.
- The relatively abrupt beginning of the out-break suggests that many people were exposed simultaneously, rather than it spreading via transmission from one case to another. The fact that no cases arise beyond one incubation period following the termination of the exposure also supports this conclusion.

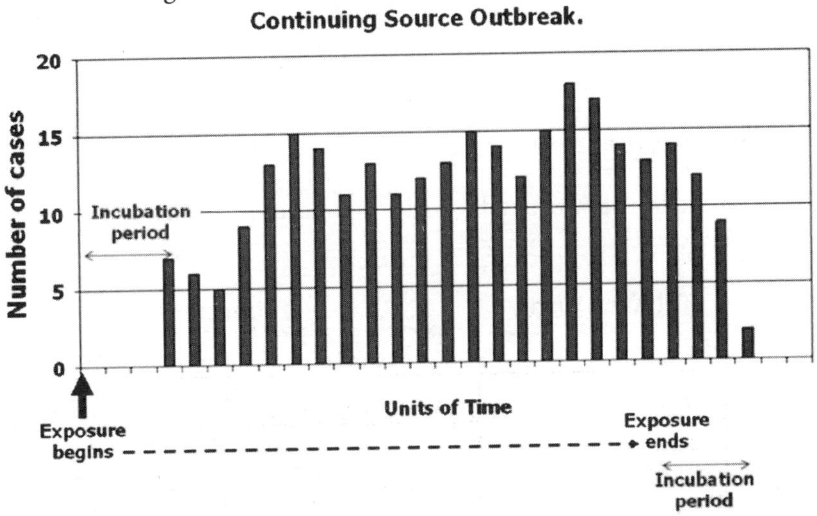

Ans. (D) i.e., 2 only

7. **Which one of the following experiments/trials is NOT a part of non randomized trial?**

(a) Uncontrolled trial
(b) Risk factor trial
(c) Natural experiment
(d) Before and after comparison studies

EXPLANATION

Non randomized trial/NRT is a clinical trial in which the participants are not assigned by chance to different treatment groups. Participants may choose which group they want to be in, or they may be assigned to the groups by the researchers. These NRT are uncontrolled trials, natural experiments & before and after trials.

Ans. (B) i.e., Risk factor trial

8. **What is the relative risk of developing tuberculosis among tobacco users as per the information given below?**

Tobacco user	Tuberculosis		Total
	Yes	No	
Yes	40	80	120
No	10	70	80
Total	50	150	200

(a) 0.48
(b) 1.33
(c) 2.67
(d) 3.90

EXPLANATION

Relative risk/risk ratio is the ratio of incidence of the disease among exposed and the incidence of the disease among unexposed (RR = IE/IO)

IE is calculated as number of subjects developing the disease out of the total exposed.

IE = 40/120 = 0.333

IO is calculated as number of subjects developing the disease out of the total unexposed.

IO = 10/80 = 0.125

RR = 0.333/0.125 = 2.664

Relative Risk Calculation

$$RR = \frac{a/(a+b)}{c/(c+d)}$$ where

Exposure	Cancer ✔	Cancer ✘
✔	a	b
✘	c	d

Ans. (C) i.e., 2.67

9. **What is the attributable risk of tobacco for developing tuberculosis as per the information given below?**

Tobacco user	Tuberculosis		Total
	Present	Absent	
Yes	40	80	120
No	10	70	80
Total	50	150	200

(a) 50.5%
(b) 62.5%
(c) 70.6%
(d) 80.6%

EXPLANATION

Attributable risk/AR is the ratio of risk difference/RD and the incidence of the disease among exposed, often expressed as percentage.

AR = RD/IE

RD = IE - IO

IE is calculated as number of subjects developing the disease out of the total exposed.

IE = 40/120 = 0.333

IO is calculated as number of subjects developing the disease out of the total unexposed.

IO = 10/80 = 0.125

RD = IE – IO = 0.208

AR = 0.208/0.333 = 62.46%

$$AR\% = \frac{CI_{exposed} - CI_{unexposed}}{CI_{exposed}} \times 100$$

$$AR\% = \frac{\frac{A}{A+B} - \frac{C}{C+D}}{\frac{A}{A+B}} \times 100$$

$$AR\% = \frac{\frac{200}{1400} - \frac{100}{1300}}{\frac{200}{1400}} \times 100$$

AR% = 46%

Ans. (B) i.e., 62.5%

2018

10. What is the sensitivity of EEG for detecting brain tumours as per the information given below?

EEG Result	Brain Tumour Absent	Brain Tumour Present
Positive	54,000	36
Negative	3,06,000	4
Total	3,60,000	40

(a) 90% (b) 85% (c) 0.07% (d) 99.99%

EXPLANATION

Sensitivity is the ability of a test to correctly identify those having the disease, i.e. true positives (% of the disease persons, showing the test result positive)

Sensitivity = a × 100/a + c

Where a is number of patients showing positive test in the presence of disease and c is number of patients showing test negative in the presence of disease (so a+c is the total number of the subjects with disease).

Sensitivity = 36000/40 = 90%

Ans. (A) i.e., 90%

11. Which sign is most important in deciding severe pneumonia in a child?

(a) Fast breathing (b) Nasal flaring (c) Chest indrawing (d) Grunting

EXPLANATION

Signs of serious illness (severe pneumonia) include:

- Chest indrawing: the inferior thoracic wall depresses on inspiration as the superior abdomen expands
- Fast breathing (may be absent if child is exhausted)
- Cyanosis (lips, oral mucosa, fingernails) or $SpO_2 < 90\%$
- Nasal flaring
- Altered consciousness (child is abnormally sleepy or difficult to wake)
- Stridor (hoarse noise on inspiration)
- Grunting (a short repetitive noise produced by a partial closure of the vocal cords) on expiration
- Refusal to drink or feed
- Children under 2 months
- Severe malnutrition

Ans. (C) i.e., Chest indrawing

2018

12. Varicella Zoster Immunoglobulin (VZIG) is NOT recommended for which of the exposed susceptible individuals?

(a) Newborn (b) HIV/AIDS positive (c) Healthy sibling (d) Pregnant women

EXPLANATION

VZIG is given for those, who are at risk such as young close contacts. High risk contacts are those with impaired immunity, malignant disease, newborn and pregnant mother contacts.

Ans. (C) i.e., Healthy sibling

13. Carriers of avirulent organism are called:

(a) Incubatory carriers (b) Convalescent carriers (c) Healthy carrier (d) Pseudo carriers

EXPLANATION

Carriers of avirulent organisms are called pseudo carriers. They are not important epidemiologically.

Ans. (D) i.e., Healthy carrier

14. A cohort study was conducted among 200 men aged 20–30 years in Rampur village. Out of 200, 120 men were tobacco users and rest 80 didn't take any form of tobacco. At the end of one year, 40 men among tobacco users and 10 men among non tobacco users developed tuberculosis. The incidence of tuberculosis among tobacco users is:

(a) 12.5 per 100 men/year (b) 25.0 per 100 men/year
(c) 30.0 per 100 men/year (d) 33.3 per 100 men/year

EXPLANATION

Incidence rate of the disease among exposed =

$$\frac{\text{Number of persons developing the disease after exposure (a)} \times 1000}{\text{Total number of persons exposed/at risk (a + b)}}$$

Incidence among tobacco users = 40 × 1000/120 = 33.3 per 100 men/year

Cohort study — Cumulative incidence

Risk or protection factor	DIS	NDIS	
Exposure	A	B	A+B
Non exposure	C	D	C+D
	A+C	B+D	A+B+C+D

Re = A/(A + B)

Ro = C/(C + D)

RR = Re/Ro

ARR = Re – Ro

RRR = (Re – Ro)/Ro

ExpAR = (RR – 1)/RR

PopAR = (Prev – Re)/Prev.

Ans. (D) i.e., 33.3 per 100 men/year

15. The data regarding two exposures A and B, associated with a disease X in a community is given below:

	Exposure A	Exposure B
Relative risk	5	10
Attributable risk	80%	90%
Population attributable risk	70%	50%

Which one of the following assertions and the reasons given is correct?

(a) Preference to control exposure B as it has a higher relative risk

(b) Preference to control exposure A, because it has a higher population attributable risk

(c) Preference to control exposure B, because it has a higher attributable risk

(d) Cannot decide, as the precedence of exposure in the community has not been mentioned

EXPLANATION

Attributable Risk/AR suggests the amount of disease that might be eliminated, if exposure/risk factor is controlled. In other words, higher the AR, greater the reduction in the incidence of the disease by elimination of that risk factor.

Ans. (C) i.e., Preference to control exposure B, because it has a higher attributable risk

16. Which of the following types of study designs will be most appropriate to find out the association between mobile phone radiation exposure and cancer?

(a) Cross sectional

(b) Case control

(c) Single arm interventional

(d) Case series

EXPLANATION

Case control studies are often used to identify factors that may contribute to a medical condition by comparing subjects who have that condition/disease (the "cases") with patients who do not have the condition/disease but are otherwise similar (the "controls"). They require fewer resources but provide less evidence for causal inference than a randomized controlled trial. We only get odds ratio from a case control study which measure the strength of the association between the disease and the suspected factor.

2018

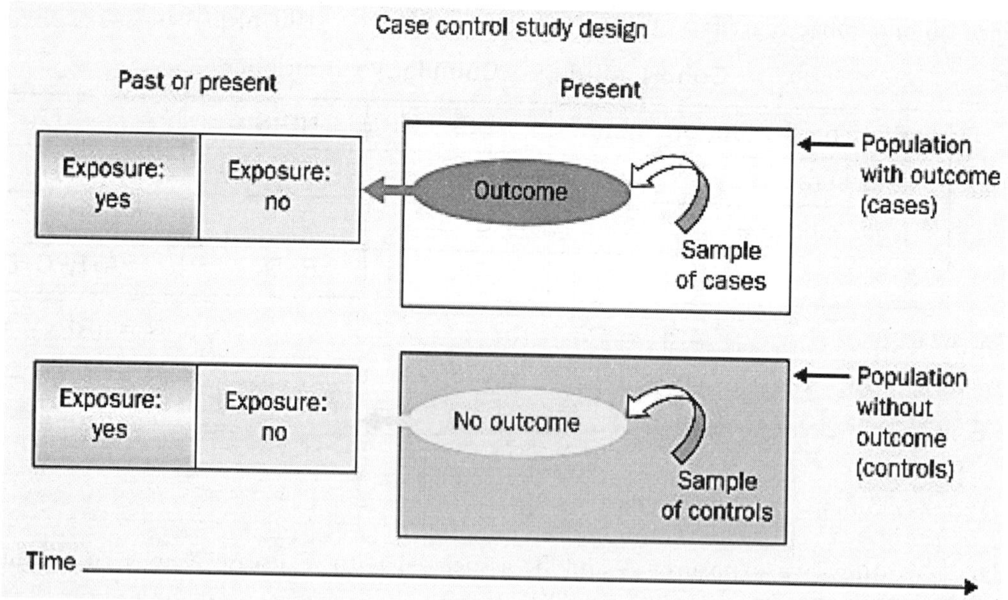

Ans. (B) i.e., Case control

2018

17. The villages A and B have the following age compositions:

Age (years)	Mid year population (Village A)	Mid year population (Village B)
0–4	8000	4000
5–9	4000	2000
10–19	5000	3000
20–39	7000	8000
40–59	6000	6000
60 and above	7000	10000

Which of the following is the best indicator for comparing the death rates of these two villages?

(a) Crude death rate
(b) Age standardized death rate
(c) Specific death rate
(d) Proportional mortality rate

EXPLANATION

The age standardized mortality rate is a weighted average of the age specific mortality rates per 100,000 persons, where the weights are the proportions of persons in the corresponding age groups of the WHO standard population.

Ans. (B) i.e., Age standardized death rate

18. Which of the following is/are suggested by rising incidence rates of any disease?

1. Need for a new disease control programme
2. Improvement in reporting practices
3. Change in the etiology of the disease

Select the correct answer using the codes given below:

(a) 1 and 3 only (b) 1 only (c) 1, 2 and 3 (d) 2 and 3 only

EXPLANATION

Incidence in epidemiology is a measure of the **probability** of occurrence of a given medical condition in a population within a specified period of time. Although sometimes loosely expressed simply as the number of new cases during some time period, it is better expressed as a proportion or a rate with a denominator. Need of a new disease control programme (suggest that previous programmes are not efficient in preventing occurrence of new cases), better reporting of cases (new cases would be reported) and change in etiology of the disease (number of new cases would increase) hints towards an increase in incidence rates.

Ans. (C) i.e., 1, 2 and 3

19. **What constitutes the denominator in 'Total Dependency Ratio'?**

(a) Population 15–45 years of age
(b) Mid year population
(c) Population 15–64 years of age
(d) Population less than 14 and more than 65 years of age

EXPLANATION

In economics, geography, demography and sociology, the **dependency ratio** is an age **population ratio** of those typically not in the labor force (the dependent part ages 0 to 14 and 65+) and those typically in the labor force (the productive part ages 15 to 64). It is used to measure the pressure on productive **population**.

$$\text{Total (Age) Dependency Ratio} = \frac{(\text{Population 0-14} + \text{Population 64>})}{\text{Working age population 15-64}} \times 100$$

$$\text{Child Dependency Ratio} = \frac{\text{Population 0-14}}{\text{Working age population 15-64}} \times 100$$

$$\text{Old Age Dependency Ratio} = \frac{\text{Population 64>}}{\text{Working age population 15-64}} \times 100$$

Ans. (C) i.e., Population 15–64 years of age

20. **A pregnant woman in 2nd trimester of pregnancy from North Eastern State has been diagnosed with uncomplicated *P. falciparum*. She should be treated with:**

(a) Artemether and Lumefantrine
(b) Artesunate and Sulphadoxine
(c) Artesunate, Sulphadoxine and Pyrimethamine
(d) Chlorine and Primaquine

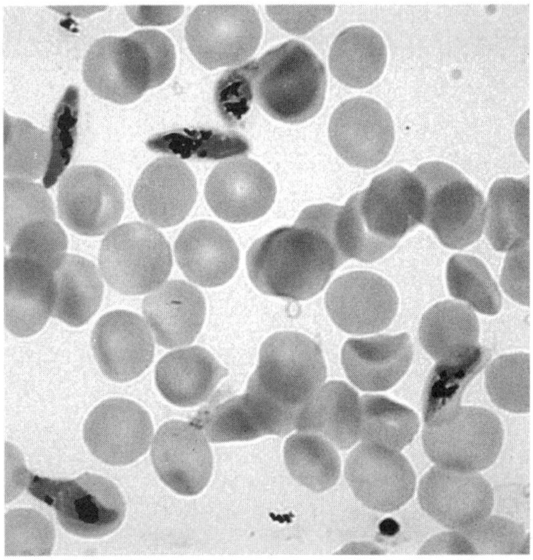

EXPLANATION

For ***pregnant*** women diagnosed with uncomplicated malaria caused by chloroquine resistant P. ***falciparum*** infection, women in the second and third trimesters can be treated with artemether lumfantrine, and for all trimesters, mefloquine or a combination of quinine sulfate and clindamycin is recommended.

Ans. (A) i.e., Artemether and Lumefantrine

21. By which one of the following studies can relative risk be best calculated?

(a) Cohort study
(b) Correlation study
(c) Case control study
(d) Randomised control trial

EXPLANATION

In cohort study, strength of association is estimated by relative risk & attributable risk.

Ans. (A) i.e., Cohort study

22. Orthotolidine (OT) test is done for determining residual free chlorine quantitatively and qualitatively. What is the colour of the solution after adding OT which indicates presence of free chlorine?

(a) Red (b) Yellow (c) Blue (d) Green

EXPLANATION

Orthotolidine (OT) test

- Enables Total, free and combined chlorine in water to be determined with speed and accuracy.
- The reagent is 'analytical grade Orthotolidine', dissolved in 10% solution of HCl.
- When this reagent is added to the water containing chlorine, it turns yellow.

Ans. (B) i.e., Yellow

23. Consider the following in respect of Navjat Shishu Suraksha Karyakram (NSSK):

1. **It is a programme aimed to train health personnel in basic newborn care and resuscitation**
2. **It addresses care at birth issue (i.e prevention of hypothermia, prevention of infection, early initiation of breastfeeding and basic newborn resuscitation)**
3. **The objective is to have a trained health person in basic newborn care and resuscitation unit at every delivery point**

Which of the statements given above are correct?

(a) 1 and 2 only (b) 1 and 3 only (c) 1, 2 and 3 (d) 2 and 3 only

EXPLANATION

"Navjaat Shishu Suraksha Karyakram" a new programme on Basic Newborn Care and Resuscitation, is being launched by the Ministry of Health and Family Welfare to address important interventions of care at birth i.e. Prevention of Hypothermia, Prevention of Infection, Early initiation of Breast feeding and Basic Newborn Resuscitation. Newborn care and resuscitation is an important starting point for any neonatal program that is required to ensure the best possible start in life. The objective of this new initiative is to have persons trained in Basic newborn care and resuscitation available at every delivery. The implementation of this programme will help prevent a significant number of newborn deaths and ensure newborn survival.

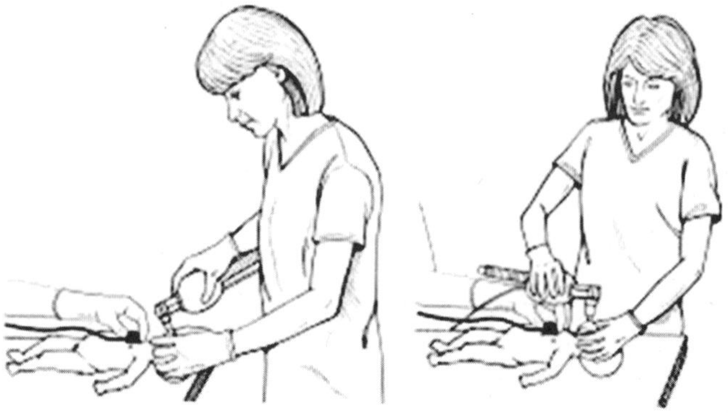

Ans. (C) i.e., 1, 2 and 3

24. **The most important indicator for assessment of impact in Salt Iodization Programme is:**

(a) Testing Iodine content of salt at consumer level
(b) Testing Iodine content of salt at production level
(c) Testing median urinary Iodine excretion
(d) Testing serum Iodine levels

EXPLANATION

The iodization of salt used in households and food processing is the most effective and sustainable strategy for IDD (iodine deficiency disorder) control. The impact of salt iodization programmes is best assessed through the measurement of urinary **iodine concentrations** (UIC) in populations.

Ans. (C) i.e., Testing median urinary Iodine excretion

25. **Caisson's disease is usually seen in which group of workers?**

(a) Cotton field agricultural workers
(b) Construction workers under sea level
(c) Workers in manufacture of gas
(d) Workers in radiation units

EXPLANATION

Decompression sickness (DCS; also known as **divers' disease, the bends, aerobullosis,** or **caisson disease**) describes a condition arising from dissolved gases coming out of solution into bubbles inside the body on depressurisation. DCS most commonly refers to problems arising from underwater diving decompression (i.e., during ascent), but may be experienced in other depressurisation events such as emerging from a caisson, flying in an unpressurised aircraft at altitude, and extravehicular activity from spacecraft. DCS and arterial gas embolism are collectively referred to as decompression illness.

Ans. (B) i.e., Construction workers under sea level

26. **These toxic effects like abdominal colic, obstinate constipation, loss of appetite, anaemia, stippling of red cells and blue line on gums are due to exposure to:**

(a) Carbon monoxide (b) Asbestos (c) Lead (d) Radiation

EXPLANATION

Chronic lead poisoning usually presents with symptoms affecting multiple systems, but is associated with three main types of symptoms: gastrointestinal, neuromuscular, and neurological. Signs of chronic exposure include loss of short term memory or concentration, depression, nausea, abdominal pain, loss of coordination, and numbness and tingling in the extremities. Fatigue, problems with sleep, headaches, stupor, slurred speech, and anemia are also found in chronic lead poisoning. A "lead hue" of the skin with pallor and/or lividity is another feature. A blue line along the gum with bluish black edging to the teeth, known as a Burton line, is another indication of chronic lead poisoning.

Ans. (C) i.e., Lead

27. **Which one of the following conditions can be screened during neonatal screening by biochemical tests?**

(a) Congenital dislocation of hip
(b) Congenital hypothyroidism
(c) Chromosomal abnormalities
(d) Congenital rubella

EXPLANATION

Newborn screening (NS) for congenital hypothyroidism (CH) is one of the major achievements in preventive medicine. Most neonates born with CH have normal appearance and no detectable physical signs. Hypothyroidism in the newborn period is almost always overlooked, and delayed diagnosis leads to the most severe outcome of CH, mental retardation, emphasizing the importance of NS. Blood spot thyroid stimulating hormone (TSH) or thyroxine (T4) or both can be used for CH screening.

Ans. (B) i.e., Congenital hypothyroidism

28. **Which of the following is NOT a mass approach in health communication?**

(a) Folk methods (b) Role play (c) Posters (d) Health exhibition

EXPLANATION

Mass approach

- **Meant to educate the whole community**
- Useful in transmitting messages to people even in remotest places
- Number of people reached is in millions
- High returns for the time and money involved
- One way communication
- Generally inadequate in changing behavior
- Useful for creating a political will in favor of health, raising health consciousness of people

Ans. (B) i.e., Role play

29. **Which of the following are non modifiable risk factors for hypertension?**

1. Age 2. Sex 3. Genetic factors

Select the correct answer using the code given below:

(a) 1 only (b) 1 and 2 only (c) 1, 2 and 3 (d) 2 and 3 only

EXPLANATION

Non modifiable risk factors of hypertension include age, gender, genetic factors (if both the parents are hypertensive, offspring have 45% possibility of developing HTN and if both the parents are normotensive, offspring have 3% possibility of developing HTN) and ethnicity (higher BP levels among black people than among whites).

Ans. (C) i.e., 1, 2 and 3

30. **What is the correct daily dose of Iron and Folic acid to be prescribed to a child aged 12 years?**

(a) 20 mg elemental Iron and 100mcg folic acid

(b) 30 mg elemental Iron and 250mcg folic acid

(c) 60 mg elemental Iron and 300mcg folic acid

(d) 100 mg elemental Iron and 500mcg folic acid

EXPLANATION

Under RCH programme, 20 mg elemental Iron and 100 mcg folic acid is prescribed to childrens.

Ans. (A) i.e., 20mg elemental Iron and 100mcg folic acid

31. **When should breastfeeding be initiated to an infant born via a normal delivery?**

(a) Within half an hour
(b) Within one hour of birth
(c) Within 2–4 hours of birth
(d) After 4 hours of birth

EXPLANATION

Breastfeeding should be initiated within half an hour of normal vaginal delivery and around four hours following delivery by Cesarean section.

Ans. (A) i.e., Within half an hour

32. **As per biomedical waste management rule 2016 the metallic body implants should be discarded in which of the following?**

(a) Yellow colored non chlorinated plastic bag
(b) Red colored non chlorinated plastic bag
(c) Card board box with blue colored marking
(d) Separate collection system

EXPLANATION

CATEGORIES OF BIOMEDICAL WASTE SCHEDULE – I

Category	Type of Waste	Type of Bag or container to be used	Treatment and Disposal Option
Blue	**Glassware:** Broken or discarded and contaminated glass including medicine vials and ampoules except those contaminated with cytotoxic wastes Metallic Body Implants	Cardboard boxeswith blue colored marking	Disinfection (by soaking the washed glass waste after cleaning with detergent and Sodium Hypochlorite treatment) or through autoclaving or microwaving or hydroclaving and then sent for recycling.

Ans. (C) i.e., Card board box with blue colored marking

33. **Which of the following is NOT a quantitative method in the management of health services?**

(a) Network analysis
(b) Management by objectives
(c) System analysis
(d) Planning programming budgeting system

EXPLANATION

Quantitative method in the management of health services (Those based on budgeting and operational research):

1. Model
2. System analysis
3. Network analysis PERT and CPM
4. Planning programming budgeting system
5. Work sampling
6. Decision taking

Ans. (B) i.e., Management by objectives

34. **India is in which stage of the demographic cycle?**

(a) High stationary
(b) Early expanding
(c) Late expanding
(d) Low stationary

2018

EXPLANATION

Stage of demographic cycle	Meaning	Countries
First stage	High stationary	-
Second stage	Early expanding	-
Third stage	Late expanding	E.g. India
Fourth stage	Low stationary	E.g. UK, Denmark, Sweden, Belgium
Fifth stage	Stage of decline	E.g. Germany, Hungary

Ans. (C) i.e., Late expanding

35. **Manual Vacuum Aspiration (MVA) that has been introduced in primary health centres helps in reducing which of the following indices?**

(a) Infant mortality (b) Neonatal mortality
(c) Preterm mortality (d) Maternal mortality

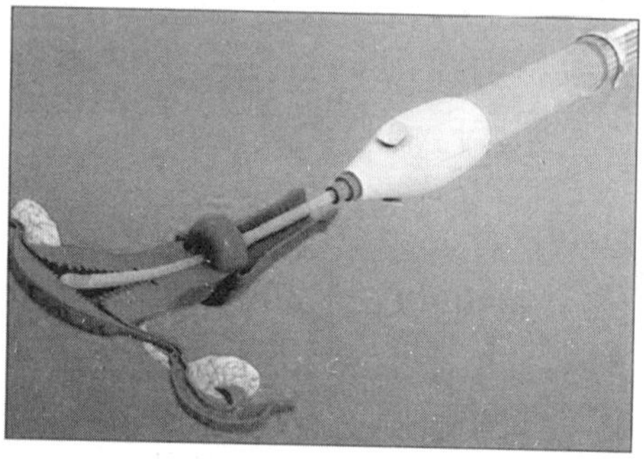

EXPLANATION

A ***Manual Aspiration*** Abortion is a safe, gentle and effective surgical ***procedure*** that is often considered to be the optimal way to end and early pregnancy of 3–7 weeks.

Ans. (D) i.e., Maternal mortality

36. **The agreement (yes/no) between two observers is statistically measured by:**

(a) Specificity (b) Sensitivity
(c) Correlation coefficient (d) Kappa coefficient

EXPLANATION

Cohen's kappa coefficient (κ) is a statistic which measures inter rater agreement for qualitative (categorical) items. It is generally thought to be a more robust measure than simple percent agreement calculation, as $\hat{e}$ takes into account the possibility of the agreement occurring by chance.

Ans. (D) i.e., Kappa coefficient

37. **How many post natal visits should be made by the ANM to the house of a low birth weight baby?**

(a) 2 (b) 4 (c) 6 (d) 8

EXPLANATION

Postnatal check up schedule

- **First visit** - If the delivery has not happened in the health centre, the first visit is to be within 24 hours of delivery.
- **Second visit** - 3rd day after delivery
- **Third visit** - 7th day after delivery
- **Fourth visit** - 6 weeks after delivery

There should be three additional visits in the case of babies with low birth weight, on days 14, 21 and 28 (as per the Integrated Management of Neonatal and Childhood Illness [IMNCI] guidelines).

Ans. (C) i.e., 6

38. **The difference between Type A and Type B sub centre as per Indian Public Health standards is in terms of:**

(a) Labour room or delivery facility
(b) Staffing pattern
(c) Location
(d) Availability of drugs

EXPLANATION

Keeping in view the current varied situation of Sub centres in different parts of the country, Sub centres have been categorized into 2 Types (Types A and B) taking into consideration various factors namely catchment area, health seeking behavior, case load, location of other facilities like PHC/CHC/FRU/Hospitals in the vicinity of the Sub centre.

Type A Sub Centre will provide all recommended services except that the facilities for conducting delivery will not be available here. If the requirement for delivery services goes up , 2 Indian Public Health Standards (IPHS) Guidelines for Sub Centres the sub centre may be considered for upgradation to Type B.

Type B Sub centre, will provide all recommended services including facilities for conducting deliveries at the Sub centre itself.

Ans. (A) i.e., Labour room or delivery facility

39. **Which of the following Screening methods for Disease is the least useful?**

(a) Mass screening
(b) High risk group screening
(c) Multiphasic screening
(d) Selective screening

EXPLANATION

Mass screening means, the screening of a whole population or a subgroup. It is offered to all, irrespective of the risk status of the individual. For example, night blood smear examination for microfilariae of every individual in hyperendemic area of filariasis. However, this is not an useful preventive measure unless it is backed up by the treatment and followup.

Ans. (A) i.e., Mass screening

40. **Which one of the following is an indicator for evaluation of impact of family planning?**

(a) Family size
(b) Number of postpartum services availed
(c) Change in behaviour of people
(d) Community needs assessment

EXPLANATION

Evaluation of impact of family planning:

- Family size (number of living children)
- Birth interval
- Age of the mother at birth of the first child and last child
- Birth order
- Number of abortions
- Changes in the birth rate and growth rate

Ans. (A) i.e., Family size

41. **Consider the following hemodynamic changes occurring during pregnancy:**

1. **Increase in cardiac output**
2. **Increase in stroke volume**
3. **Increase in colloid oncotic pressure**
4. **Increase in pulse rate**

Which of the statements given above are correct?

(a) 1, 3 and 4
(b) 1, 2 and 4
(c) 1, 2 and 3
(d) 2, 3 and 4

EXPLANATION

Cardiopulmonary Physiology in Pregnancy

- By the early second trimester, circulating blood volume increases 40–50%. This is due to an increase in both the circulation red cell mass and an even larger increase in the plasma volume.
- The larger increase in plasma volume leads to a dilutional anemia and a decrease in the serum colloid oncotic pressure.
- The cardiac output also increases by about 30–45% by the early second trimester.
- Estrogen mediates this rise in cardiac output by increasing the pre load and stroke volume, mainly via a higher overall blood volume (which increases by 40–50%)
- The heart rate increases, but generally not above 100 beats/minute.

Ans. (B) i.e., 1, 2 and 4

42. Which of the following are the hypotheses for the onset of Labor?

1. **Uterine distension**
2. **Activation of fetal hypothalamic pituitary adrenal axis**
3. **Increase in prostaglandins**
4. **Increase in serum calcium levels**

Select the correct answer using the code given below:

(a) 1, 2 and 3 (b) 1, 2 and 4 (c) 1 and 3 only (d) 2, 3 and 4

EXPLANATION

Activated fetal hypothalamic pituitary adrenal (HPA) axis leads to a surge in adrenal cortisol production. Fetal cortisol stimulates activity of placental 17 α hydroxylase/17, 20 lyase (CYP 17) enzyme, which catalyzes the conversion of pregnenolone to estradiol. The altered ratio of progesterone: estrogen in favor of later, up regulates the synthesis of uterine prostaglandins (PG) and labour.

2018

Ans. (A) i.e., 1, 2 and 3

43. Which of following statements regarding Puerperal sepsis are correct?

1. **Multiple per vaginal examinations increase the risk**
2. **The responsible microorganisms are group A and B beta haemolytic *Streptococcus***
3. **Retained bits of placenta and membrane predispose**
4. **Vaginal packing can decrease the risk**

Select the correct answer using the code given below:

(a) 1, 2 and 3 (b) 2, 3 and 4 (c) 1, 3 and 4 (d) 1, 2 and 4

EXPLANATION

Risk factors of puerperal sepsis include Cesarean section (C section), the presence of certain bacteria such as group B streptococcus in the vagina, premature rupture of membranes, multiple vaginal exams, manual removal of the placenta, and prolonged labour among others. Retained bits of placenta and membrane also predispose.

Ans. (A) i.e., 1, 2 and 3

44. In case of Labour complicated with cord prolapse, which of the following statements are correct?

1. **Reposition the patient in exaggerated Sims position**
2. **To replace the cord in the vagina**

3. To replace the cord inside the uterus
4. Early amniotomy can prevent cord prolapse

Select the correct answer using the code given below:

(a) 1, 2, 3 and 4 (b) 1 and 2 only

(c) 1, 2 and 3 only (d) 3 and 4 only

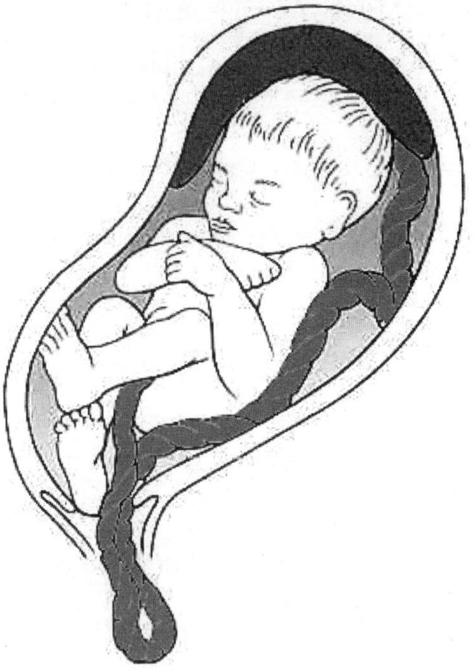

EXPLANATION

There are several measures to relieve cord compression which should be carried out till CS/Cesarean section is performed. These measures include manual elevation of the fetal presenting part using two fingers or the whole hand through the vagina, the positioning of the patient in steep Trendelenburg, exaggerated Sim's position or knee chest position, filling the bladder with 500–700cc or more of saline and the now out of favor method of cord replacement. Care should be exercised not to excessively manipulate the cord as this can result in umbilical artery vasospasm and do more harm than good.

Ans. (C) i.e., 1, 2 and 3 only

45. The following are the contents of broad ligament except:

(a) Fallopian tube

(b) Uterine and ovarian arteries with their branches

(c) Ovarian ligament

(d) Internal iliac artery

EXPLANATION

MNEMONIC for contents of broad ligament

F = Fallopian tube

U = Uterine vessels and nerves

R = Round ligament of uterus

R = Round ligament of ovary

O = Ovarian vessels and nerves

P = Paroophoron

E = Epoophoron

Ans. (D) i.e., Internal iliac artery

46. Which one of the following is true regarding normal menstrual physiology?

(a) Ovulation occurs after 48 hours of LH surge

(b) Oestradiol levels peak at 48 hours prior to ovulation

(c) Ovulation occurs after 12 hours of LH peak

(d) Threshold of LH surge generally persists for 48 hours

EXPLANATION

An LH surge is a rapid increase of the luteinizing hormone (LH) in a woman's bloodstream that occurs 24–48 hours prior to ovulation.

Ans. (C) i.e., Ovulation occurs after 12 hours of LH peak

47. **Which one of the following is NOT a feature of Candida Vaginitis?**
    (a) Pruritus is out of proportion to discharge
    (b) Discharge is thick and curdy
    (c) Yeast buds and pseudohyphae forms can be seen under the microscope
    (d) Metronidazole is the treatment of choice

EXPLANATION

Treatment of candidal vaginitis is with an antifungal medication. This may be either as a cream such as clotrimazole or with oral medications such as fluconazole.

Ans. (D) i.e., Metronidazole is the treatment of choice

48. **Which of the following is NOT a high risk factor for developing endometrial carcinoma?**
    (a) Delayed menopause (b) Hypertension (c) Multiparity (d) Obesity

EXPLANATION

Risk factors for endometrial cancer include obesity, diabetes mellitus, breast cancer, use of tamoxifen, never having had a child, late menopause, high levels of estrogen, and increasing age.

Ans. (C) i.e., Multiparity

2018

49. **All of the following are the features of functional ovarian cyst except:**
    (a) Usually < 7 cm in diameter
    (b) Spontaneous regression occurs
    (c) Unilocular
    (d) Usually symptomatic

EXPLANATION

The **follicular cyst of ovary**, or *graafian follicle cyst*, or *follicular cyst* is a type of functional, simple cyst, and is the most common type of ovarian cyst. Usually, these cysts produce no symptoms and disappear by themselves within a few months.

Ans. (D) i.e., Usually symptomatic

50. **Gestational trophoblastic disease is a spectrum comprising which of the following entities?**
    1. Complete Hydatidiform mole
    2. Partial Hydatidiform mole
    3. Invasive mole
    4. Chorio carcinoma

    Select the correct answer using the code given below:
    (a) 1, 2 and 3 only (b) 2, 3 and 4 only (c) 1, 2, 3 and 4 (d) 1 and 4 only

EXPLANATION

GTD is the common name for five closely related tumours (one benign tumour, and four malignant tumours):

- The benign tumour
  - o Hydatidiform mole (two subtypes of hydatidiform mole: complete hydatidiform mole, and partial hydatidiform mole.
- The four malignant tumours
  - o Invasive mole
  - o Choriocarcinoma
  - o Placental site trophoblastic tumour
  - o Epithelioid trophoblastic tumour

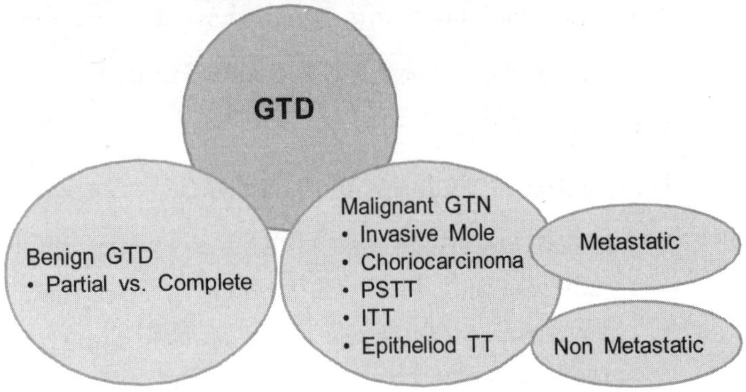

Ans. (C) i.e., 1, 2, 3 and 4

51. **Which of the following is NOT a component of Fothergill's operation as a conservative surgery for uterovaginal prolapse?**
    (a) Amputation of cervix
    (b) Plication of Mackenrodt's ligaments
    (c) Anterior colporrhaphy
    (d) Cervicopexy

EXPLANATION

Steps in Fothergill's operation:

1. Preliminary dilatation and curettage
2. Amputation of cervix
3. Strengthening the cervix by suturing cut end of Mackenrodt ligament in front of cervix
4. Anterior colporrhaphy
5. Posterior colpoperineorrhaphy

Ans. (D) i.e., Cervicopexy

52. **Which one of the following statements is NOT true regarding general physiological changes after delivery?**
    (a) Pulse may be raised on first day
    (b) Temperature should not be above 99°F
    (c) Blood volume returns to normal by second week
    (d) Cardiac output remains unchanged after delivery

EXPLANATION

Cardiac output rises soon after delivery to about 80% above the prelabor value but slowly returns to the normal within 1 week.

Ans. (D) i.e., Cardiac output remains unchanged after delivery

53. **Consider following statements regarding Beta Thalassemia in pregnancy:**
    1. There is low MCH and MCV
    2. Total Iron binding capacity may be elevated or normal
    3. HbA_2 more than 3.5% is seen in Haemoglobin Electrophoresis

2018

Which of the statements given above is/are correct?

(a) 1 only (b) 1 and 2 only (c) 2 and 3 only (d) 1, 2 and 3

EXPLANATION

Hematological findings in thalassemia:

- There is low MCV and MCH but normal MCHC (in iron deficiency anemia, all are low)
- Serum iron and TIBC are normal or elevated
- Hb electrophoresis shows raised concentration of HbA_2 (apha2, delta2) to more than 3.5% with normal to raised HbF (alpha2, gamma2).

Ans. (D) i.e., 1, 2 and 3

54. **A 20-year old Primigravida, comes at 35 weeks of gestation with complaints of swelling of feet. On examination her blood pressure is 170/110 mm Hg on 2 occasions; urine examination shows proteinuria. Which one of the following statements regarding her management is NOT true?**

(a) Can be labelled as Preeclampsia
(b) Requires urgent admission
(c) Injection Dexamethasone is to be given for fetal lung maturity
(d) Both maternal and fetal monitoring are required

EXPLANATION

Management of preeclampsia

- Admission in hospital & rest
- Antihypertensives (methyldopa, labetalol)
- Fetal well being assessment.
- Adequate protein in diet (100 g)
- Progress chart

Ans. (C) i.e., **Injection Dexamethasone is to be given for fetal lung maturity**

2018

55. **A 25-year old, $G_2P_1L_1$ came with amenorrhoea of two and half months followed by bleeding PV and pain abdomen. On examination cervical OS is open with slight bleeding. The uterus is 10 weeks size with no tenderness in the fornices. The probable clinical diagnosis is:**

(a) Ectopic pregnancy (b) Incomplete abortion
(c) Missed abortion (d) Inevitable abortion

EXPLANATION

Incomplete miscarriage

- It is the most common type of miscarriage met amongst women, hospitalized for miscarriage complications
- Continuation of pain in lower abdomen
- Uterus is smaller than period of amenorrhoea (in question, it is of 10 weeks, though the pregnancy is of 2.5 months)
- Patulous cervical os often admitting tip of the finger

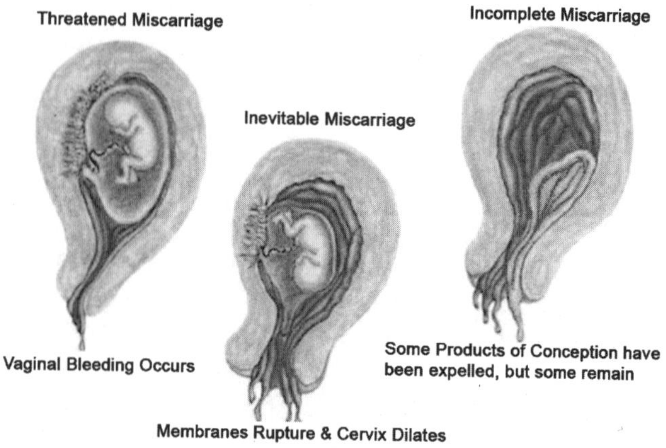

Ans. (B) i.e., **Incomplete abortion**

56. Which one of the following statements regarding intrauterine growth restriction is NOT correct?

(a) Defined according to biparietal diameter

(b) Doppler studies are indicated

(c) There is danger of fetal asphyxia during delivery

(d) Generally not seen in women with gestational diabetes

EXPLANATION

IUGR is seen in pregestational diabetes & gestational diabetes.

Ans. (D) i.e., Generally not seen in women with gestational diabetes

57. A 15-year old girl comes to the gynac casualty with a relative with complains of amenorrhoea 2 months. The urine pregnancy test is positive, ultrasound confirms 8 weeks pregnancy. The attendants are not willing to file a police case. What should the treating doctor do?

(a) Take consent for abortion and proceed

(b) Inform the police and make MLC

(c) Take parents consent for MTP

(d) None of these

EXPLANATION

When the pregnancy is caused by rape, both in cases of major or minor and in mentally imbalanced women, MTP is indicated. Pregnancy in a minor girl (below the age of 18 years) or lunatic cannot be terminated without written consent of the parents or legal guardian.

Ans. (C) i.e., Take parents consent for MTP

58. Which of the following is an absolute contraindication for use of oral contraceptive pills?

(a) Epilepsy (b) Smoking (c) Focal Migraine (d) Bronchial Asthma

EXPLANATION

Absolute contraindications for use of OCP include :

- **Thrombophlebitis** or thromboembolic disorders.
- Cerebrovascular or coronary artery disease.
- Carcinoma of the **breast** or other estrogen dependent neoplasia.
- Undiagnosed abnormal genital **bleeding.**
- Known or suspected **pregnancy.**
- Benign or malignant liver tumor.
- Diabetes with vascular complications
- Focal migraine
- Severe hypercholesterolemia

Ans. (C) i.e., Focal Migraine

59. The amount of Ethinyl Estradiol in third generation combined oral contraceptive pills is:

(a) 10–20 mcg (b) 20–30 mcg (c) 30–35 mcg (d) 35–50 mcg

EXPLANATION

Generations of OCPs

- The first generation contraceptive pill had a higher concentration of the both oestrogen and progestin. The artificial versions of the hormone progesterone found in the first generation pills included norethynodrel, norethindrone, lynestrenol and ethynodiol diacetate.
- The next generation of pills came into use in the 1970s, and had a much lower amount of hormones. They contain progestins such as levonorgestrel and norethisterone.
- Around a decade after the release of second generation pills came third generation pills. This group of pills uses progestins such as norgestimate, desogestrel, gestodene and cyproterone acetate. Amount of ethinyl estradiol is 20–30 microgram.
- The most recent type of combined oral contraceptives contain progestins such as drospirenone, nomegestrol acetate or dienogest.

Ans. (B) i.e., 20–30mcg

60. Which one of the following clinical situations is NOT ideal to perform female sterilization procedure?

(a) Postmenstrual period
(b) 7 days postpartum
(c) Concurrent with MTP
(d) 3 months post abortion

EXPLANATION

Sterilization can be done during puerperium (puerperal). If the patient is otherwise healthy, the operation can be done 24–48 hours following delivery. Its chief advantage is technical simplicity. Hospital stay and rest at home following delivery are enough to help patient to recover simultaneously from the two events, i.e. delivery and sterilization operation.

Ans. (B) i.e., 7 days postpartum

2018

61. Cardiac diseases in pregnancy which have major risk of maternal mortality are

1. Pulmonary hypertension

2. Aortic coarctation with valvular involvement

3. Atrial septal defect

4. Mitral stenosis

Select the correct answer using the code given below:

(a) 1 and 4
(b) 2 and 3
(c) 1 and 2
(d) 3 and 4

EXPLANATION

Heart disease with major risk (maternal mortality of 25–50%)

- Pulmonary hypertension
- Marfan syndrome (aortic involvement)
- Aortic coarctation with valvular involvement

Ans. (C) i.e., 1 and 2

62. Pregnancy can be terminated at any gestation if the fetus is diagnosed to have:

(a) Duodenal atresia
(b) Bilateral talipes
(c) Anencephaly
(d) Hydrocephalus

EXPLANATION

MTP is done on eugenic grounds under the provision of 'substantial risk of the childhood being born with serious physical and mental abnormalities so as to be handicapped in life'. The indications are structural (Anencephaly), chromosomal (Down's syndrome) or genetic (Hemophilia) abnormalities of the fetus.

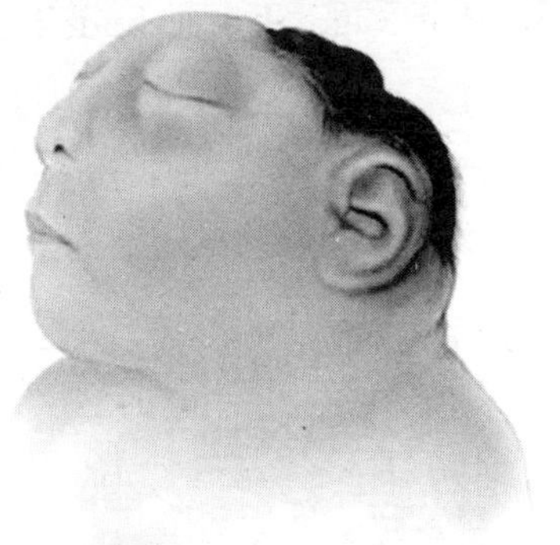

Ans. (C) i.e., Anencephaly

63. **Which one of the following is NOT a cause of recurrent spontaneous abortion?**

(a) Chromosomal abnormality
(b) Antiphospholipid syndrome
(c) Rubella infection
(d) Inherited thrombophillia

EXPLANATION

Recurrent miscarriage, habitual abortion, or **recurrent pregnancy loss** (RPL)

- It is three or more consecutive pregnancy losses.
- A balanced translocation or Robertsonian translocation in one of the partners leads to unviable fetuses that are miscarried. This explains why a karyogram is often performed in both partners if a woman has experienced repeated miscarriages.
- The antiphospholipid syndrome is an autoimmune disease that is a common cause of recurrent pregnancy loss. Around 15% of the women who have recurrent miscarriages have high levels of antiphospholipid antibodies.
- An important example of RPL is the possible increased risk of miscarriage in women with thrombophilia (propensity for blood clots). The most common problem is the factor V Leiden and prothrombin G20210A mutation.

Ans. (C) i.e., Rubella infection

2018

64. **The congenital abnormality which is invariably lethal is:**

1. **Anencephaly**
2. **Transposition of great vessel**
3. **Down Syndrome**

Select the correct answer using the code given below:

(a) 1 only
(b) 1 and 3
(c) 1 and 2
(d) 2 and 3

EXPLANATION

Lethal congenital disorders

- **Anencephaly** is the absence of a major portion of the brain, skull, and scalp that occurs during embryonic development. It is a cephalic disorder that results from a neural tube defect that occurs when the rostral (head) end of the neural tube fails to close, usually between the 23rd and 26th day following conception.
- **Transposition of the great vessels** (TGV) is a group of congenital heart defects involving an abnormal spatial arrangement of any of the great vessels: superior and/or inferior venae cavae, pulmonary artery, pulmonary veins, and aorta.

Ans. (C) i.e., 1 and 2

65. For vaginal breech delivery, ideal selection criteria would include:

1. Fetus not compromised
2. Adequate pelvis
3. Extended breech presentation
4. Estimated fetal weight < 3.5 kg

Select the correct answer using the code given below:

(a) 1, 2 and 3 only
(b) 1, 2, 3 and 4
(c) 1, 3 and 4 only
(d) 2 and 4 only

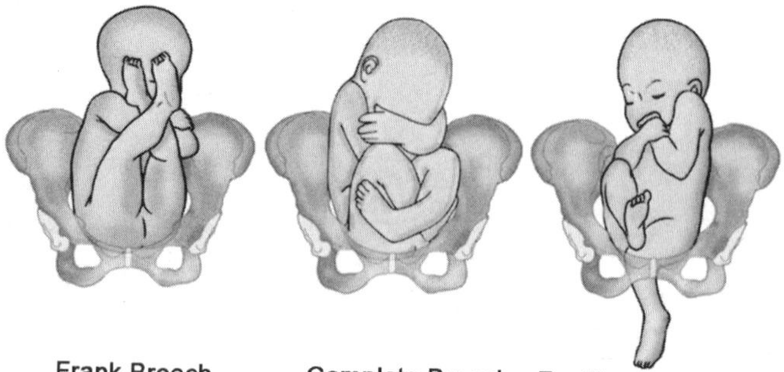

EXPLANATION

Criteria for Vaginal breech delivery

- Fetus not compromised
- Adequate pelvis
- Extended/frank breech
- Average fetal weight (1.5kg and 3.5kg)

Ans. (B) i.e., 1, 2, 3 and 4

66. Consider the following presentations:

1. Brow presentation
2. Left mento anterior position
3. Occipito posterior position
4. Breech presentation

In which of the above Vaginal delivery is NOT possible?

(a) 1, 2 and 3 (b) 1 and 3 only (c) 1 only (d) 4 only

EXPLANATION

There is no mechanism of labor in brow presentation, in an average size baby with normal pelvis. However if the baby is small and the pelvis is roomy with good uterine contractions, delivery can occur in mento-anterior brow position.

Ans. (A) i.e., 1, 2 and 3

67. The blood supply of uterus is from:

1. Uterine artery 2. Ovarian artery 3. Pudendal artery 4. Superior vesical artery

Select the correct answer using the code given below:

(a) 1 and 2 (b) 2 and 4 (c) 1 and 3 (d) 3 and 4

EXPLANATION

The uterus is supplied by arterial blood both from the uterine artery and the ovarian artery.

Ans. (A) i.e., 1 and 2

68. Which one of the following regarding amniotic fluid is true?

(a) The volume is highest at 28 weeks
(b) It reveals information about fetal lung maturity and wellbeing
(c) It is decreased in duodenal atresia in baby
(d) It is decreased in gestational diabetes

EXPLANATION

Study of amniotic fluid provides useful information about the well being and also maturity of the fetus.

Ans. (B) i.e., It reveals information about fetal lung maturity and wellbeing

69. **Consider the following statements regarding changes in pregnancy:**

    1. **Plasma volume increases up to 30–50%**
    2. **Pregnancy is a hypercoagulable state**
    3. **Hematocrit is decreased**
    4. **Total plasma proteins increases**

    Which of the statements given above is/are correct?

    (a) 1 only (b) 1, 2, 3 and 4 (c) 1 and 2 only (d) 3 and 4 only

EXPLANATION

Hematological changes in pregnancy

- Plasma volume: Increase by 30–40%
- Fibrinogen: Increase by 50%
- Hematocrit: Decrease by 6%
- Total plasma proteins: Increase by 30%

Ans. (B) i.e., 1, 2, 3 and 4

70. **Which one of the following statements regarding anatomy of fetal head is NOT true?**

    (a) Coronal suture separates frontal bones from parietal bones
    (b) Lambdoid suture separates the two parietal bones
    (c) Frontal suture separates the two frontal bones
    (d) Bregma is a diamond shaped space at junction of coronal and sagittal sutures

EXPLANATION

Sagittal suture separates the two parietal bones.

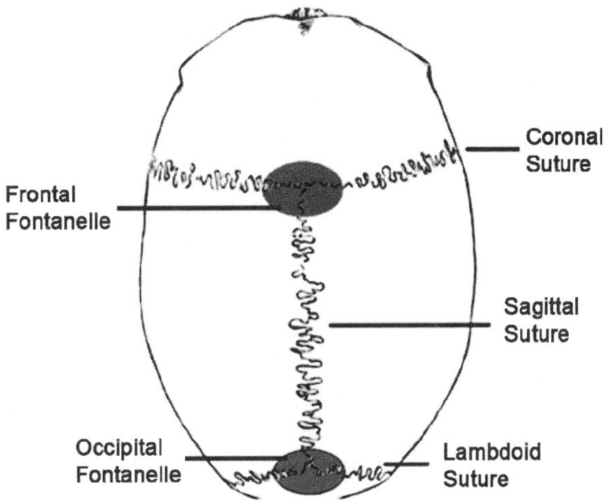

Ans. (B) i.e., Lambdoid suture separates the two parietal bones

71. A 30-year old lady, mother of 3 children presents with mass descending per vaginum. On examination it is found to have stage 3 prolapse, moderate cystocele, no posterior vaginal wall prolapse. The recommended surgery would be:

2018

1. Cystocele repair
2. Rectocele repair
3. Manchester operation
4. Vaginal hysterectomy

Select the correct answer using the codes given below:

(a) 1 and 3 only (b) 1, 2 and 3 (c) 3 only (d) 1, 2 and 4

EXPLANATION

The **Manchester operation** or simply "Fothergill **operation** is an **operation** for uterine prolapse. Its purpose is to reduce the cystourethrocele and to reposition the uterus within the pelvis.

Ans. (C) i.e., 3 only

72. A 50-year old post menopausal woman comes with complaints of bleeding per vaginum. Which one of the following investigations is NOT required?

(a) Endometrial biopsy
(b) Diagnostic laparoscopy
(c) Hysteroscopy
(d) Pap smear

EXPLANATION

Evaluation of post menopausal bleeding

- Abnormal endometrium may have to be investigated by a hysteroscopy with a biopsy or a dilation and curettage.
- Pap smear is done to rule out carcinoma cervix

Ans. (B) i.e., Diagnostic laparoscopy

2018

73. Which of the following statements regarding β Human chorionic Gonadotropin are NOT correct?

1. It is a glycoprotein hormone.
2. Serum levels increase in pregnancy, germ cells tumor and gestational trophoblastic disease
3. Its levels are same in single and multiple pregnancy
4. It has common and Alpha subunit with other hormones FSH, LH and TSH.

Select the correct answer using the codes given below:

(a) 1, 2 and 4 (b) 1, 2 and 3 (c) 2, 3 and 4 (d) 1, 3 and 4

EXPLANATION

High levels of hCG could be detected in multiple pregnancy (levels are not same in single pregnancy and multiple pregnancy).

Ans. (A) i.e., 1, 2 and 4

74. Which one of the following is NOT an emergency contraception method?

(a) Levenorgestrel
(b) Norplant
(c) Intrauterine contraceptive device
(d) High dose oral contraceptive pill

EXPLANATION

Levonorgestrel releasing implant/Norplant is 99% – 99.95% effective at preventing pregnancy, and is one of the most reliable, though not the most available, forms of birth control. Levonorgestrel releasing implant prevents pregnancy through multiple methods: by preventing ovulation, which means that no eggs are released for fertilization; by thickening the mucus of the cervix, which prevents sperm from entering; and by thinning the lining of the uterus, which makes implantation of an embryo less likely.

Ans. (B) i.e., Norplant

75. **All of the following statements are correct about vasectomy except:**

(a) No Scalpel Vasectomy (NSV) was first developed in China.

(b) It increases the incidence of testicular cancer

(c) It is less time consuming than tubectomy

(d) Addition contraception should be used for 3 months after vasectomy

EXPLANATION

There is no increase in prostate or testicular cancer or heart disease after NSV.

VASECTOMY

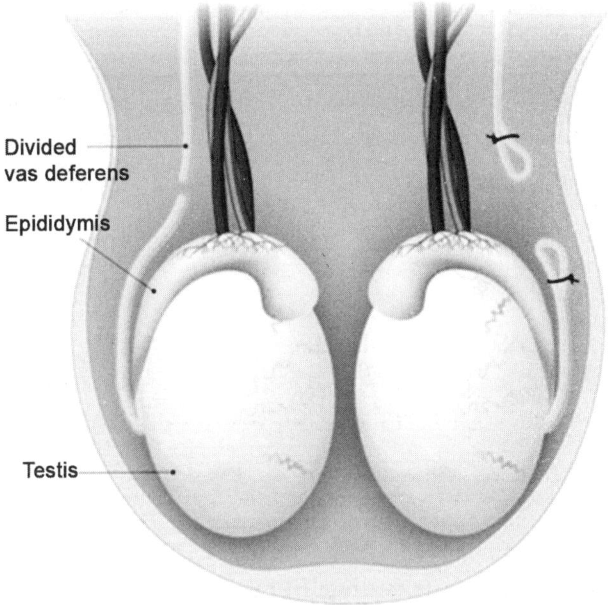

Ans. (B) i.e., It increases the incidence of testicular cancer

76. **Which of the statement regarding anemia in pregnancy is NOT true?**

(a) Iron deficiency anemia is most common in Tropics

(b) Faulty dietary habit is one of the factors responsible for anemia

(c) Mild anemia is most common

(d) If mother is severely anemic, the fetus is also severely anemic

EXPLANATION

Baby born at term, to severely anemic mother will not be anemic at birth, but as there is little or no reserve iron, anemia develops in neonatal period.

Ans. (D) i.e., If mother is severely anemic, the fetus is also severely anemic

77. **Which one of the following statements about male sterilization is NOT true?**

(a) It is safer and less expensive

(b) Most men develop antisperm antibodies

(c) It has a low failure rate
(d) It is performed under general anaesthesia

EXPLANATION

NSV is done under local anaesthesia.

Ans. (D) i.e., It is performed under general anaesthesia

78. Which of the following is NOT a method of second Trimester abortion?

(a) Mifepristone and PGE_1
(b) PGE_2 analog
(c) Intraamniotic KCl instillation
(d) Hysterotomy

EXPLANATION

Surgical methods of midtrimester termination of pregnancy include intraamniotic instillation of hypertonic saline 20% or hyperosmotic urea.

Ans. (C) i.e., Intra-amniotic KCl instillation

79. In the process of MTP (Medical Termination of Pregnancy) done by suction and evacuation, it was realized that perforation of uterus occurred with cannula. The next step should be:

(a) Laparotomy with exploration of bowel
(b) Manual vacuum aspiration
(c) Wait and watch
(d) Complete the evacuation with currette

EXPLANATION

If perforation is caused by suction cannula, diagnostic laparoscopy is helpful to assess the size and site of perforation and the amount of hemorrhage. Operative laparoscopy or Laparotomy may be needed to tackle the situation. One should not forget to inspect the intestine or omentum for evidence of injury.

Ans. (A) i.e., Laparotomy with exploration of bowel

2018

80. Consider the following statements regarding MTP (Medical Termination of Pregnancy):

1. Suction and evacuation can be done up till 12 weeks.

2. Medical methods can be used up till 10 weeks

3. Manual vacuum aspiration (MVA) syringe can be used up to 6 weeks

Which of the statements given above is/are correct?

(a) 1 only
(b) 2 and 3
(c) 2 only
(d) 1 and 3

EXPLANATION

Suction evacuation is a surgical method for MTP in first trimester (up to 12 weeks). Though it is not suitable with bigger size uterus of more than 10 weeks as chance of retained products is more.

Ans. (A) i.e., 1 only

81. Cellulitis is:

(a) A suppurative invasive infection of skin and subcutaneous tissues
(b) A nonsuppurative invasive infection of tissues
(c) Infection caused by Gram negative bacilli
(d) Infection caused by anaerobic *Streptococci*

EXPLANATION

Cellulitis is a bacterial infection involving the inner layers of the skin. It specifically affects the dermis and subcuta-neous fat. The bacteria most commonly involved are streptococci and *Staphylococcus aureus.*

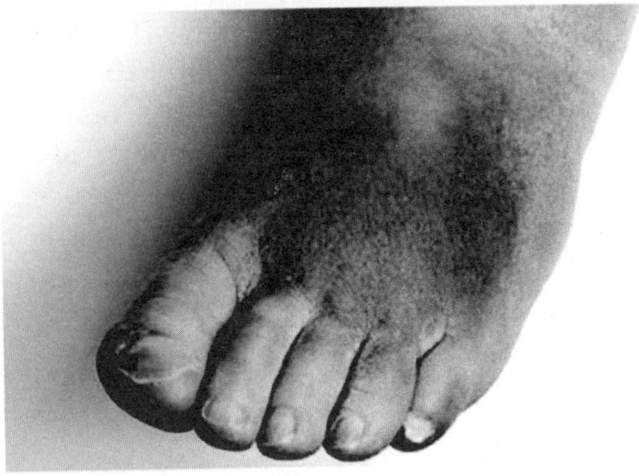

Ans. (C) i.e., Infection caused by Gram negative bacilli

82. **Following are the factors for increased risk of wound infection except:**

(a) Malnutrition
(b) Good blood supply
(c) Metabolic diseases (diabetes, uraemia)
(d) Immunosuppression

EXPLANATION

Poor blood supply results in delayed wound healing.

Ans. (B) i.e., Good blood supply

83. **A 25-year old lady underwent exploratory laparotomy for bowel injury which happened while she underwent medical termination of pregnancy 2 days back. 24 hours after exploratory laparotomy her pulse is 106/m, respiratory rate 26/m, total leucocyte count 14000/cumm with blood urea 84mg% and serum creatinine 2.0mg/dL. The lady is having:**

(a) Wound infection
(b) Systematic inflammatory response syndrome
(c) Sepsis syndrome
(d) Multisystem organ failure (MSOF)

EXPLANATION

Systemic inflammatory response syndrome

Finding	Value
Temperature	<36°C (96.8°F) or >38°C (100.4°F)
Heart rate	>90/min
Respiratory rate	>20/min or PaCO2<32 mmHg (4.3 kPa)
WBC	<4×10⁹/L (<4000/mm³), >12×10⁹/L (>12,000/mm³), or 10% bands

Ans. (B) i.e., Systematic inflammatory response syndrome

84. **A 22-year old young man came with history of occasional bleeding per rectum. On colonoscopy, numerous sessile polyps were seen in descending and sigmoid colon. On family history his elder brother was operated for thyroid malignancy. The young man should be advised:**

(a) Prophylactic panproctocolectomy
(b) Prophylactic anterior resection
(c) Surveillance colonoscopy every 6 months
(d) Colonoscopic removal of all polyps

EXPLANATION

Cowden syndrome (also known as **Cowden's disease** and multiple hamartoma syndrome)

- It is an autosomal dominant inherited condition characterized by benign overgrowths called hamartomas as well as an increased lifetime risk of breast, thyroid, uterine, and other cancers.
- The most common malignancies associated with the syndrome are adenocarcinoma of the breast (20%), followed by adenocarcinoma of the thyroid (7%), squamous cell carcinomas of the skin (4%), and the remaining from the colon, uterus, or others (1%).
- Polyps are extremely common as they are found in about 95% of Cowden syndrome patients undergoing a colonoscopy. They are numerous ranging from a few to hundreds, usually of the hamartomatous subtype, and distributed across the colon as well as other areas within the gastrointestinal tract.
- Colonoscopy, starting at age 35 years, then every 5 years or more frequently if patient is symptomatic or polyps found.

Ans. (C) i.e., Surveillance colonoscopy every 6 months

85. A 47-year old post menopausal lady was on adjuvant hormonal treatment with Tamoxifen for 3 years for Carcinoma Breast. She came to Outpatient Department with history of passing blood clots per vagina. She is probably suffering from:

(a) Carcinoma Vulva
(b) Carcinoma Vagina
(c) Carcinoma Endometrium
(d) Uterine fibroid

EXPLANATION

Tamoxifen increases the incidence of uterine carcinoma.

Ans. (C) i.e., Carcinoma Endometrium

2018

86. Which of the following regarding blood supply of rectum is NOT true?

(a) Superior rectal artery is a direct continuation of Inferior mesenteric artery
(b) Middle rectal artery arises from external iliac artery and passes through the lateral ligaments into rectum
(c) Inferior rectal artery arises from internal pudendal artery
(d) Inferior rectal artery traverses the Alcock's canal into rectum

EXPLANATION

Arterial supply of rectum

- Superior rectal artery: Terminal branch of inferior mesenteric artery
- Middle rectal artery: Branch of internal iliac artery
- Inferior rectal artery: Branch of the internal pudendal artery

Arterial Supply

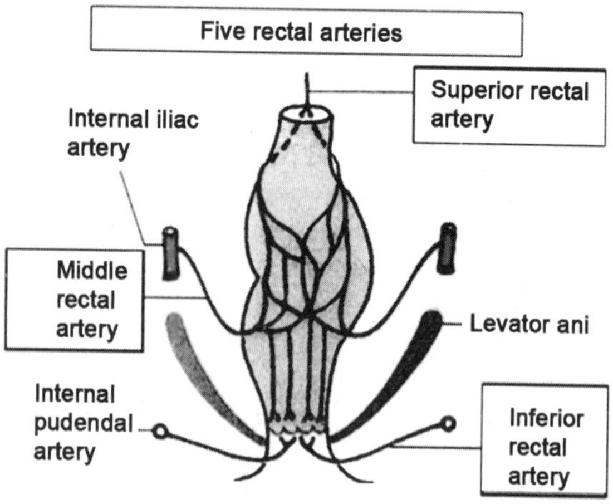

Ans. (B) i.e., Middle rectal artery arises from external iliac artery and passes through the lateral ligaments into rectum

87. Gastric conduit after oesophageal resection is based upon:

(a) Right Gastroepiploic artery
(b) Short gastric vessels and Vasa brevia
(c) Left gastric artery
(d) Right gastric artery

EXPLANATION

The most important consideration in an esophageal anastomosis is the blood supply of the conduit. Replacement of the esophagus requires a conduit with a sufficient blood supply to heal an anastomosis at its most ischemic extreme. In contrast to the segmental blood supply of the native esophagus, the interposition graft must provide its own axial blood supply. For example, the stomach interposition graft is based on the gastroepiploie artery.

Ans. (A) i.e., Right Gastroepiploic artery

88. A 70-year old male having comorbidities present with benign appearing parotoid tumour. The best option is:

(a) Tumour enucleation
(b) Superficial Parotidectomy
(c) Aspiration biopsy confirmation
(d) Radiotherapy

EXPLANATION

FNAC is very important and diagnostic in pleomorphic adenoma.

Ans. (C) i.e., Aspiration biopsy confirmation

89. Fine Needle Aspiration Cytology (FNAC) is NOT conclusive in which one of the following thyroid swellings?

(a) Papillary carcinoma thyroid
(b) Follicular carcinoma thyroid
(c) Medullary carcinoma thyroid
(d) Thyroiditis

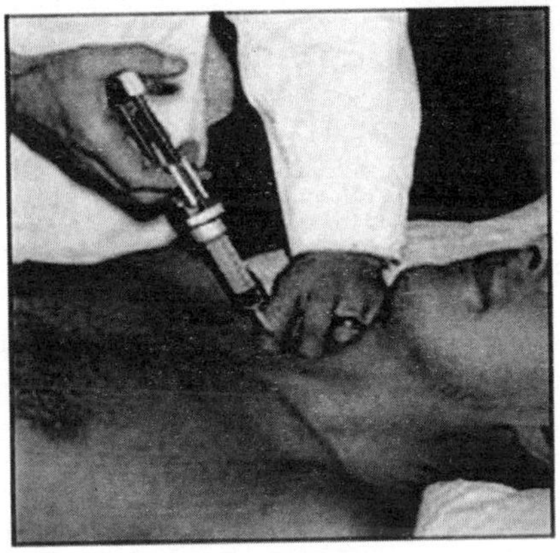

EXPLANATION

FNAC is not reliable at present in follicular carcinoma of thyroid as capsular and vascular invasions cannot be found.

Ans. (B) i.e., Follicular carcinoma thyroid

90. Patients with phlebographically confirmed deep vein thrombosis of the calf:

(a) can expect asymptomatic recovery if treated promptly with anticoagulant
(b) may be effectively treated with low dose heparin
(c) may be effectively treated with pneumatic compression stockings
(d) are at risk for significant pulmonary embolism

EXPLANATION

Pulmonary embolism can occur in 15% of DVT cases.

Ans. (D) i.e., are at risk for significant pulmonary embolism

91. Herceptin (Trastuzumab) is an immunotherapeuctic agent used for:

(a) Carcinoma prostrate
(b) Carcinoma breast
(c) Carcinoma rectum
(d) Ovarian malignancy

EXPLANATION

Trastuzumab, sold under the brand name **Herceptin** among others, is a monoclonal antibody used to treat breast cancer. Specifically it is used for breast cancer that is HER2 receptor positive.

Ans. (B) i.e., Carcinoma breast

92. Mainstay of an accurate diagnosis of pancreatic injury following blunt abdominal trauma is:

(a) Computed Tomogram
(b) Diagnostic peritoneal lavage
(c) USG abdomen
(d) MRI abdomen

EXPLANATION

High resolution CT scan is diagnostic for pancreatic injury.

Ans. (A) i.e., Computed Tomogram

93. Pancreatic pseudocysts developing complications are best managed by:

(a) Conservative treatment
(b) Radiologically guided interventions
(c) External drainage
(d) Surgery

EXPLANATION

Management of uncomplicated pancreatic pseudocysts include conservative treatment (watchful monitoring), surgical internal drainage (open or laparoscopic), or endoscopic internal drainage.

Ans. (D) i.e., Surgery

94. Which one of the following regarding absorbable meshes is NOT true?

(a) They are made of polygycolic acid fibre
(b) They are used in temporary abdominal wall closure
(c) They are used to buttress sutured repair
(d) They show very good results as collagen deposition is maximum

EXPLANATION

The polyglycolic acid absorbable meshes are not widely used as there are mixed views as to whether ingowth of fibrous tissue into the mesh is sufficient to achieve permanent repair.

Ans. (D) i.e., They show very good results as collagen deposition is maximum

95. Which one of the following is NOT a surgical modality for management of femoral hernia?

(a) Lotheissen's (Inguinal) operation
(b) The high approach (Mc Evedy)
(c) The low approach (Lockwood)
(d) The canal ring narrowing operation (Lytle's)

EXPLANATION

Lytle's repair is done for indirect inguinal hernia.

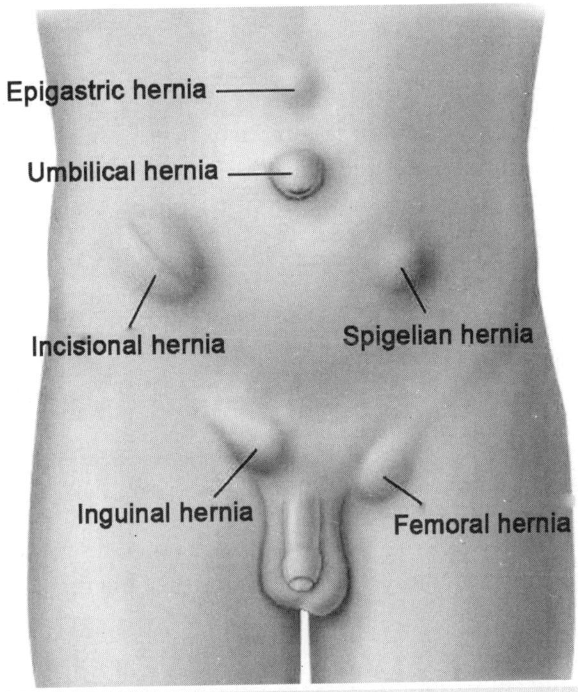

Ans. (D) i.e., The canal ring narrowing operation (Lytle's)

96. "Triangle of Doom" dissected and seen during Laparoscopic inguinal hernia repair is bounded by all except:

(a) Vas deference
(b) Cord structures
(c) Peritoneal fold
(d) Inferior epigastric artery

EXPLANATION

The **Triangle of Doom** is an anatomical triangle defined by the vas deferens medially, spermatic vessels laterally and peritoneal fold inferiorly. This triangle contains external iliac artery and vein, the deep circumflex iliac vein, the genital branch of genitofemoral nerve and hidden by fascia, the femoral nerve.

It bears significance in laparoscopic repair of groin hernia. Surgical staples are avoided here.

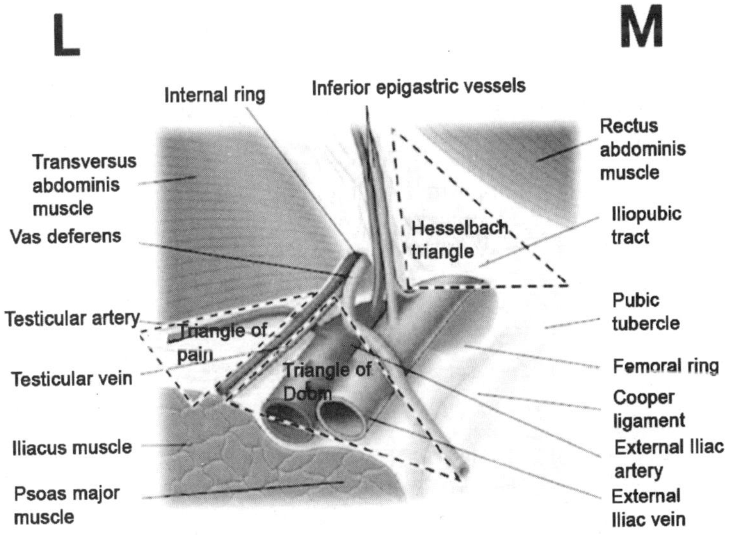

Note: base of hesselbacks triangle is formed by inguinal ligament...

Note: Base of triangle of doom and pain is formed by "peritoneal reflection"

Ans. (D) i.e., Inferior epigastric artery

97. Antrochonal polyp always arises from:

(a) Maxillary sinus
(b) Posterior ethmoidal cells
(c) Posterior end of the septum
(d) Nasopharynx

EXPLANATION

Antrochoanal polyps (ACP) are benign lesions that arise from the mucosa of the maxillary sinus, grow into the maxillary sinus and reach the choana, and nasal obstruction being their main symptom.

Ans. (A) i.e., Maxillary sinus

98. Paralytic ileus is a type of:

(a) Dynamic obstruction
(b) Adynamic obstruction
(c) Inflammatory obstruction
(d) Drug induced obstruction

EXPLANATION

Ileus is a disruption of the normal propulsive ability of the gastrointestinal tract. Although *ileus* originally referred to any lack of digestive propulsion, including bowel obstruction, upto date medical usage restricts its meaning to those disruptions caused by the failure of peristalsis, rather than by mechanical obstruction.

Ans. (B) i.e., Adynamic obstruction

99. Indication of Coronary artery bypass grafting (CABG) is:

(a) More than 25% stenosis of critical left main stem
(b) More than 25% stenosis of proximal left anterior interventricular artery
(c) Triple vessel disease
(d) Deranged Stress Echocardiography report

EXPLANATION

The 1999 Guidelines for CABG Surgery developed by the American College of Cardiology and the American Heart Association list the following 6 conditions as indications for CABG in patients with stable angina:

1. Significant left main coronary artery stenosis.
2. Left main equivalent: significant (70 percent) stenosis of the proximal left anterior descending (LAD) and proximal left circumflex arteries.
3. Three vessel disease.
4. Two vessel disease with significant proximal LAD stenosis and either ejection fraction <0.50 or demonstrable ischemia on non invasive testing.
5. One- or 2-vessel stenosis without significant proximal LAD stenosis, but with a large area of viable myocardium and high risk criteria on non invasive testing.
6. Disabling angina despite maximal non invasive therapy, when surgery can be performed with acceptable risk.

Ans. (C) i.e., Triple vessel disease

100. Normal anatomical narrowing of ureter are present in all except:

(a) Ureteropelvic junction
(b) Crossing the abdominal aorta
(c) Entering bladder wall
(d) Ureteric orifice

EXPLANATION

The ureter has a diameter of 3 mm but there are three constrictions, which are the most common sites of renal calculus obstruction:

- At the pelviureteric junction (PUJ) of the renal pelvis and the ureter
- As the ureter enters the pelvis (brim of pelvis) and crosses over the common iliac artery bifurcation
- At the vesicoureteric junction (VUJ) as the ureter obliquely enters the bladder wall

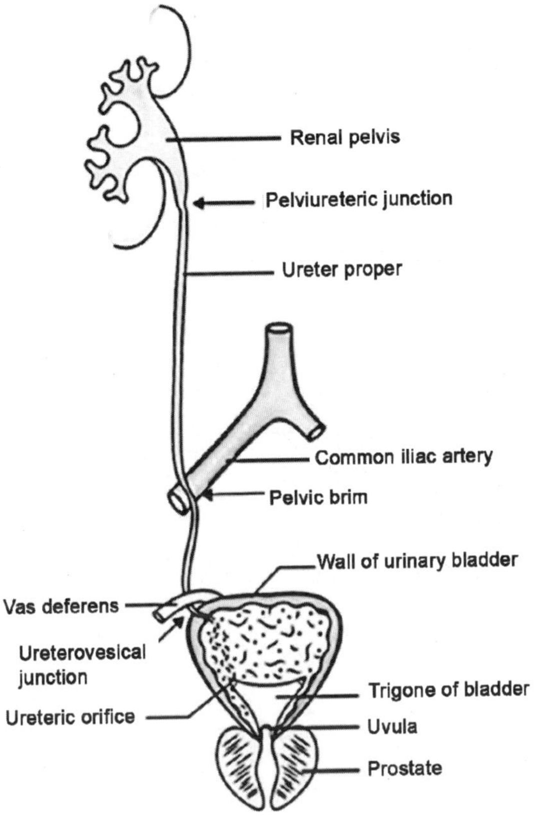

Ans. (B) i.e., Crossing the abdominal aorta

101. Which one of the following is NOT correct regarding Adenocarcinoma of the kidney?

(a) It is also called Grawitz tumour

(b) It always presents with haematuria

(c) It may be associated with Pyrexia of unknown origin

(d) Renal vein extention may embolize to lungs

EXPLANATION

Hematuria is the presenting complaint of Renal Cell Carcinoma/RCC in only 30% of cases.

Ans. (B) i.e., It always presents with haematuria

102. Which one of the following regarding abdominal paediatric surgery is correct?

(a) Transverse abdominal incision is always used

(b) Incision can be closed with absorbable suture

(c) Bowel must be always anastomosed in double layer

(d) Skin over abdomen can never be closed with subcuticular sutures

EXPLANATION

Intestinal anastomosis with one layer of suture is as safe as anastomosis with two layers in children, and the time spent for completion of the procedure is significantly less with one plane of suture. For those reasons, it is the method of choice for intestinal anastomosis in children.

Ans. (C) i.e., Bowel must be always anastomosed in double layer

103. Genetic disorder predisposing patients to develop Berry aneurysm includes all except:

(a) Adult polycystic kidney
(b) Fibromuscular dysplasia
(c) Neurofibromatosis Type II
(d) Marfan's syndrome

EXPLANATION

Genetic conditions associated with connective tissue disease may also be associated with the development of aneurysms. This includes:

- Autosomal dominant polycystic kidney disease,
- Neurofibromatosis type I,
- Marfan syndrome,
- Multiple endocrine neoplasia type I,
- Pseudoxanthoma elasticum,
- Hereditary hemorrhagic telangiectasia and
- Ehlers Danlos syndrome types II and IV.

Ans. (C) i.e., Neurofibromatosis Type II

104. Which one of the following regarding Nasal polyps is NOT true?

(a) Nasal polyps are very painful to touch
(b) Simple polyps are bilateral
(c) Bleeding polyp may indicate malignancy
(d) Meningocele must be excluded in children with polyps

EXPLANATION

Nasal polyps (NP) are noncancerous growths within the nose or sinuses. Symptoms include trouble breathing through the nose, loss of smell, decreased taste, post nasal drip, and a runny nose.

Ans. (C) i.e., Bleeding polyp may indicate malignancy

105. Allen's test is used in Cardiac surgery:

(a) To select finger prick for blood glucose estimation
(b) When radial artery harvest is planned
(c) For evaluation of AV fistula
(d) To check warmth of hands

EXPLANATION

The modified Allen's test is also performed prior to heart bypass surgery. The radial artery is occasionally used as a conduit for bypass surgery, and its patency lasts longer in comparison to the saphenous veins. Prior to heart bypass surgery, the test is performed to assess the suitability of the radial artery to be used as a conduit.

Ans. (B) i.e., When radial artery harvest is planned

106. In a lateral facial wound, if facial nerve injury is suspected, it should be:

(a) Left alone

(b) Skin and subcutaneous flaps to be raised to cover the cut ends

(c) Primary repair should be attempted

(d) Secondary repair using microscope gives best result

EXPLANATION

Primary neuropathy of facial nerve at the time of injury should be managed by interpositional graft by using sural or greater auricular nerve grafts.

Ans. (C) i.e., Primary repair should be attempted

107. Radiologic views used for fracture Mandible (body and Ramus) are all except:

(a) Orthopantomogram (b) Lateral obliques (c) Lower occlusal (d) Submentovertex

EXPLANATION

Submentovertical view is primarily taken to demonstrate sphenoid sinuses.

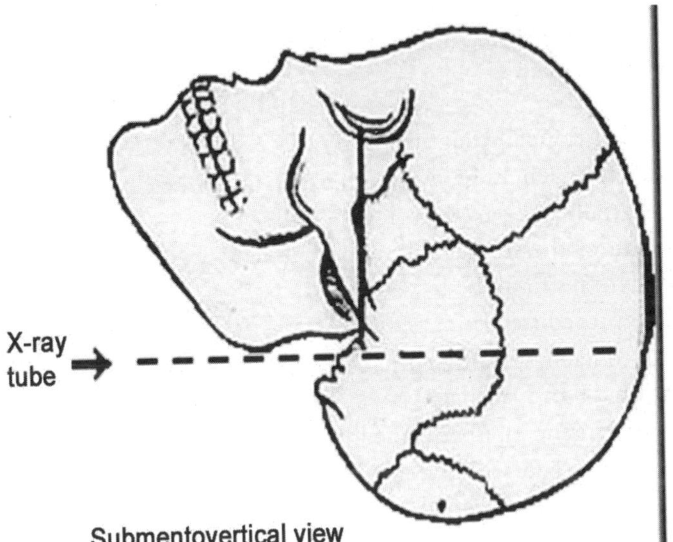

Submentovertical view

Ans. (D) i.e., Submentovertex

108. Mallory Weiss tear causing haematemesis is seen over:

(a) Oesophagus

(b) Gastroesophageal junction

(c) Anterior wall of stomach

(d) Fundus of stomach

EXPLANATION

Mallory Weiss syndrome or **gastroesophageal laceration syndrome** refers to bleeding from a laceration in the mucosa at the junction of the stomach and esophagus. This is usually caused by severe vomiting because of alcoholism or bulimia, but can be caused by any condition which causes violent vomiting and retching such as food poisoning. The syndrome presents with hematemesis. The laceration is sometimes referred to as a *Mallory Weiss tear*.

Ans. (B) i.e., Gastroesophageal junction

2018

2018

109. Which one of the following factors is NOT involved in the pathogenesis of Systematic inflammatory response syndrome (SIRS)?

(a) Increased cytokine production
(b) Abnormal nitric oxide synthesis
(c) Free radical production
(d) Microvascular occlusion

EXPLANATION

SIRS, independent of the etiology, has the same pathophysiology with minor differences in inciting cascades. Many consider the syndrome as a self defense mechanism, which uses inflammation as the body's response to nonspecific insults that arise from chemical, traumatic or infectious stimuli. The inflammatory cascade is complex and involves humoral and cellular responses, complement and the cytokine cascades.

Ans. (D) i.e., Microvascular occlusion

110. Sleeve Gastrectomy done for Morbid obesity is a:

(a) Restrictive procedure
(b) Reversible procedure
(c) Mildly restrictive and mainly malabsorptive
(d) Malabsorptive procedure only

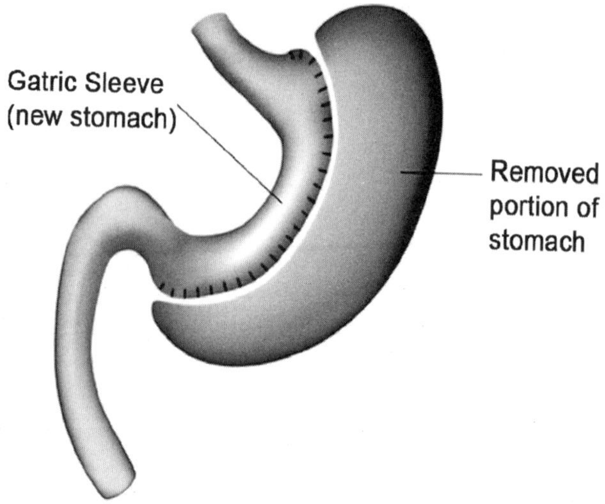

EXPLANATION

Sleeve gastrectomy is a surgical weight loss procedure in which the stomach is reduced to about 15% of its original size, by surgical removal of a large portion of the stomach along the greater curvature. The result is a sleeve or tube like structure. The procedure permanently reduces the size of the stomach, although there could be some dilatation of the stomach later on in life. The procedure is generally performed laparoscopically and is irreversible. It's a restrictive weight loss surgical procedure.

Ans. (A) i.e., Restrictive procedure

111. Preoperative Nutrition Screening in a patient with morbid obesity planned for Gastric Bypass includes all except:

(a) Serum Magnesium (b) Serum Calcium (c) Serum Vitamin B_{12} (d) Serum Insulin

EXPLANATION

Calcium supplements, iron supplements, protein supplements, multivitamins (sometimes prenatal vitamins are best), and vitamin B_{12} (cyanocobalamin) supplements are all very important to the post operative bypass patient.

Ans. (D) i.e., Serum Insulin

112. In postoperative care the long term risks after Bariatric Surgery include all except:

(a) Protein Calorie Malnutrition
(b) Deep Vein Thrombosis
(c) Vitamin and Micronutrient depletion syndromes
(d) Weight regain

EXPLANATION

After surgery, patients feel fullness after ingesting only a small volume of food, followed soon thereafter by a sense of satiety and loss of appetite. Total food intake is markedly reduced.

Ans. (D) i.e., Weight regain

113. Hilton's method of Incision and drainage of abscess has the advantage of:

(a) Complete drainage of pus

(b) Avoids injury to underlying vessels and nerves

(c) Provides irrigation

(d) Heals without scar

EXPLANATION

Depending upon the site of abscess, incisions are made along the line of blood vessels and nerves and not across it. Where possible natural skin crease is selected in a dependent area. Most often the point where it fluctuates the most may be utilised. The length of the incision will depend upon the width and depth of the abscess. Generally, incision is made through most of the width of the abscess.

Once skin incision is made, drainage is done as follows:

An opening is made into the abscess using a sinus forceps or a closed blunt hemostat and when the abscess is entered open the jaws of the sinus forceps or hemostat allowing the purulent material to escape (Hilton's method).

Ans. (B) i.e., Avoids injury to underlying vessels and nerves

114. Indications of computed tomography after head injury include all except:

(a) Glasgow Coma Scale < 13 at any point

(b) Open depressed fracture

(c) Mild head injury in a 50-year old man

(d) Amnesia > 30 minutes

EXPLANATION

CT scan in head injuries

A. Exclusion criteria (cases in which rules cannot be applied and in which head imaging is typically pursued)
   1. Neurologic deficit
   2. Seizure
   3. Oral Anticoagulant use or other Bleeding Diathesis

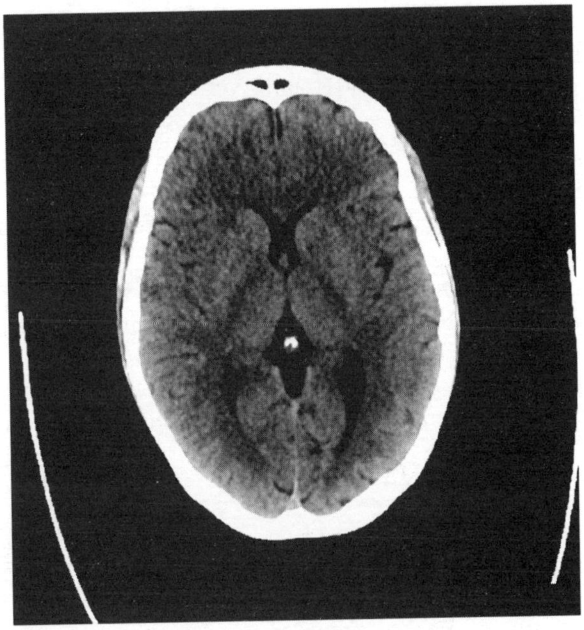

B. High risk indications for Head CT
   1. Glasgow Coma Scale <15 at 2 hours after injury
   2. Open or depressed Skull Fracture
   3. Vomiting (Two or more episodes)
   4. Age 65 years or over
   5. Basal Skull Fracture signs
      a. Hemotympanum
      b. Periorbital Bruising (Raccoon's Eyes)

c. Mastoid process Ecchymosis (Battle's Sign)
d. Cerebrospinal fluid leakage from ear or nose

C. Moderate risk indications for Head CT

1. Pre trauma amnesia lasting longer than 30 minutes
2. High risk mechanism of injury
   a. Pedestrian in Motor Vehicle Accident
   b. Passenger ejected from vehicle
   c. Fall from height over 3 feet or 5 stairs

Ans. (C) i.e., Mild head injury in a 50-year old man

115. Mondor's disease is:

(a) Thrombophlebitis of superficial veins of the breast and anterior chest wall
(b) Other name for tuberculosis of breast
(c) Rare type of chronic intramammary abscess
(d) Named after the scientist who first coined the term "Actinomycosis of Breast"

EXPLANATION

Mondor's disease (also known as "Mondor's syndrome of superficial thrombophlebitis") is a rare condition which involves thrombophlebitis of the superficial veins of the breast and anterior chest wall.

Ans. (A) i.e., Thrombophlebitis of superficial veins of the breast and anterior chest wall

2018

116. Sengstaken Blakemore tube is used to control bleeding in:

(a) Renal trauma
(b) Bleeding varices
(c) Splenic injury in portal hypertension
(d) Duodenal ulcer bleed

EXPLANATION

A **Sengstaken–Blakemore tube** is a medical device inserted through the nose or mouth and used occasionally in the management of upper gastrointestinal hemorrhage due to esophageal varices (distended and fragile veins in the esophageal wall, usually a result of cirrhosis).

Ans. (B) i.e., Bleeding varices

117. Which one of the following regarding Pancreatic effusion is correct?

(a) Free fluid collection in Pleural cavity
(b) Never associated with abdominal collection
(c) Pancreatic stenting is to be done
(d) Percutaneous drainage under image guidance is necessary

EXPLANATION

Treatment of pancreatic ascites is controversial but includes conservative medical therapy or endoscopic transpapillary pancreatic duct stenting (by ERCP) or surgery.

Ans. (C) i.e., Pancreatic stenting is to be done

118. Which one of the following bone is affected in Keinbock's disease?

(a) Lunate bone
(b) Capitellum of the humerus
(c) Metatarsal
(d) Navicular bone

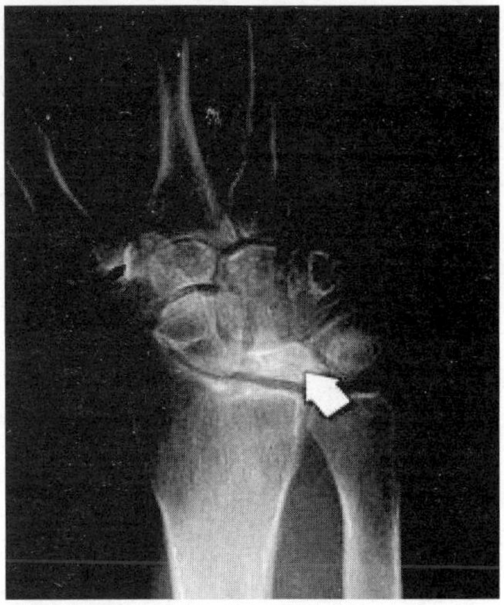

EXPLANATION

Kienbock's disease, also known as avascular necrosis of the lunate, is a condition in which the lunate bone, one of eight small bones in the wrist, loses its blood supply, leading to death of the bone. The lunate is a central bone in the wrist that is important for proper movement and support of the joint

Ans. (A) i.e., Lunate bone

119. Which one of the following regarding management of acute wounds is NOT true?

(a) The whole patient should be examined according to ATLS principles
(b) Wounds should be examined, taking into consideration site and structures damaged
(c) Bleeding wounds should be elevated and a pressure pad applied
(d) Clamps should be used to stop all bleeding vessels

EXPLANATION

Advanced trauma life support (ATLS) is a training program for medical providers in the management of acute trauma cases, developed by the American College of Surgeons. The premise of the ATLS program is to treat the greatest threat to life first. It also advocates that the lack of a definitive diagnosis and a detailed history should not slow the application of indicated treatment for life threatening injury, with the most time critical interventions performed early.

Ans. (A) i.e., The whole patient should be examined according to ATLS principles

120. Risk Scoring System which can be used post operatively is:

(a) ASA → American Society of Anaesthesiologist
(b) MET → Metabolic Equivalent Task
(c) RCRI → Revised Cardiac Risk Index
(d) POSSUM → Physiologic and Operative Severity Score for enUmeration of Mortality and Morbidity

EXPLANATION

The **Metabolic Equivalent of Task** (MET), or **metabolic equivalent**, is the objective measure of the energy expended by an individual while performing some specific physical activity compared to a reference, set by convention at 3.5 ml of oxygen per kilogram per minute, which is roughly equivalent to the energy expended when sitting quietly.

Ans. (B) i.e., MET → Metabolic Equivalent Task

CHAPTER 2

CMS EXAMINATION 2018

PAPER - 1

1. **Most common valve involved in Carcinoid syndrome is:**

   (a) Mitral valve
   (b) Tricuspid valve
   (c) Aortic valve
   (d) Pulmonary valve

   EXPLANATION

   The vast majority of patients with **cardiac** involvement in carcinoid syndrome present with signs of right **heart** failure secondary to severe dysfunction of the tricuspid and pulmonary valves

   Ans. (B) i.e., Tricuspid valve.

2. **A 70-year old man reports to the emergency with acute chest pain. ECG shows inferior wall Myocardial Infarction (MI). He has recently been discharged 7 days back following thrombolysis with streptokinase for Acute Anterior wall MI. What will be the appropriate management?**

   (a) Aspirin, Sublingual nitroglycerin, Clopidogrel, Primary PCI
   (b) Aspirin, Sublingual nitroglycerin, Clopidogrel, Streptokinase
   (c) Aspirin, Sublingual nitroglycerin, Clopidogrel, Heparin
   (d) Aspirin, Sublingual nitroglycerin, Clopidogrel, Beta blockers

   EXPLANATION

   Management of MI

   - For people who have already had a heart attack or stroke, taking aspirin daily for two years prevented 1 in 50 from having a cardiovascular problem (heart attack, stroke, or death), but also caused non fatal bleeding problems to occur in 1 of 400 people.
   - Improved myocardial oxygen demand vs oxygen delivery ratio (on administering sublingual nitroglycerine) leads to the following therapeutic effects during episodes of angina pectoris: subsiding of chest pain, decrease of blood pressure, increase of heart rate, and orthostatic hypotension.
   - Clopidogrel is used to prevent heart attack and stroke in people who are at high risk of these events, including those with a history of myocardial infarction and other forms of acute coronary syndrome, stroke, and those with peripheral artery disease.
   - **Percutaneous coronary intervention**/PCI may be appropriate for patients with stable coronary artery disease if they meet certain criteria, such as having any coronary stenosis greater than 50 percent or having angina symptoms that are unresponsive to medical therapy.

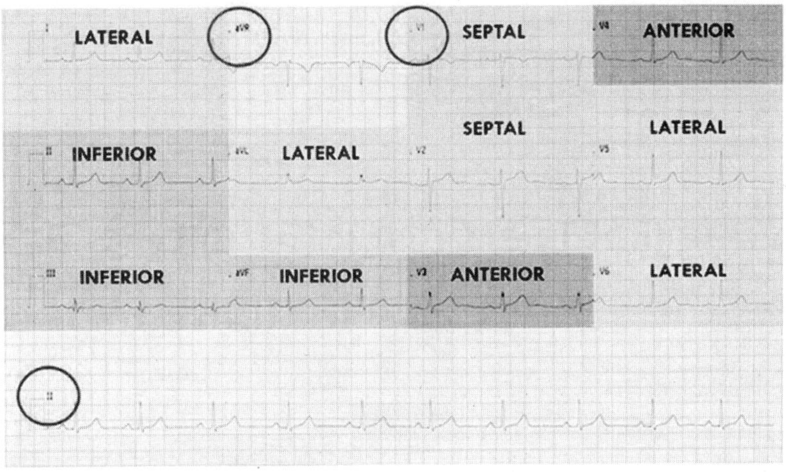

Ans. (A) i.e., Aspirin, Sublingual nitroglycerin, Clopidogrel, Primary PCI.

3. **The presence of a fusion beat on an Electrocardiogram is diagnostic of:**

(a) Atrial Fibrillation
(b) Ventricular Tachycardia
(c) Supraventricular Tachycardia
(d) Sinus Bradycardia

EXPLANATION

Fusion beat/Ventricular *fusion beats* can occur when the heart's natural *rhythm* and the impulse from a pacemaker coincide to activate the same part of a ventricle at the same time, causing visible variation in configuration and height of the QRS complex of an *electrocardiogram* reading of the heart's activity.

Lead MCL1

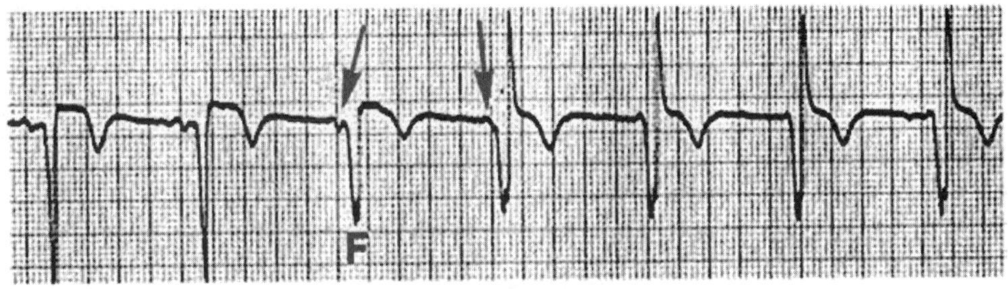

Isochronic ventricular rhythm
F = fusion beat
Arrows point at dissociated P waves

Ans. (B) i.e., Ventricular Tachycardia

4. **A 64-year old man presents with chest pain of 24 hours duration. His ECG reveals ST elevation, Anterior Wall Myocardial Infarction. The preferred treatment modality for him is:**

(a) Primary percutaneous coronary intervention
(b) Thrombolysis with Alteplase
(c) Thrombolysis with Streptokinase
(d) Nitroglycerin infusion, Aspirin and Beta blockers

EXPLANATION

Indications for thrombolysis with streptokinase include MI with ST elevation in the ECG, more than 0.1mV (1mm) in two or more contiguous leads within 12 hours of onset of symptoms.

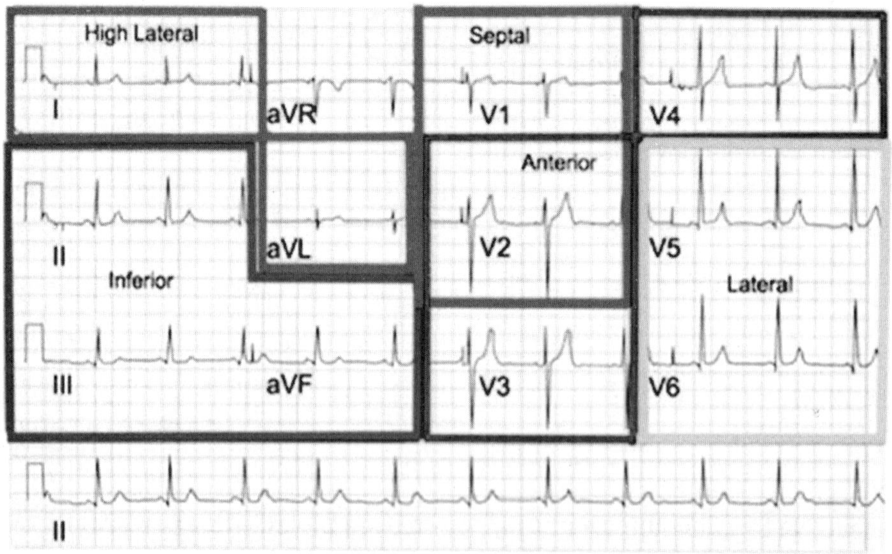

Ans. (B) i.e., Thrombolysis with Alteplase

5. **The preferred anti hypertensive drug for a 74-year old male with benign prostatic hypertrophy is:**

(a) Amlodepine (b) Hydrochlorothiazide (c) Prazosin (d) Atenolol

EXPLANATION

Alpha 1 blockers are ideal for older men with benign prostatic hypertrophy.

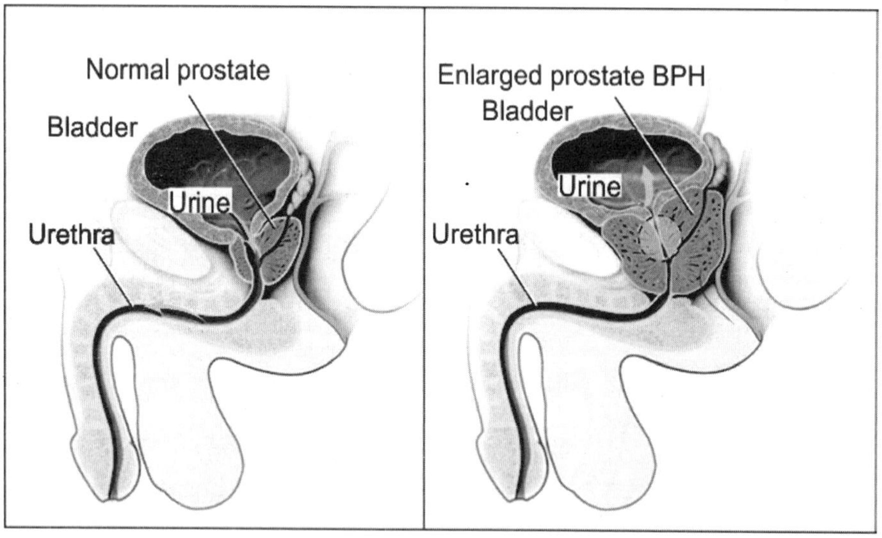

Ans. (C) i.e., Prazosin

6. **The treatment of choice for a 32-year old male patient of severe mitral stenosis (Rheumatic) with thickened and calcified valves on echocardiography is:**

(a) Balloon mitral valvuloplasty/BMV (b) Mitral valve replacement/MVR

(c) Medical management only (d) Mitral valvotomy/MV

EXPLANATION

Though initially only ideal pliable valves were taken up for BMV, with technical improvements and expertise, especially with newer devices like Cribier Commissurotome, patients with calcification and mild to moderate mitral regurgitation are also being taken up for BMV with good results.

2018

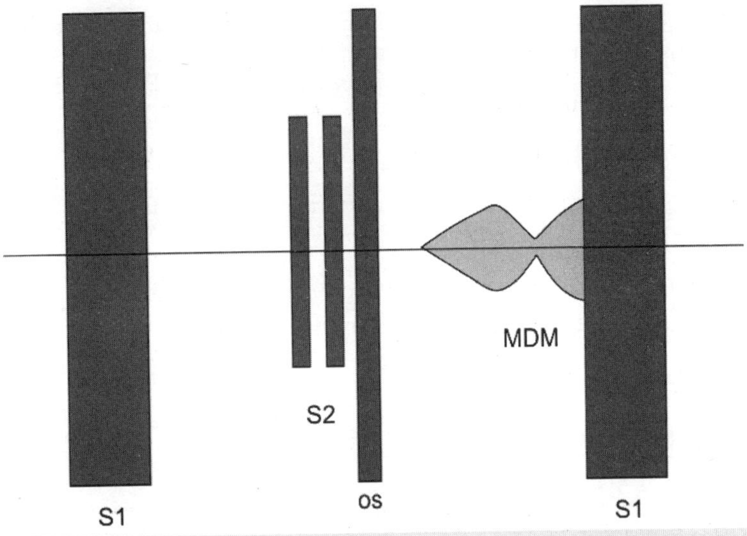

Ans. (A) i.e., Balloon mitral valvuloplasty/BMV

7. **Which one of the following is an example of Type IV respiratory failure?**

(a) Bronchial asthma (b) Pulmonary embolism (c) COPD (d) Shock

EXPLANATION

Type IV respiratory failure ensues when the circulation fails and resolves when shock is corrected, as long as one of the other types of respiratory failure has not supervened.

Ans. (D) i.e., Shock

8. **All of the following are seen in Polyarteritis Nodosa except:**

(a) Glomerulonephritis
(b) Peripheral Neuropathy
(c) Bowel Infarction
(d) Pericarditis

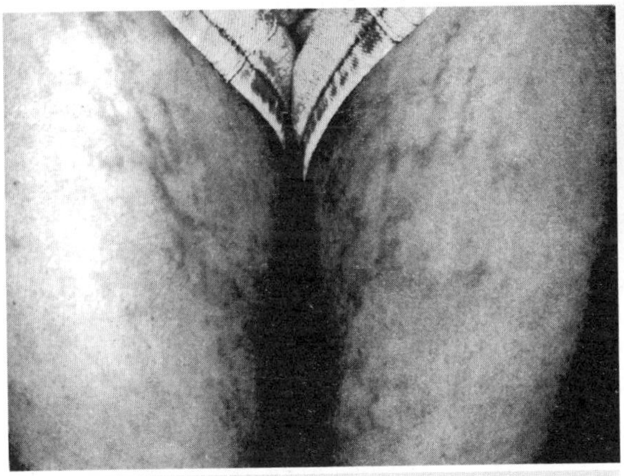

EXPLANATION

PAN may affect nearly every organ system and thus it can present with a broad array of signs and symptoms. These manifestations result from ischemic damage to affected organs, often the skin, heart, kidneys, and nervous system.

Ans. (C) i.e., Bowel Infarction

9. **All of the following are the pointers to organic cause of psychiatric disease except:**

(a) Late age of onset of psychiatric illness

(b) No previous history of psychiatric illness

(c) Family history of psychiatric illness

(d) No apparent psychological precipitant

EXPLANATION

Aspects of the history that may indicate the presence of an organic psychiatric disorder (including psychoactive substance abuse) include:

- History of presenting illness – the patient may complain of psychological dysfunction (such as difficulties in cognitive functioning).
- Family history – of an organic disorder with a genetic component.
- Personal history – e.g. birth injury, childhood infections.
- Past medical history – physical disorders, operations and medication (interactions, side effects and toxicity, e.g. steroid psychosis).
- Drug history – alcohol (e.g. Korsakov's syndrome), tobacco (e.g. carcinoma of the bronchus with cerebral metastases), illicit drugs (e.g. amphetamine psychosis).
- Premorbid personality – change in personality, e.g. in the frontal lobe syndrome.

Ans. (D) i.e., No apparent psychological precipitant

10. All of the following are Long Acting Beta Agonists (LABA) except:

(a) Levo salbutamol (b) Salmeterol (c) Formoterol (d) Indacaterol

EXPLANATION

Levosalbutamol, also known as **levalbuterol** is a short acting β_2 adrenergic receptor agonist used in the treatment of asthma and chronic obstructive pulmonary disease (COPD).

Ans. (A) i.e., Levo salbutamol

11. Deficiency of which immune function results in tubercular infections?

(a) Defective phagocytic function (b) Defect in T cell function
(c) Defect in B cell function (d) Defect in antibody productivity

EXPLANATION

T-lymphocytes play a major role in conferring immunity against M. tuberculosis.

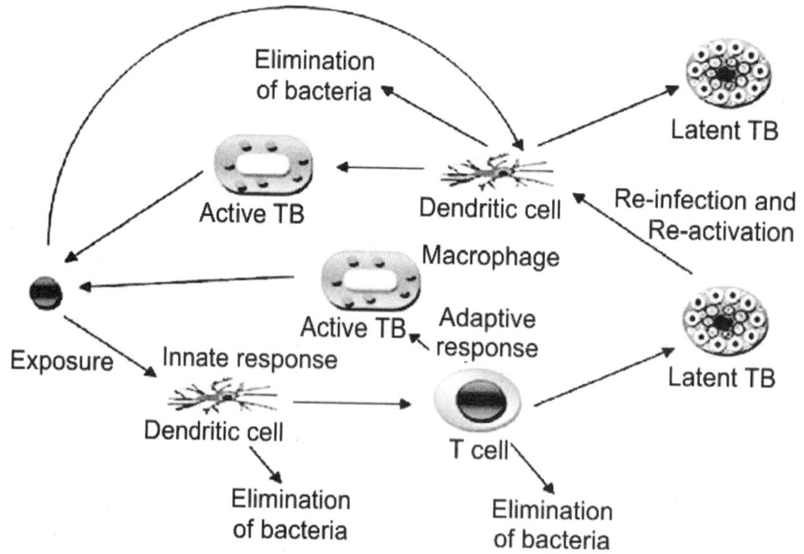

Ans. (B) i.e., Defect in T cell function

12. The most common agent responsible for community acquired pneumonia is:

(a) Streptococcus pneumoniae (b) Mycoplasma pneumoniae
(c) Staphylococcus aureus (d) Legionella haemophilia

EXPLANATION

50–80% cases of community acquired pneumonia are caused by pneumococcus.

Community Acquired Pneumonia
Definition: • Community acquired Pneumonia (CAP) is an alveolar infection that develops in the outpatient setting or within 48 hours of admission to a hospital. • CAP is not acquired in a hospital, long-term care facitlity, or other recent contact with the health care system, for 14 days before presentation of the acute illness.

Ans. (A) i.e., Streptococcus pneumoniae

13. A 26-year old woman presents with fever, arthralgia and erythema nodosum. Her chest X-ray reveals bilateral hilar lymphadenopathy. Her mantoux test is negative. The most likely diagnosis is:

(a) Tuberculosis
(b) Allergic bronchopulmonary aspergillosis
(c) Sarcoidosis
(d) Pulmonary thromboembolism

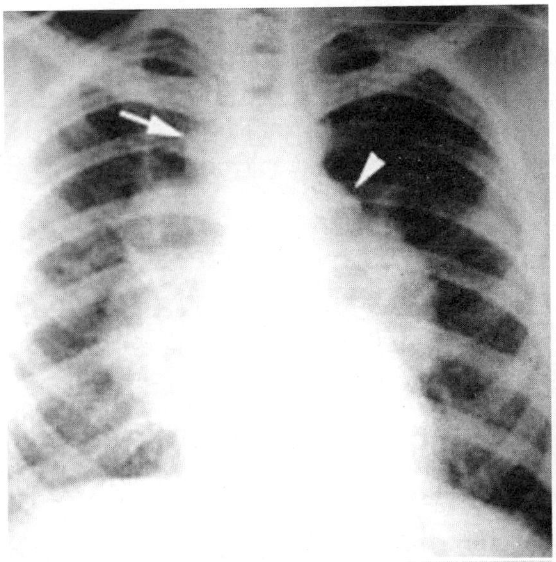

EXPLANATION

The most common presentation of sarcoidosis is as bilateral hilar lymphadenopathy with associated fever and erythema nodosum.

Ans. (C) i.e., Sarcoidosis

2018

14. Which of the following are the characteristics of Exudative pleural effusion?

1. Pleural fluid protein/serum protein > 0.5
2. Pleural fluid protein/serum protein < 0.5
3. Pleural fluid LDH/serum LDH > 0.6
4. Pleural fluid LDH/serum LDH < 0.6

Select the correct answer using the code given below:

(a) 1 and 3 (b) 1 and 4 (c) 2 and 3 (d) 2 and 4

EXPLANATION

Light's Criteria: Exudative **Effusions** will have at least one or more of the following:

- **Pleural fluid** protein/Serum protein >0.5.
- **Pleural fluid** LDH/Serum LDH >0.6.
- **Pleural fluid** LDH > 200 U/Lit (2/3 of Serum LDH Upper Limit of Normal).

Light's criteria (Sensitivity 99%, Specificity 98%)

Criteria	Transudate	Exudate
Pleural fluid protein : Serum : protein ratio	≤0.5	>0.5
Pleural fluid LDH : Serum LDH	≤0.6	>0.6
Pleural fluid LDH	≤200	>200

Ans. (A) i.e., 1 and 3.

15. **All of the following are seen in Whipple's disease except:**

(a) Weight loss
(b) Migratory arthropathy
(c) Dementia
(d) Hemolytic anemia

EXPLANATION

Whipple's disease primarily causes malabsorption but may affect any part of the body including the heart, brain, joints, skin, lungs and the eyes. Weight loss, diarrhea, joint pain, and arthritis are common presenting symptoms, but the presentation can be highly variable and approximately 15% of patients do not have these classic signs and symptoms. Of those affected by Whipple's disease, 10–40% of people have problems related to the involvement of the brain; the symptoms relate to the part of the brain that is affected. The most common problems are dementia, memory loss, confusion, and decreased level of consciousness.

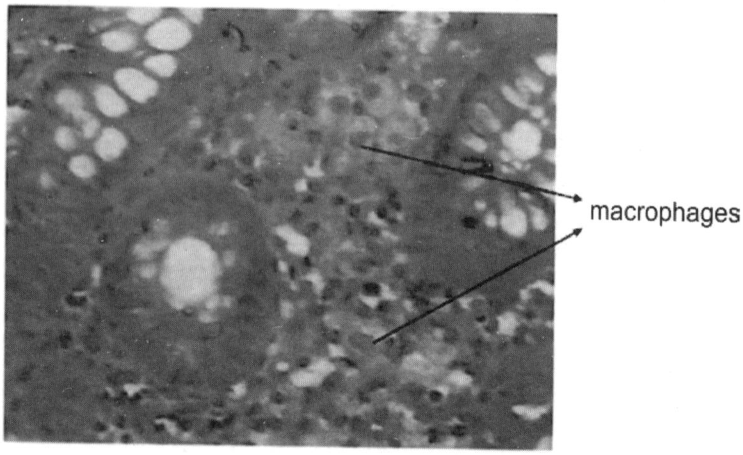

Microscopy showing sheets of foamy macrophages in the lamina propria of the small intestine (original magnification × 40, H&E)

Ans. (D) i.e., Hemolytic anemia

16. **A middle aged patient with chronic liver disease presents with pain abdomen and distension. He also has diarrhoea and fever since one day. On examination, he is hemodynamically stable with fever of 100°F. There is jaundice, pallor, pedal edema and ascites. A diagnostic paracentesis is done. Ascitic fluid protein is 0.8gm%, sugar 100mg%, total count 500/mm^3 of which 85% are polymorphonuclear leaukocytes and 15% lymphocytes. Most likely diagnosis is:**

(a) Spontaneous bacterial peritonitis
(b) Secondary bacterial peritonitis
(c) Perforation peritonitis
(d) T B peritonitis

EXPLANATION

Bacterial peritonitis

- Spontaneous bacterial peritonitis is diagnosed if the fluid contains neutrophils at greater than 250 cells per mm^3 (equals a cell count of 250 × 10^6/L) fluid in the absence of another reason for this (such as inflammation of one of the internal organs or a perforation).
- The crux of this algorithm is *Runyon's Criteria* for secondary bacterial peritonitis, which requires two of these three features: total protein >1g/dL, glucose <50mg/dL (2.8mM), and lactate dehydrodgenase above the upper limit of normal for serum.

Ans. (A) i.e., Spontaneous bacterial peritonitis

17. **Herald patch followed by rash is characteristic of:**

(a) Psoriasis
(b) Lichen planus
(c) Pityriasis rosea
(d) Dermatophytosis

EXPLANATION

Pityriasis rosea is a type of skin rash. Classically, it begins with a single red and slightly scaly area known as a "herald patch". This is then followed, days to weeks later, by a pink whole body rash. It typically lasts less than three months and goes away without treatment.

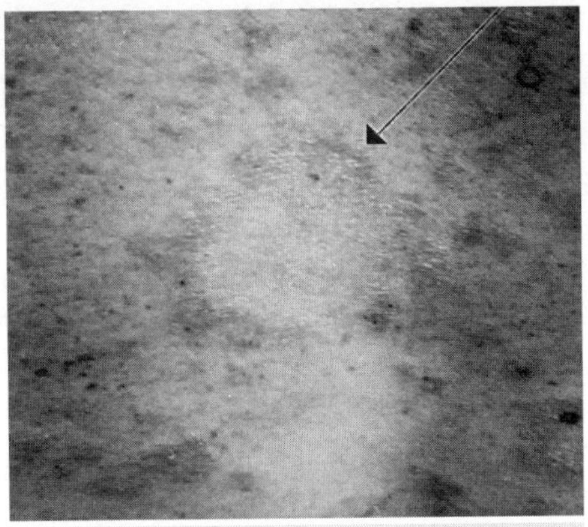

Ans. (C) i.e., Pityriasis rosea

18. **A young male comes to the OPD with history of jaundice since many years. He has noted that the jaundice may fluctuate but is often aggravated when he is fasting. There is no history of hospitalisation, no drug use, alcoholism or blood transfusion. Family history is not significant. Clinical examination is unremarkable except for mild scleral icterus. What is the likely diagnosis?**

(a) Dubin Johnson syndrome
(b) Crigler Najjar syndrome type I
(c) Gilbert's syndrome
(d) Rotor syndrome

EXPLANATION

Gilbert's syndrome (GS) is a mild liver disorder in which the liver does not properly process bilirubin. Many people never have symptoms. Occasionally a slight yellowish color of the skin or sclera may occur. Episodes of jaundice may be triggered by stress such as exercise, menstruation, or not eating.

Types of Jaundice	Prehepatic	Hepatic	Post hepatic
Type of bilirubin elevated	Unconjugated bilirubin	Both conjugated and unconjugated bilirubin	Conjugated bilirubin
Serum bilirubin Van den Bergh test	Indirect positive	Biphasic	Direct positive
Urine			
✓ Conj. Bilirubin	Absent	++	+++
✓ Urobilinogen	+++	+ early, obst, -dec.	Absent
✓ Bile salt	Absent	+	++
Urine color	Normal-Acholuric	Dark-Choluric	Dark-Choluric
Stool color	Dark brown color	N/decreased	Clay colored stools
AST and ALT	Normal	Very high	Inc.
ALP Levels	Normal	2–3 times increased	10–12 times inc.

Ans. (C) i.e., Gilbert's syndrome

19. **All of the following are causes of anemia in a case of chronic kidney disease except:**

(a) Decreased red blood cell survival
(b) Hemoglobinopathy
(c) Erythropoietin deficiency
(d) Gastrointestinal blood loss

2018

EXPLANATION

Hemoglobinopathy is a kind of genetic defect that results in abnormal structure of one of the globin chains of the hemoglobin molecule. Hemoglobinopathies are inherited single gene disorders; in most cases, they are inherited as autosomal codominant traits. Common hemoglobinopathies include sickle cell disease.

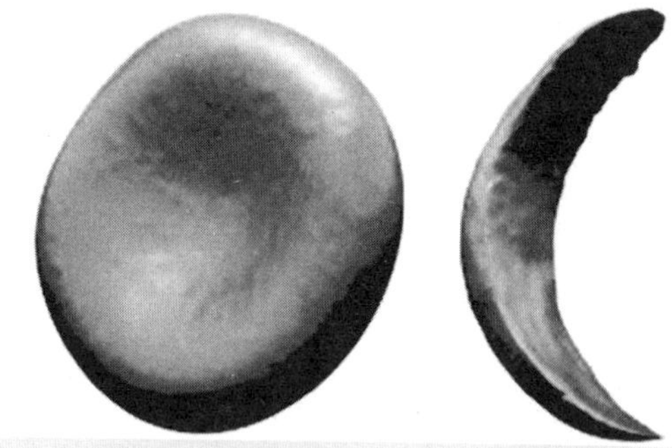

Ans. (B) i.e., Hemoglobinopathy

20. **Characteristic feature of upper motor neuron lesion includes:**

(a) Fasciculations (b) Hyporeflexia (c) Clonus (d) Muscle wasting

EXPLANATION

Clonus (from the Greek for "violent, confused motion") is a series of involuntary, rhythmic, muscular contractions and relaxations. Clonus is a sign of certain neurological conditions, particularly associated with upper motor neuron lesions involving descending motor pathways, and in many cases is, accompanied by spasticity (another form of hyperexcitability).

Ans. (C) i.e., Clonus

21. **Which one of the following arteries is involved in causation of lateral medullary syndrome?**

(a) Anterior superior cerebellar artery (b) Anterior inferior cerebellar artery
(c) Posterior superior cerebellar artery (d) Posterior inferior cerebellar artery

EXPLANATION

Lateral medullary syndromeis a neurological disorder causing a range of symptoms due to ischemia in the lateral part of the medulla oblongata in the brainstem. The ischemia is a result of a blockage in the posterior inferior cerebellar artery or one of its branches. Lateral medullary syndrome is also called Wallenberg syndrome or posterior inferior cerebellar artery syndrome.

Ans. (D) i.e., Posterior inferior cerebellar artery

22. **A right handed 70-year old man has a brain scan which reveals a lesion that has damaged his left angular and supramarginal gyrus. On examination, one would expect the following except:**

(a) Difficulty with left to right discrimination (b) Inappropriate affect
(c) Finger agnosia (d) Inability to write

EXPLANATION

The angular gyrus is the part of the brain associated with complex language functions (i.e. reading, writing and interpretation of what is written). Lesion to this part of the brain shows symptoms of the Gerstmann syndrome: effects include finger agnosia, alexia (inability to read), acalculia (inability to use arithmetic operations), agraphia (inability to copy), and left right confusion.

Ans. (B) i.e., Inappropriate affect

23. **Total iron binding capacity of more than 360μg/dl is seen in anemia due to:**

(a) Chronic inflammation (b) Hemoglobinopathies
(c) Sideroblastic anemia (d) Iron deficiency anaemia

EXPLANATION

Anemia and parameters

Condition	Serum iron (highly variable)	Transferrin and TIBC	Percent transferrin saturation
Iron deficiency anemia	Low	High. The liver produces more transferrin, presumably attempting to maximize use of the little iron that is available.	Low, as there is insufficient iron
Anemia of chronic disease	Low, as the body holds iron intra-cellularly with ferritin.	Low. The body produces less transferrin (but more erritin), presumably to keep iron away from pathogens that require it for their metabolism. This is mainly regulated by increased hepcidin production.	Normal

Ans. (D) i.e., Iron deficiency anaemia

24. **Escape behaviour with paroxysmal occurrence is seen in:**

(a) Phobic disorder
(b) Anxiety disorder
(c) Obsessive compulsive disorder
(d) Panic disorder

EXPLANATION

When total avoidance is impossible, escape behaviors may be used as a means of dealing with feared situations. Escape involves leaving or escaping from a feared social or performance situation. Some examples of escape include

- Leaving a gathering early
- Walking out in the middle of a speech
- Hiding in the restroom during a dinner party

Ans. (A) i.e., Phobic disorder

2018

25. **Which of the following conditions are associated with prolonged prothrombin time?**

1. **Factor VIII deficiency**
2. **Factor VII deficiency**
3. **Heparin anticoagulation**
4. **Warfarin anticoagulation**

EXPLANATION

Select the correct answer using the code given below:

(a) 1 and 4
(b) 1 and 3
(c) 2 and 3
(d) 2 and 4

EXPLANATION

The prothrombin time can be prolonged as a result of deficiencies in vitamin K, warfarin therapy, malabsorption, or lack of intestinal colonization by bacteria (such as in newborns). In addition, poor factor VII synthesis (due to liver disease) or increased consumption (in disseminated intravascular coagulation) may prolong the PT.

Coagulation Factor Activation

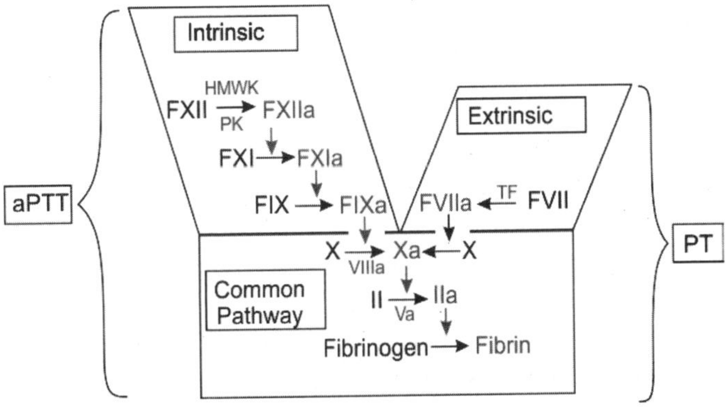

Ans. (D) i.e., 2 and 4.

26. **Syndrome X includes:**

(a) Hyperlipidemia, Obesity, Type 2 DM
(b) Obesity, CAD, COPD
(c) Hyperlipidemia, Hyperuricemia with CAD
(d) Hyponatremia, Hyperlipidemia with type 2 DM

EXPLANATION

Metabolic syndrome, sometimes known as Syndrome X, is a clustering of at least three of the five following medical conditions: central obesity, high blood pressure, high blood sugar (type 2 diabetes mellitus), high serum triglycerides, and low serum high density lipoprotein (HDL).

Ans. (A) i.e., Hyperlipidemia, Obesity, Type 2 DM

27. **Growth hormone secretion is inhibited by:**

(a) Arginine (b) Glucose (c) Clonidine (d) L Dopa

EXPLANATION

Inhibitors of GH secretion include:

- GHIH (*somatostatin*) from the periventricular nucleus
- Circulating concentrations of GH and IGF 1 (negative feedback on the pituitary and hypothalamus)
- Hyperglycemia
- Glucocorticoids
- Dihydrotestosterone

Ans. (B) i.e., Glucose

2018

28. **Which one of the following drugs causes hypercalcemia?**

(a) Phenytoin (b) Heparin (c) Lithium (d) Furosemide

EXPLANATION

Most cases of hypercalcemia are due to primary hyperparathyroidism or cancer. Other causes include sarcoidosis, tuberculosis, Paget disease, multiple endocrine neoplasia (MEN), vitamin D toxicity, familial hypocalciuric hypercalcaemia, and certain medications such as lithium and hydrochlorothiazide.

Ans. (C) i.e., Lithium

29. **All of the following insulins are longer acting except:**

(a) Glargine (b) Degludec (c) Glulisine (d) Detemir

EXPLANATION

longer acting insulin includes the analogues *glargine* and *detemir*, each of which begins working within 1 to 2 hours and continues to be active, without major peaks or dips, for about 24 hours, although this varies in many individuals. Currently only ultra longer acting insulin includes the analogue *degludec*, which begins working within 30 to 90 minutes and continues to be active for greater than 24 hours.

Ans. (A) i.e., Glargine

30. The presence of vitiligo on examination suggests an associated:

(a) Autoimmune disease
(b) Degenerative disease

(c) Infection
(d) Malignancy

EXPLANATION

The exact cause of vitiligo is unknown. It is believed to be due to genetic susceptibility that is triggered by an environmental factor such that an autoimmune disease occurs.

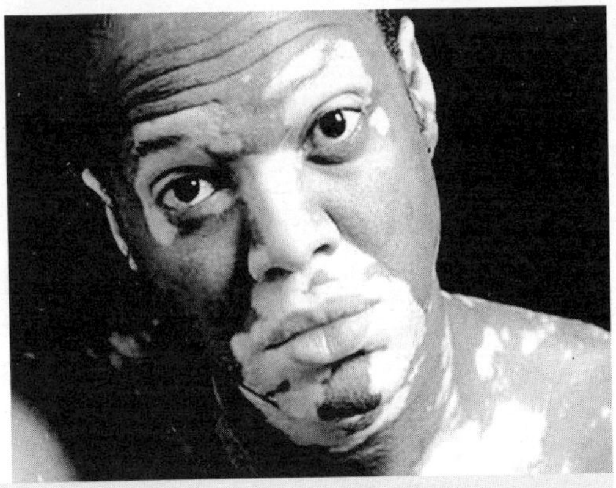

Ans. (A) i.e., Autoimmune disease

31. **A mildy elevated TSH (5–20 mU/L) along with a normal T3 and normal T4 levels is suggestive of:**
(a) Primary hypothyroidism
(b) Subclinical hypothyroidism
(c) Artefact
(d) Thyroid hormone resistance

EXPLANATION

TSH	T4	Interpretation
Normal	Normal	Normal thyroid function
Elevated	Low	Overt hypothyroidism
Normal/low	Low	Central hypothyroidism
Elevated	Normal	Subclinical hypothyroidism

Ans. (B) i.e., Subclinical hypothyroidism

32. **Which one of the following suggests patient to be prediabetic?**
(a) HbA1c 5.6%, FPG 126mg/dL
(b) HbA1c 6%, FPG 130mg/dL
(c) HbA1c 6.2%, FPG 105mg/dL
(d) HbA1c 6.6%, FPG 115mg/dL

EXPLANATION

Usually, prediabetes is diagnosed with a blood test:
- Fasting blood sugar (glucose) level of:
- 110 to 125mg/dL (6.1mM/L to 6.9mM/L) – WHO criteria
- 100 to 125mg/dL (5.6mM/L to 6.9mM/L) – ADA criteria
- Two hour glucose tolerance test after ingesting the standardized 75gm glucose solution the blood sugar level of 140 to 199mg/dL (7.8 to 11.0mM)
- Glycated haemoglobin between 5.7 and 6.4 percent.

Ans. (C) i.e., HbA1c 6.2%, FPG 105mg/dL

33. **Cutaneous manifestations of tuberculosis includes:**
(a) Erythema nodosum and lupus vulgaris
(b) Erythema marginatum and lupus vulgaris
(c) Phyctenular conjunctivitis and erythema multiforme
(d) Pyoderma gangrenosum and Dactylitis

EXPLANATION

Lesion associated with TB

- Erythema nodosum (EN), also known as subacute migratory panniculitis of Vilanova and Piñol, is an inflammatory condition characterized by inflammation of the fat cells under the skin, resulting in tender red nodules or lumps that are usually seen on both shins.
- Lupus vulgaris (also known as tuberculosis luposa) are painful cutaneous tuberculosis skin lesions with nodular appearance, most often on the face around the nose, eyelids, lips, cheeks, ears and neck. It is the most common *Mycobacterium tuberculosis* skin infection.

Ans. (A) i.e., Erythema nodosum and lupus vulgaris

34. Treatment of scrub typhus is:

(a) Ciprofloxacin (b) Clindamycin (c) Penicillin (d) Azithromycin

EXPLANATION

The drug most commonly used drug for scrub typhus is doxycycline or tetracycline, but chloramphenicol is an alternative. Strains that are resistant to doxycycline and chloramphenicol have been reported in northern Thailand. Rifampicin and azithromycin are alternatives.

Ans. (D) i.e., Azithromycin

35. Which one of the following is NOT correct regarding Clostridum tetani?

(a) Anaerobic
(b) Non motile
(c) Gram positive
(d) Spore bearing

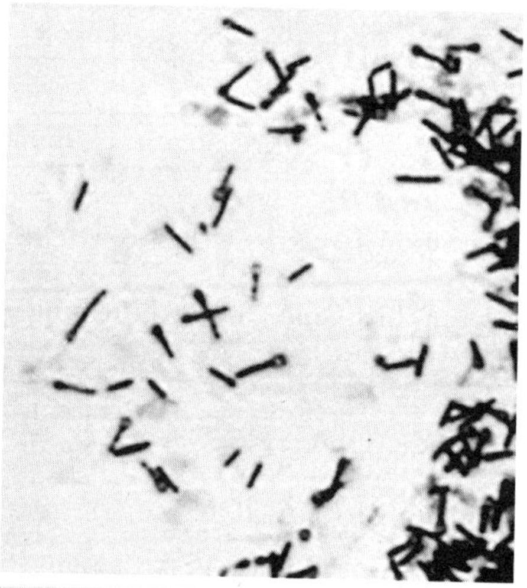

EXPLANATION

C. tetani is a rod shaped Gram positive bacterium, typically up to 0.5 micrometers wide and 2.5 micrometers long. It is motile by way of various flagellae that surround its body. *C. tetani* is an anaerobe and cannot survive in the presence of oxygen. It grows best at temperatures ranging from 33°C to 37°C.

Ans. (B) i.e., Non motile

36. All of the following are extrapulmonary manifestations of mycoplasma infection except:

(a) Arthritis
(b) Guillain Barre syndrome
(c) Stevens Johnson syndrome
(d) Dementia

EXPLANATION

Extra articular manifestations of mycoplasma:

- Neurologic: Meningo encephalitis, encephalitis, Guillain Barre syndrome and aseptic meningitis.
- Dermatologic: Skin rashes including erythema multiforme major (Steven Johnson syndrome)
- Rheumatologic: Reactive arthritis

Ans. (D) i.e., Dementia

37. A 'slapped cheek rash' is characteristic of infection with:

(a) Rubella
(b) Parvovirus B19
(c) Human herpesvirus 6
(d) Measles

2018

EXPLANATION

Erythema infectiosum or **fifth disease** is one of several possible manifestations of infection by parvovirus B19. The name "fifth disease" comes from its place on the standard list of rash causing childhood diseases, which also includes measles (first), scarlet fever (second), rubella (third), Dukes' disease (fourth, but is no longer widely accepted as distinct), and roseola (sixth).

The bright red rash of fifth disease most commonly appears in the face, particularly the cheeks. This is a defining symptom of the infection in children (hence the name "slapped cheek disease").

Ans. (B) i.e., Parvovirus B19

38. A 34 week pregnant nurse comes in contact with a patient with chickenpox at her workplace. She has never had chickenpox in the past and is unvaccinated. The best option for her is:

(a) Varicella zoster immunoglobulin to be given within 7 days

(b) Vaccinate for chicken pox

(c) Start oral acyclovir

(d) Wait and watch

EXPLANATION

Varicella (live attenuated vaccine) is not recommended in pregnancy. Varicella zoster immunoglobulin (VZIG) should be given to exposed non immune patients as it reduces the morbidity.

Ans. (A) i.e., Varicella zoster immunoglobulin to be given within 7 days

39. Which one of the following has the maximum diagnostic sensitivity for Leishmaniasis?

(a) Splenic aspirate

(b) Bone marrow aspirate

(c) Ascitic fliud aspirate

(d) Lymph node aspirate

EXPLANATION

The gold standard for diagnosis is visualization of the amastigotes in splenic aspirate or bone marrow aspirate. This is a technically challenging procedure that is frequently unavailable in areas of the world where visceral leishmaniasis is endemic.

Ans. (A) i.e., Splenic aspirate

40. Which one of the following statements regarding cryptosporidiosis is NOT correct?

(a) Infection is acquired by feco oral route

(b) It is usually a mild self limiting illness in immunocompetent patient

(c) In HIV infected persons it is a serious opportunistic infection

(d) Treatment is with metronidazole

EXPLANATION

Cryptosporidiosis

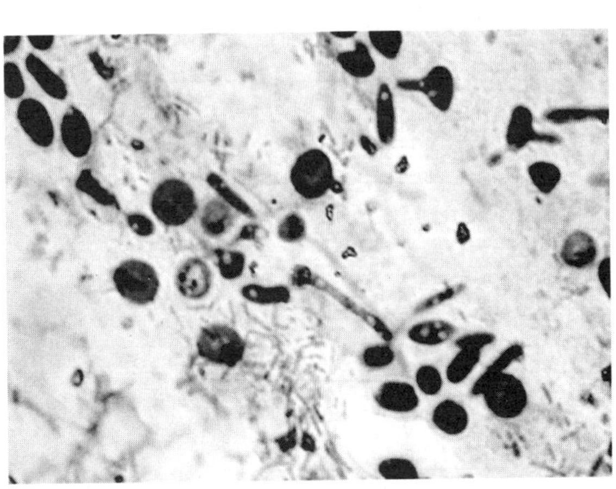

- It is primarily spread through the fecal oral route, often through contaminated water; recent evidence suggests that it can also be transmitted via fomites in respiratory secretions.
- It affects the distal small intestine and can affect the respiratory tract in both immunocompetent (i.e., individuals with a normal functioning immune system) and immunocompromised

(e.g., persons with HIV/AIDS or autoimmune disorders) individuals, resulting in watery diarrhea with or without an unexplained cough.

- In immunosuppressed individuals, the symptoms are particularly severe and can be fatal.

Ans. (C) i.e., In HIV infected persons it is a serious opportunistic infection

41. All of the following are live attenuated vaccines except:

(a) MMR (Measles, Mumps, Rubella) vaccine
(b) Rabies vaccine
(c) Oral polio vaccine
(d) BCG vaccine

EXPLANATION

The human diploid cell rabies vaccine (H.D.C.V.) was started in 1967. Human diploid cell rabies vaccines are inactivated vaccines made using the attenuated Pitman Moore L503 strain of the virus.

Ans. (B) i.e., Rabies vaccine

42. All of the following are soil transmitted nematodes except:

(a) Ancyclostoma duodenale
(b) Strongyloides stercoralis
(c) Necator americanus
(d) Ascaris lumbricoides

EXPLANATION

Soil transmitted helminths refer to the intestinal worms infecting humans that are transmitted through contaminated soil ("helminth" means parasitic worm): *Ascaris lumbricoides* (sometimes called just "*Ascaris*"), whipworm (*Trichuris trichiura*), and hookworm (*Anclostoma duodenale* and *Necator americanus*).

Ans. (B) i.e., Strongyloides stercoralis

2018

43. A veterinary doctor is bitten by a stray dog, which is classified as a category 3 bite. He has completed his preexposure prophylactic vaccination with human diploid cell Rabies vaccine with three doses administered on day 0, 7, 28 about 1 year back. Appropriate treatment would include which of the following?

1. Wound care

2. Antibiotics

3. Booster dose of Anti Rabies vaccine

4. Rabies immune globulin at wound site

Select the correct answer using the code given below:

(a) 1 only
(b) 1 and 2 only
(c) 1, 2 and 3
(d) 2, 3 and 4

EXPLANATION

In persons who have received preexposure prophylaxis, if risk of infection occurs two booster doses of the vaccine should be given on days 0 and 3. Local washing of the wound and wound toilet are absolutely necessary to reduce the risk.

Ans. (C) i.e., 1, 2 and 3

44. Loffler's syndrome is caused due to infection by:

(a) Strongyloidiasis
(b) Filariasis
(c) Cysticercosis
(d) Ascaris

EXPLANATION

Löffler's syndrome or **Loeffler's syndrome** is a disease in which eosinophils accumulate in the lung in response to a parasitic infection. The parasite can be *Strongyloides Stercoralis, Dirofilaria immitis* or *Ascaris* which can contaminate the body through contact with the soil.

Ans. (A & D) i.e., Strongyloidiasis & Ascaris

45. Which of the following is/are the common infectious syndrome(s) associated with klebsiella pneumoniae?

1. Pneumonia 2. Intra abdominal infections 3. Hepatitis

Select the correct answer using the code given below:

(a) 1 only (b) 1 and 2 only (c) 1, 2 and 3 (d) 2 only

EXPLANATION

The range of clinical diseases caused by Klebsiella pneumoniae includes pneumonia, thrombophlebitis, urinary tract infection, cholecystitis, diarrhea, upper respiratory tract infection, wound infection, osteomyelitis, meningitis, and bacteremia and septicemia.

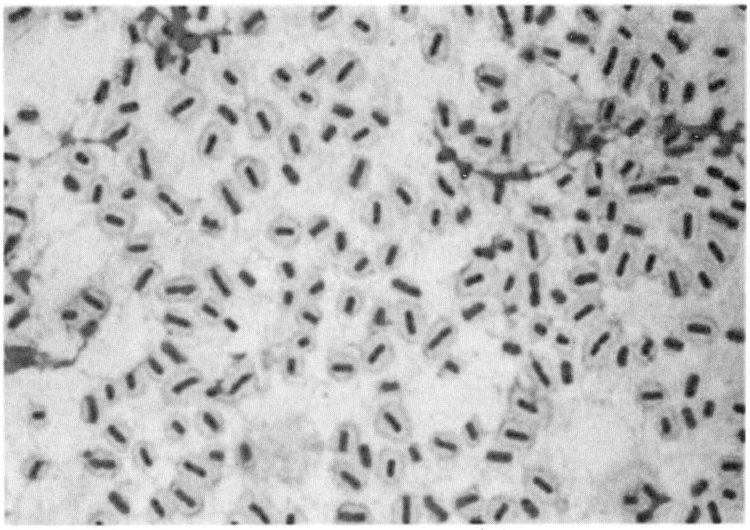

Ans. (C) i.e., 1, 2 and 3

46. Differential diagnosis of dysenteric syndrome includes which of the following?

1. Salmonella infection 2. Campylobacter infection

3. Shigella infection 4. Clostridium infection

Select the correct answer using the code given below:

(a) 1, 2 and 4 only (b) 2, 3 and 4 only (c) 1 and 3 only (d) 1, 2, 3 and 4

EXPLANATION

Dysentery can have a number of causes. Bacterial infections are by far the most common causes of dysentery. These infections include *Shigella, Campylobacter, E. coli,* and *Salmonella* species of bacteria.

Ans. (D) i.e., 1, 2, 3 and 4

47. Antifungal agent of choice for the treatment of mucormycosis is:

(a) Voriconazole (b) Intraconazole

(c) Amphotericin B (d) Fluconazole

2018

EXPLANATION

If mucormycosis is suspected, amphotericin B therapy should be immediately administered due to the rapid spread and high mortality rate of the disease.

Ans. (C) i.e., Amphotericin B

48. What drug therapy would be appropriate for management of UTI in a pregnant patient?

(a) Trimethoprim sulfamethoxazole
(b) Ciprofloxacin
(c) Ampicillin
(d) All of these

EXPLANATION

Co trimoxazole & fluoroquinolones are contraindicated in pregnancy.

Ans. (C) i.e., Ampicillin

49. Which one of the following conditions is NOT associated with lymphocytosis?

(a) Infectious mononucleosis
(b) Viral fevers
(c) Rickettsial fevers
(d) Leptospirosis

EXPLANATION

Lymphocytopenia, but not idiopathic CD4+ lymphocytopenia, is associated with corticosteroid use, infections with HIV and other viral, bacterial, and fungal agents etc.

Ans. (B) i.e., Viral fevers

50. Which of the following is NOT a diagnostic criterion of Kwashiorkor?

(a) Serum albumin < 2.8g/dl
(b) Triceps skinfold thickness < 3mm
(c) Easy hair pluckability
(d) Edema

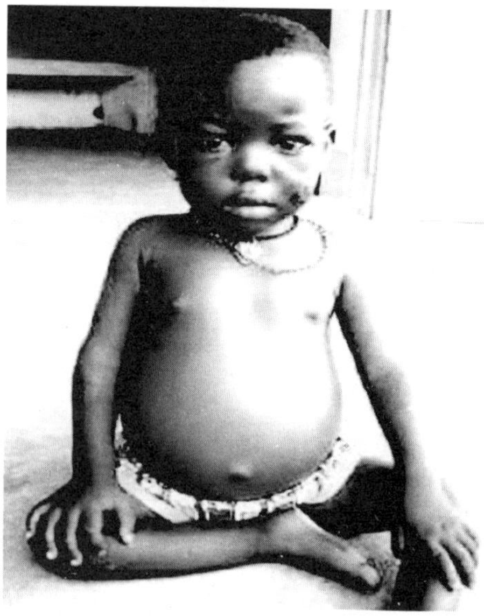

EXPLANATION

Kwashiorkor is a form of severe protein malnutrition characterized by edema, and an enlarged liver with fatty infiltrates. Sufficient calorie intake, but with insufficient protein consumption, distinguishes it from marasmus.

Ans. (B) i.e., Triceps skinfold thickness < 3 mm

51. Which one of the following drugs does NOT have any action against Salmonella typhi?

(a) Erythromycin
(b) Amoxicillin
(c) Cotrimoxazole
(d) Doxycycline

EXPLANATION

Typhoid fever (caused by Salmonella typhii), when properly treated, is not fatal in most cases. Antibiotics, such as ampicillin, chloramphenicol, trimethoprim sulfamethoxazole, amoxicillin, and ciprofloxacin, have been commonly used to treat typhoid fever in microbiology.

Ans. (D > A) i.e., Doxycycline > Erythromycin

52. **All of the following drugs are used for the treatment of influenza except:**

(a) Zanamivir (b) Rimantadine (c) Oseltamivir (d) Tenofovir

EXPLANATION

The two classes of antiviral drugs used against influenza are neuraminidase inhibitors (oseltamivir, zanamivir, laninamivir and peramivir) and M2 protein inhibitors (adamantane derivatives). The antiviral drugs amantadine and rimantadine inhibit a viral ion channel (M2 protein), thus inhibiting replication of the influenza A virus.

Ans. (D) i.e., Tenofovir

53. **Diagnostic accuracy has been enhanced by the ability to detect specific DNA sequences in all of the following infectious microorganisms except:**

(a) Cytomegalovirus(CMV) (b) Human Immunodeficiency virus (HIV)
(c) Mycobacterium tuberculosis (d) Staphylococcus aureus

EXPLANATION

Polymerase Chain Reaction permits identification of non cultivatable or slow growing microorganisms such as mycobacteria, anaerobic bacteria, or viruses from tissue culture assays and animal models.

Ans. (D) i.e., Staphylococcus aureus

54. **Hip Flexor Spasm is characteristic of:**

(a) Osteomyelitis femur
(b) Septic arthritis hip joint
(c) Psoas abscess
(d) Deep vein thrombosis

EXPLANATION

An abscess in the psoas muscle of the abdomen may be caused by lumbar tuberculosis. Owing to the proximal attachments of the iliopsoas, such an abscess may drain inferiorly into the upper medial thigh and present as a swelling in the region.

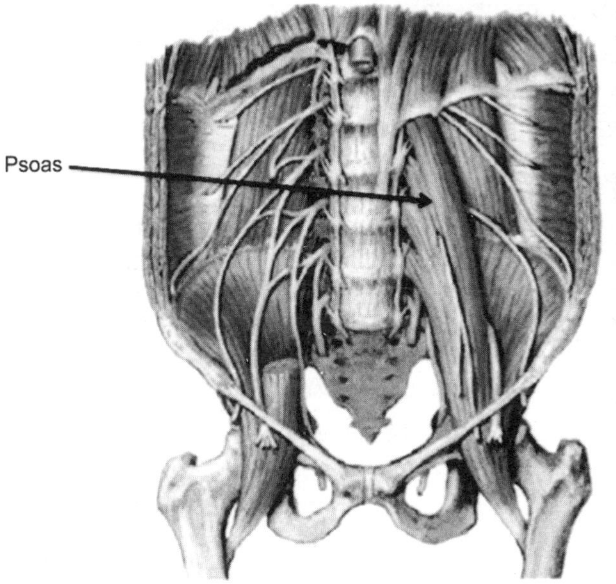

Ans. (C) i.e., Psoas abscess

55. **Gastroenteritis associated with eating raw eggs is usually attributed to:**

(a) E.coli (b) Noro virus
(c) Salmonella species (d) Clostriduim botulinum

EXPLANATION

Salmonella infection is usually caused by eating raw or undercooked meat, poultry, eggs or egg products. The incubation period ranges from several hours to two days. Most salmonella infections can be classified as stomach flu (gastroenteritis).

Ans. (C) i.e., Salmonella species

56. Which one of the following diseases is NOT caused by protozoa?

(a) Trypanosomiasis (b) Leishmaniasis (c) Amoebiasis (d) Schistosomiasis

EXPLANATION

Several pathogenic protozoans appear to be capable of sexual processes involving meiosis (or at least a modified form of meiosis). Included among these protozoans are *Plasmodium falciparum* (malaria), *Toxoplasma gondii* (toxoplasmosis), *Leishmania* species (leishmaniases), *Trypanosoma brucei* (African sleeping sickness), *Trypanosoma cruzi* (Chagas disease) and *Giardia intestinalis* (giardiasis)

Ans. (D) i.e., Schistosomiasis

57. An adult with fever and right sided chest pain is found to have a moderate right sided pleural effusion. Chest X-Ray (PA view) also shows a moderate pleural effusion. A diagnostic thoracocentesis reveals straw coloured exudates with 50 mg% of sugar and lymphocytic pleocytosis. ADA levels are borderline. What investigation would be most likely to confirm a diagnosis of tuberculosis?

(a) Needle Biopsy of the Pleura (b) Pleural Fluid Xpert MTB/RIF assay

(c) Pleural Fluid AFB smear (d) Pleural Fluid AFB culture

EXPLANATION

The gold standard for the diagnosis of TB pleuritis is detection of *M. tuberculosis* in the sputum, pleural fluid or pleural biopsy specimens, either by microscopy and/or culture, or the histological demonstration of caseating granulomas in the pleura along with acid fast bacilli (AFB)

Ans. (D) i.e., Pleural Fluid AFB culture

2018

58. Consider the following statements with regard to acute anterior poliomyelitis:

1. **It is caused by a virus belonging to picornavirus family**
2. **Muscle pain and cramps may be associated with diffuse transient fasciculations at the onset**
3. **Tonsillectomy reduces the risk of bulbar poliomyelitis**
4. **Cerebrospinal fluid may show mild pleocytosis with increase polymorphonuclear cells in early course of disease**

Which of the above statements are correct?

(a) 1, 2 and 3 (b) 2, 3 and 4 (c) 1, 2 and 4 (d) 1, 3 and 4

EXPLANATION

Polio

- **Poliovirus**, the causative agent of poliomyelitis (commonly known as **polio**), is a human enterovirus and member of the family of *Picornaviridae.*
- Virus invasion causes inflammation of the nerve cells of anterior horn cells of spinal cord, leading to damage or destruction of motor neuron ganglia. With the destruction of nerve cells, the muscles no longer receive signals from the brain or spinal cord; without nerve stimulation, the muscles atrophy, becoming weak, floppy and poorly controlled, and finally completely paralyzed. Maximum paralysis progresses rapidly (two to four days), and usually involves fever and muscle pain.
- Tonsillectomy increases the risk of bulbar poliomyelitis.
- Analysis of the patient's cerebrospinal fluid (CSF), which is collected by a lumbar puncture ("spinal tap"), reveals an increased number of white blood cells and a mildly elevated protein level.

Ans. (C) i.e., 1, 2 and 4

59. **Which one of the following is NOT seen in case of Marasmus?**

(a) Reduced triceps skinfold thickness
(b) Normal serum albumin
(c) Easy hair pluckability
(d) Decreased mid arm circumference

EXPLANATION

Marasmus is commonly represented by a shrunken, wasted appearance, loss of muscle mass and subcutaneous fat mass.

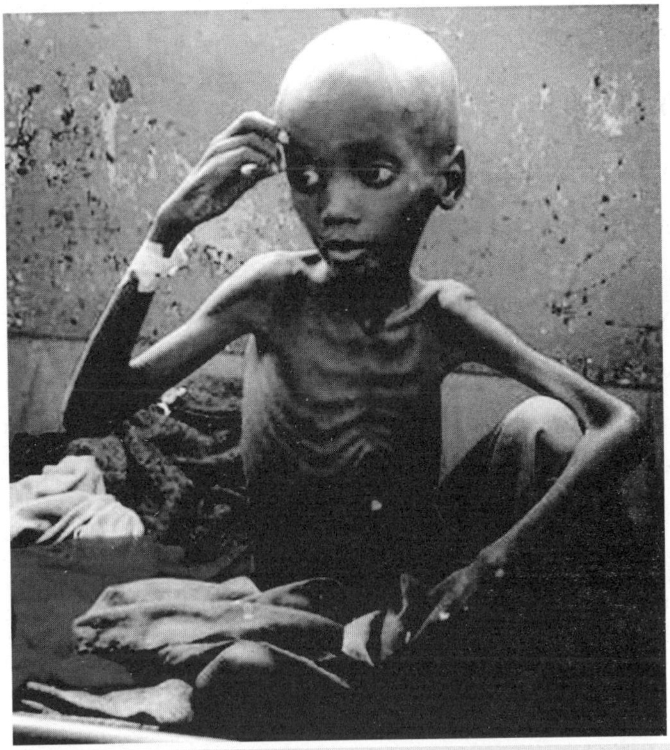

Ans. (C) i.e., Easy hair pluckability

60. **Perception of an object in absence of stimulus is:**

(a) Illusions
(b) Delusions
(c) Hallucination
(d) Psychosis

EXPLANATION

A **hallucination** is a perception in the absence of external stimulus that has qualities of real perception. Hallucinations are vivid, substantial, and are perceived to be located in external objective space.

Ans. (C) i.e., Hallucination

61. **All of the following drugs can be used for the treatment for cessation of smoking except:**

(a) Nicotine gum
(b) Clonazepam
(c) Bapropion
(d) Varenicline

EXPLANATION

Many different strategies can be used for smoking cessation, including abruptly quitting without assistance ("cold turkey"), cutting down then quitting, behavioral counseling, and medications such as bupropion, cytisine, nicotine replacement therapy, or varenicline.

Ans. (B) i.e., Clonazepam

62. **All of the following features are present in Organophosphorus poisoning except:**

(a) Bronchorrhea
(b) Hypertonia
(c) Confusion
(d) Fasciculations

EXPLANATION

Overstimulation of nicotinic acetylcholine receptors in the central nervous system, due to accumulation of ACh, results in anxiety, headache, convulsions, ataxia, depression of respiration and circulation, tremor, general weakness, and potentially coma. When there is expression of muscarinic overstimulation due to excess acetylcholine at muscarinic acetylcholine receptors symptoms of visual disturbances, tightness in chest, wheezing due to bronchoconstriction, increased bronchial secretions (bronchorrhea), increased salivation, lacrimation, sweating, peristalsis, and urination can occur. The effects of organophosphate poisoning on muscarinic receptors are recalled using the mnemonic SLUDGEM (salivation, lacrimation, urination, defecation, gastrointestinal motility, emesis, miosis).

Ans. (B) i.e., Hypertonia

63. Small sized pupils are seen in poisoning with all except:

(a) Organophosphorous compounds (b) Opioids

(c) Clonidine (d) Cocaine

EXPLANATION

Drugs causing miosis

- Opioids such as fentanyl, morphine, heroin and methadone (the notable exception being pethidine)
- Imidazolines such as clonidine, naphazoline, oxymetazoline and tetrahydrozoline
- Antipsychotics,including risperidone, haloperidol, chlorpromazine, olanzapine, quetiapine and others
- Cholinergic agents such as acetylcholine
- Acetylcholinesterase inhibitors
- Organophosphates

Ans. (D) i.e., Cocaine

2018

64. A 24-year old male presents with consumption of an unknown substance. His respiratory rate is 22/minute, pulse rate is 110/minute, BP is 150/94mmHg and he has 2 episodes of seizures. There are tremors and hallucinations. The substance ingested most likely is:

(a) Amphetamines (b) Diazepam (c) Oxycodone (d) Ethanol

EXPLANATION

Amphetamine toxicity

- Amphetamines increase the activity of the neurotransmitters dopamine and norepinephrine.
- Tachycardia and other arrhythmias are due to the sympathomimetic effects of amphetamines. Amphetamines cause tachycardia and hypertension and can cause significant cerebral blood flow which increases by 30%.
- Increased dopamine levels in the central nervous system (CNS) cause psychosis, euphoric effects, and other movement disorders. Amphetamine toxicity can also cause seizures due to neuronal death from the interaction between amphetamines and NMDA receptors.

Ans. (A) i.e., Amphetamines

65. The toxic effects of aluminium phosphide is due to the release of:

(a) Phosgene (b) Chlorine

(c) Inorganic phosphates (d) Phosphine

EXPLANATION

The toxicity of aluminium phosphide is attributed to the liberation of phosphine gas, a cytotoxic compound that causes free radical mediated injury, inhibits vital cellular enzymes and is directly corrosive to tissues.

Ans. (D) i.e., Phosphine

66. An 18-year old boy was brought to the emergency department after being bitten by a sawscaled viper. The monitoring which is most crucial in this patient is:

(a) Single breath count
(b) Neck flop
(c) Whole blood clotting time
(d) Creatine phosphokinase

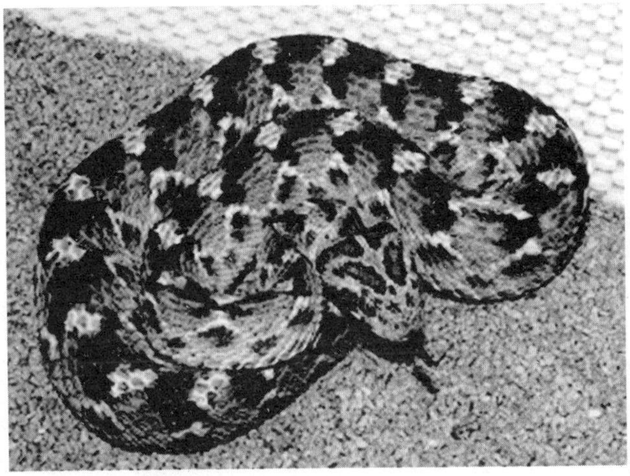

EXPLANATION

Most of saw scaled viper species have venom that contains factors that can cause a consumption coagulopathy and defibrination, which may persist for days to weeks. This may result in bleeding anywhere in the body, including the possibility of an intracranial hemorrhage. The latter classically occurs a few days following the bite.

Ans. (C) i.e., Whole blood clotting time

67. Bite of cobra is likely to result in:

(a) Flaccid paralysis (b) Coagulopathy (c) Myolysis (d) Cardiotoxicity

EXPLANATION

Cobras belong to the sub group of snakes known as **elapids**. An elapid's venom contains postsynaptic neurotoxins that spread rapidly in its victim's bloodstream, causing respiratory failure and, eventually, death.

Ans. (A) i.e., Flaccid paralysis

68. Hematuria is a prominent symptom with infection due to:

(a) Strongyloides stercoralis (b) Schistosoma hematobium
(c) Toxocara spp. (d) Gnathostomiasis

EXPLANATION

Schistosomiasis, also known as **snail fever** and **bilharzia**, is a disease caused by parasitic flatworms called schistosomes. The urinary tract or the intestines may be infected. Symptoms include abdominal pain, diarrhea, bloody stool, or blood in the urine.

Ans. (B) i.e., Schistosoma hematobium

69. Bite of the Tsetse Fly transmits:

(a) Leishmaniasis (b) Chaga's disease
(c) Dengue fever (d) African Trypanosomiasis

EXPLANATION

Tse-tse fly have a prominent economic impact in sub Saharan Africa as the biological vectors of trypanosomes, which cause human sleeping sickness and animal trypanosomiasis.

Ans. (D) i.e., African Trypanosomiasis

70. A 60-year old man with pneumonia is unconscious and has a PaO_2 of 50 mm Hg. The preferred modality of treatment for him is:

(a) Oxygen through nasal cannula
(b) Non invasive ventilation
(c) Invasive mechanical ventilation
(d) No respiratory support is indicated

EXPLANATION

Non invasive ventilation may be beneficial in those patients of pneumonia who admitted to the intensive care unit.

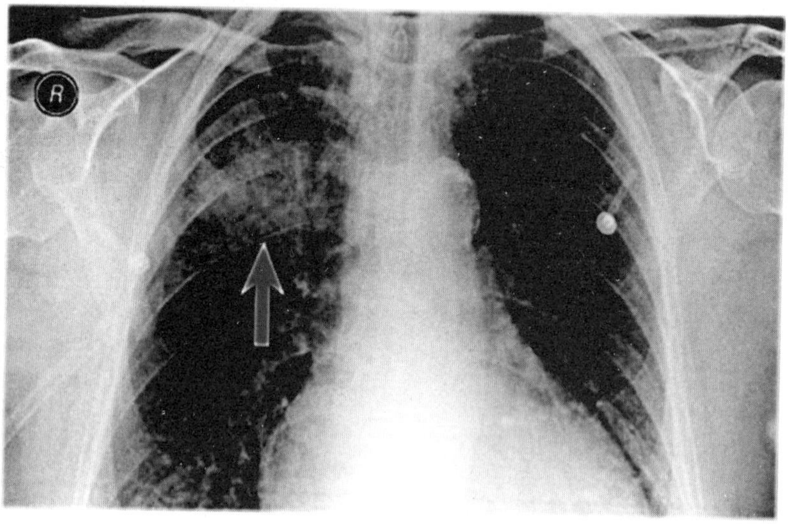

Ans. (B) i.e., Non invasive ventilation

71. Oliguria is defined as a reduction in urine output

(a) Less than 1 ml/kg/hour
(b) Less than 0.5 ml/kg/hour
(c) Less than 200 ml in 24 hours
(d) Any decrease over previous urine output

EXPLANATION

Oliguria is defined as a urine output that is less than 1 mL/kg/h in infants, less than 0.5 mL/kg/h in children, and less than 400 mL or 500 mL per 24h in adults - this equals 17 or 21 mL/hour. For example, in an adult weighing 70 kg it equals 0.24 or 0.3 mL/hour/kg. Alternatively, however, the value of 0.5 mL/kg/h is commonly used to define oliguria in adults as well.

Ans. (B) i.e., Less than 0.5 ml/kg/hour

72. All of the following are signs of Brain death except:

(a) Pupils fixed and unresponsive to light
(b) Corneal reflexes absent
(c) Bilateral planter response – Mute or Absent
(d) No gag reflex

EXPLANATION

The definitive criteria of brain stem death are:

1. Fixed pupils which do not respond to sharp changes in the intensity of incident light.

2018

2. No corneal reflex.
3. Absent oculovestibular reflexes – no eye movements following the slow injection of at least 50ml of ice cold water into each ear in turn (the caloric reflex test).
4. No response to supraorbital pressure.
5. No cough reflex to bronchial stimulation or gagging response to pharyngeal stimulation.
6. No observed respiratory effort in response to disconnection of the ventilator for long enough (typically 5 minutes) to ensure elevation of the arterial partial pressure of carbon dioxide to at least 6.0kPa (6.5kPa in patients with chronic carbon dioxide retention). Adequate oxygenation is ensured by preoxygenation and diffusion oxygenation during the disconnection (so the brainstem respiratory centre is not challenged by the ultimate, anoxic, drive stimulus). This test—the apnoea test—is dangerous – and may prove lethal.

Ans. (C) i.e., Corneal reflexes absent

73. A 35-year old man with history of alcoholism presents with ophthalmoplegia, ataxia and global confusion. The treatment of choice for this patient is:

(a) I.V. Glucose (b) I.V. Thiamine (c) I.V. Mannitol (d) I.V. Immunoglobulin

EXPLANATION

Classically, Wernicke encephalopathy is characterised by the triad – ophthalmoplegia, ataxia, and confusion. In patients suspected of WE, thiamine treatment should be started immediately. Blood should be immediately taken to test for thiamine, other vitamins and minerals levels. Following this an immediate intravenous or intramuscular dose of thiamine should be administered two or three times daily.

Ans. (B) i.e., I.V. Thiamine

2018

74. Most common form of paroxysmal supraventricular Tachycardia is:

(a) Junctional Ectopic Tachycardia
(b) AV Nodal Reentry Tachycardia (ANVRT)
(c) Accessory Pathways
(d) Accelerated junctional rhythm

EXPLANATION

AV nodal reentrant tachycardia (AVNRT), or **atrioventricular nodal reentrant tachycardia**, is a type of abnormal fast heart rhythm. It is a type of supraventricular tachycardia (SVT), meaning that it originates from a location within the heart above the bundle of His. AV nodal reentrant tachycardia is the most common regular supraventricular tachycardia.

Supraventricular Tachycardia (SVT)

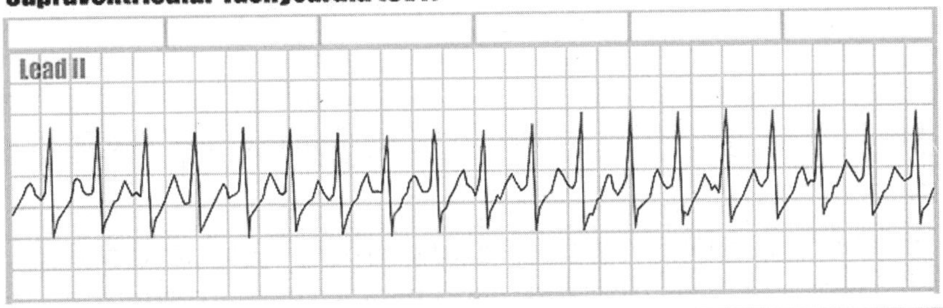

Ans. (B) i.e., AV Nodal Reentry Tachycardia (ANVRT)

75. The primary therapeutic intervention in symptomatic Sino atrial node dysfunction is:

(a) I.V. Atropine
(b) I.V. Isoprenaline
(c) Permanent pacemaker
(d) I.V. Theophylline

EXPLANATION

Sinus **node dysfunction** refers to a number of conditions causing physiologically inappropriate **atrial** rates. Symptoms may be minimal or include weakness, effort intolerance, palpitations, and syncope. Diagnosis is by ECG. **Symptomatic** patients require a pacemaker.

Ans. (C) i.e., Permanent pacemaker

76. **Which of the following are the Indications for lung transplantation?**

1. **Emphysema**
2. **Primary pulmonary hypertension**
3. **Obliterative bronchiolitis**

Select the correct answer using the code given below:

(a) 1 and 2 only (b) 2 and 3 only (c) 1 and 3 only (d) 1, 2 and 3

EXPLANATION

As of 2005, the most common reasons for lung transplantation in the United States were:

- 27% chronic obstructive pulmonary disease (COPD), including emphysema;
- 16% idiopathic pulmonary fibrosis;
- 14% cystic fibrosis;
- 12% idiopathic (formerly known as "primary") pulmonary hypertension;
- 5% alpha 1 antitrypsin deficiency;
- 2% replacing previously transplanted lungs that have since failed;
- 24% other causes, including bronchiectasis and sarcoidosis.

Ans. (A) i.e., 1 and 2 only

2018

77. **Which one of the following is used to distinguish narrowing of large airway from small airway?**

(a) Peak expiratory flow rate is measured
(b) Flow/volume loops are recorded
(c) Forced expiratory volume in one second is measured
(d) Flow/time loops are recorded

EXPLANATION

The forced expiratory volume in the first second (FEV_1) mainly reflects large airways obstruction.

Ans. (C) i.e., Forced expiratory volume in one second is measured

78. **The most common cause of chronic relapsing diarrhoea is:**

(a) Inflammatory bowel disease (b) Coeliac disease
(c) Microscopic colitis (d) Irritable bowel syndrome

EXPLANATION

Lymphocytic colitis and collagenous (components of microscopic colitis) are characterized by the presence of chronic non bloody watery diarrhea, normal appearances on colonoscopy and characteristic histopathology findings of inflammatory cells. The prognosis for both is good, and both conditions are considered to be benign. The majority of people afflicted with the conditions recover from their diarrhea, and their histological abnormalities resolve, although relapses commonly occur if maintenance treatment is not continued.

Ans. (C) i.e., Microscopic colitis

79. **The most common cause of severe acute lower gastrointestinal bleeding is:**

(a) Angiodysplasia of colon
(b) Diverticular disease
(c) Ischaemia of bowel
(d) Inlammatory bowel disease

EXPLANATION

Diverticular disease is when problems occur due to diverticulosis, a condition defined by the presence of pouches in the wall of the large intestine (diverticula). This includes diverticula becoming inflamed (diverticulitis) or bleeding.

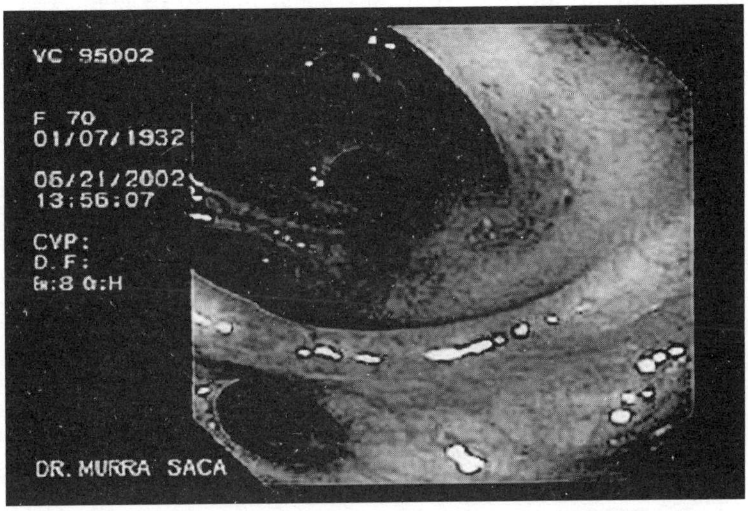

Ans. (B) i.e., Diverticular disease

80. **Risk scoring system used to stratify the patients of acute upper gastrointestinal bleeding (UGIB) to predict the need for intervention to treat bleeding is:**

(a) Modified Blatchford score
(b) Modified Child Pugh score
(c) Balthazar score
(d) Meld score

EXPLANATION

Several scoring systems have been designed for risk stratification and prediction of outcomes in UGIB. They may be endoscopic like complete Rockall score, nonendoscopic like Preendoscopy (clinical) Rockall, Glasgow Blatchford score (GBS), AIMS65, ALBI score, PALBI score.

Ans. (A) i.e., Modified Blatchford score

81. **Corkscrew hairs are seen due to deficiency of:**

(a) Vitamin A (b) Vitamin E (c) Vitamin K (d) Vitamin C

EXPLANATION

Initial symptoms of fatigue, mood changes, and other constitutional symptoms are nonspecific, leading to a delay in diagnosis of vitamin C deficiency. Cutaneous manifestations include follicular hyperkeratosis associated with coiled or "corkscrew" hairs.

Ans. (D) i.e., Vitamin C

82. **Which of the following are the indications of Renal biopsy?**

1. **Chronic Kidney disease with normal sized kidney**
2. **Nephrotic syndrome in adults**

3. Nephrotic syndrome in children with atypical features

Select the correct answer using the code given below:

(a) 1 and 2 only (b) 2 and 3 only (c) 1 and 3 only (d) 1, 2 and 3

EXPLANATION

The following are examples of the most common reasons for native kidney biopsy:

- Haematuria: While renal biopsy is not indicated in all cases of haematuria, it may be performed in those with glomerular haematuria (blood that is thought to come from damage to the glomerulus) or when combined with features of progressive renal disease (e.g. increasing proteinuria, elevated blood pressure and kidney failure). One example is the nephritic syndrome.
- Proteinuria (or protein in the urine) occurs in many renal conditions. Renal biopsy is usually reserved for patients with high or increasing levels of proteinuria, or for patients who have proteinuria along with other signs of renal dysfunction. One example is the nephrotic syndrome.
- Kidney failure (or impaired kidney function due to kidney injury) can occur abruptly (acute kidney failure) or progress over a period of time (chronic kidney disease). The cause of acute kidney failure can usually be determined without kidney biopsy. Biopsy is performed in those instances where the cause is uncertain.

Ans. (D) i.e., 1, 2 and 3

2018

83. Which of the following are common risk factors for contrast Induced Nephrotoxicity?

1. Use of high osmolality, ionic contrast media

2. Diabetes Mellitus

3. Myeloma

Select the correct answer using the code given below:

(a) 1 and 2 only (b) 2 and 3 only (c) 1 and 3 only (d) 1, 2 and 3

EXPLANATION

There are multiple risk factors of contrast induced nephropathy, whereof a review in 2016 emphasized chronic kidney disease, diabetes mellitus, high blood pressure, reduced intravascular volume, use of contrast agents with high osmolality (limited use today) and/or old age.

Ans. (D) i.e., 1, 2 and 3

84. Presence of Dysmorphic Erythrocytes in urine analysis is suggestive of:

(a) Pyelonephritis

(b) Nephritis

(c) Renal stone disease

(d) Renal tract infection

EXPLANATION

There are two types of **erythrocytes** in urine sediment: isomorphic (indicating non glomerular hematuria) and **dysmorphic** (indicating glomerular hematuria).

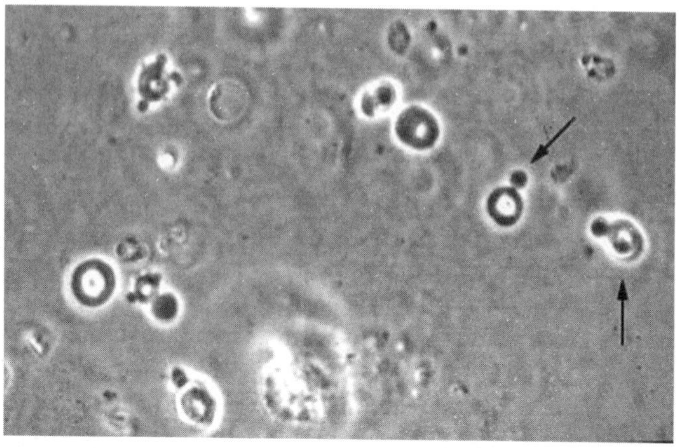

Ans. (B) i.e., Nephritis

85. **Syndrome of Inappropriate ADH secretion (SIADH) is usually associated with:**

(a) Small cell lung cancer
(b) Squamous cell lung cancer
(c) Large cell lung cancer
(d) Adenocarcinoma lung cancer

EXPLANATION

Due to its high grade neuroendocrine nature, small cell lung carcinomas can produce ectopic hormones, including adrenocorticotropic hormone (ACTH) and antidiuretic hormone (ADH). Ectopic production of large amounts of ADH leads to syndrome of inappropriate antidiuretic hormone hypersecretion (SIADH).

Ans. (A) i.e., Small cell lung cancer

86. **A silent, resonant Hemithorax on examination is suggestive of:**

(a) Large Pleural effusion (b) Pneumothorax (c) Bronchial asthma (d) Consolidation

EXPLANATION

Upon physical examination in a case of pneumothorax, breath sounds (heard with a stethoscope) may be diminished on the affected side, partly because air in the pleural space dampens the transmission of sound. Measures of the conduction of vocal vibrations to the surface of the chest may be altered. Percussion of the chest may be perceived as hyper resonant (like a booming drum), and vocal resonance and tactile fremitus can both be noticeably decreased.

Ans. (B) i.e., Pneumothorax

87. **Gower's sign is positive in:**

(a) Peroneal muscle atrophy
(b) Duchenne's dystrophy
(c) Friedreich ataxia
(d) Cerebellar disease

EXPLANATION

Gowers' sign indicates weakness of the proximal muscles, namely those of the lower limb. The sign describes a patient that has to use their hands and arms to "walk" up their own body from a squatting position due to lack of hip and thigh muscle strength. Gowers' sign is classically seen in Duchenne muscular dystrophy where it is mostly evident at 4–6 years, but also presents itself in centronuclear myopathy, myotonic dystrophy and various other conditions associated with proximal muscle weakness, including Becker muscular dystrophy, dermatomyositis and Pompe disease.

Gowers sign

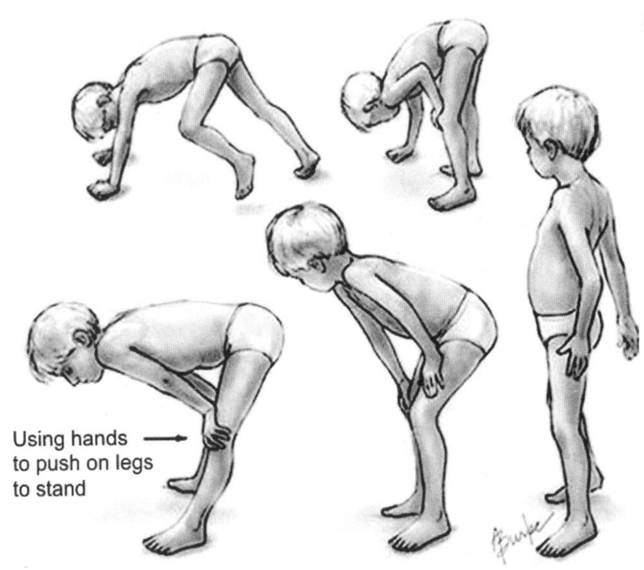

Ans. (B) i.e., Duchenne's dystrophy

88. **All of the following are the indications of renal replacement therapy except:**

(a) Metabolic Acidosis (pH < 7.25)
(b) Hypercalcemia
(c) Hyperkalemia ($K^+ > 6$mmol/L)
(d) Fluid overload

EXPLANATION

Indications for dialysis/renal replacement therapy in the patient with acute kidney injury/AKI are summarized with the vowel mnemonic of "AEIOU":

1. Acidemia from metabolic acidosis in situations in which correction with sodium bicarbonate is impractical or may result in fluid overload.
2. Electrolyte abnormality, such as severe hyperkalemia, especially when combined with AKI.
3. Intoxication, that is, acute poisoning with a dialyzable substance. These substances can be represented by the mnemonic SLIME: salicylic acid, lithium, isopropanol, magnesium containing laxatives and ethylene glycol.
4. Overload of fluid not expected to respond to treatment with diuretics
5. Uremia complications, such as pericarditis, encephalopathy, or gastrointestinal bleeding.

Ans. (B) i.e., Hypercalcemia

89. All of the bacterial diseases are exotoxin mediated except:

(a) Botulism (b) Diphtheria (c) Typhoid (d) Tetanus

EXPLANATION

Well known exotoxins include: botulinum toxin produced by *Clostridium botulinum*; *Corynebacterium diphtheriae* toxin, produced during life threatening symptoms of diphtheria; tetanospasmin produced by Clostridium tetani.

Ans. (C) i.e., Typhoid

90. The following substances can cause dilated pupils except:

(a) Tricyclic Antidepressants (b) Cocaine
(c) Clonidine (d) Amphetamines

EXPLANATION

Imidazolines such as clonidine, naphazoline, oxymetazoline and tetrahydrozoline causes miosis.

Ans. (C) i.e., Cocaine

91. Which one of the following drugs can cause Pulmonary Eosinophilia?

(a) Nitrofurantoin (b) Valproate (c) Enalapril (d) Amoxycillin

EXPLANATION

Allergic reactions to drugs are a common cause of eosinophilia, with manifestations ranging from diffuse maculopapular rash, to severe life threatening drug reactions with eosinophilia and systemic symptoms (DRESS). Drugs that has allopurinol, nonsteroidal anti inflammatory drugs (NSAIDs), some antipsychotics such as risperidone, and certain antibiotics. Phenibut, an analogue of the neurotransmitter GABA, has also been implicated in high doses. There are a number of reports of nitrofurantoin **causing** pulmonary disease with **eosinophilia.**

Ans. (A) i.e., Nitrofurantoin

92. CA 19-9 is a tumour marker used for the diagnosis of:

(a) Lung cancer (b) Prostate cancer
(c) Ovarian cancer (d) Pancreatic cancer

EXPLANATION

CA 19-9 (**carbohydrate antigen 19-9**, also called **cancer antigen 19-9** or **sialylated Lewis (a) antigen**) is a tumor marker that is used primarily in the management of pancreatic cancer.

Ans. (C) i.e., Ovarian cancer

93. Tinea versicolor is caused by:

(a) Candida albicans (b) Trichophyton (c) Streptococci (d) Malassezia furfur

EXPLANATION

Tinea versicolor is a condition characterized by a skin eruption on the trunk and proximal extremities. The majority of tinea versicolor is caused by the fungus *Malassezia globosa*, although *Malassezia furfur* is responsible for a small number of cases.

Ans. (D) i.e., Malassezia furfur

94. Osborn wave in ECG is characteristic of:

(a) Hypothyroidism
(b) Hypovolemia
(c) Hypothermia
(d) Hypocalcemia

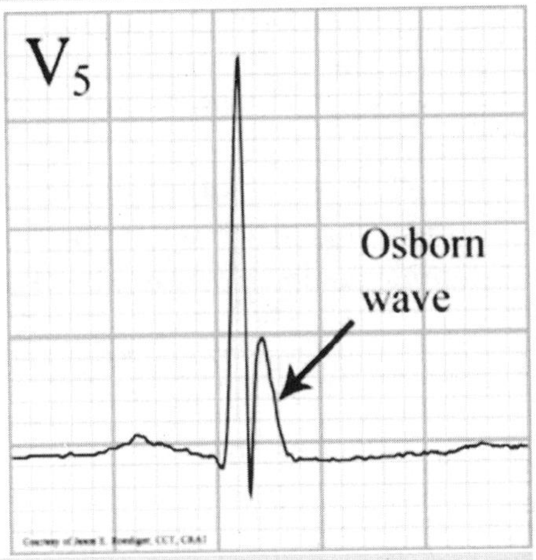

EXPLANATION

A J wave — also known as **Osborn wave, camel hump sign, late delta wave, hathook junction, hypothermic wave, K wave, H wave** or **current of injury** — is an abnormal electrocardiogram finding.

Ans. (C) i.e., Hypothermia

95. Disease modifying agent of choice for the peripheral manifestations of ankylosing spondylitis is:

(a) Methotrexate (b) Hydroxychloroquine
(c) Sulfasalazine (d) Leflunomide

EXPLANATION

There is no cure for ankylosing spondylitis. Treatments may improve symptoms and prevent worsening. This may include medication, exercise, and surgery. Medications used include NSAIDs, steroids, DMARDs such as sulfasalazine, and biologic agents such as infliximab.

Ans. (C) i.e., Sulfasalazine

96. Drug of choice for treating hypertensive emergency in a case of Aortic dissection is:

(a) Phentolamine (b) Prazosin (c) Nitroprusside (d) Amlodipine

EXPLANATION

Beta blockers are the first line treatment for patients with acute and chronic aortic dissection. In acute dissection, fast acting agents which can be given intravenously and have doses that are easier to adjust (such as esmolol, propranolol, or labetalol) are preferred. Vasodilators such as sodium nitroprusside can be considered for people with ongoing high blood pressure, but they should never be used alone, as they often stimulate a reflexive increase in the heart rate.

Ans. (C) i.e., Nitroprusside

97. A 5-year old boy is brought to the Emergency Room following a crushing injury. The ECG reveals peaked T waves, prolonged PR interval and widened QRS complexes. Which of the following treatments should be administered immediately?

(a) Sodium bicarbonate infusion
(b) Intravenous bolus procainamide
(c) Insulin infusion
(d) Intravenous magnesium sulphate

EXPLANATION

With mild to moderate hyperkalemia, there is prolongation of the PR interval and development of peaked T waves. Severe hyperkalemia results in a widening of the QRS complex, and the ECG complex can evolve to a sinusoidal shape. Insulin (e.g. intravenous injection of 10–15 units of regular insulin along with 50 ml of 50% dextrose to prevent the blood sugar from dropping too low) leads to a shift of potassium ions into cells, secondary to increased activity of the sodium potassium ATPase. Its effects last a few hours, so it sometimes must be repeated while other measures are taken to suppress potassium levels more permanently. The insulin is usually given with an appropriate amount of glucose to prevent hypoglycemia following the insulin administration.

Ans. (C) i.e., Insulin infusion

2018

98. **A child with Acute Lymphoblastic Leukemia is started on chemotherapy. After 2 days he develops vomiting, decreased urine output abdominal pain and tetanic spasms. The ECG reveals QT_C prolongation. Which one of the following therapies will be detrimental to his management?**

(a) Normal maintenance intravenous fluid
(b) Oral phosphate binders
(c) Intravenous rasburicase
(d) None of these

EXPLANATION

Tumor lysis syndrome (TLS) is a group of metabolic abnormalities that can occur as a complication during the treatment of cancer, where large amounts of tumor cells are killed off (lysed) at the same time by the treatment, releasing their contents into the bloodstream. This occurs most commonly after the treatment of lymphomas and leukemias. Tumor lysis syndrome is characterized by high blood potassium (hyperkalemia), high blood phosphate (hyperphosphatemia), low blood calcium (hypocalcemia), high blood uric acid (hyperuricemia), and higher than normal levels of blood urea nitrogen (BUN) and other nitrogen containing compounds (azotemia). People about to receive chemotherapy for a cancer with a high cell turnover rate, especially lymphomas and leukemias, should receive prophylactic oral or IV allopurinol (a xanthine oxidase inhibitor, which inhibits uric acid production) as well as adequate IV hydration to maintain high urine output (> 2.5 L/day). Rasburicase is an alternative to allopurinol and is reserved for people who are high risk in developing TLS. **Phosphate binders** are medications used to reduce the absorption of phosphate and taken with meals and snacks.

Ans. (D) i.e., None of these

99. **Which of the following treatment modalities is NOT recommended for worsening respiratory distress in a child suspected to be suffering from acute croup?**

(a) Sedation
(b) Intravenous antibiotics
(c) Nebulised racemic epinephrine
(d) Intramuscular dexamethasone

EXPLANATION

Croup can be caused by a number of viruses including parainfluenza and influenza virus. Since croup is usually a viral disease, antibiotics are not used unless secondary bacterial infection is suspected.

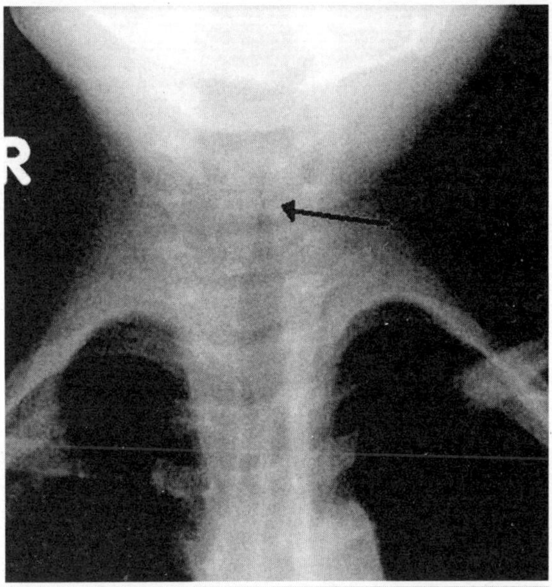

Ans. (B) i.e., Intravenous antibiotics

100. Which of the following developmental skills will you expect a child to have acquired by 9 months?

(a) Cruising around the furniture
(b) Mature pincer grasp
(c) Waves 'bye-bye'
(d) Refers to mother as 'ma-ma'

EXPLANATION

Pincer grasp wherein the pointer finger and the thumb squeeze to grasp an object. Children are usually able to use a pincer grasp by the age of 9 to 10 months.

Ans. (B) i.e., Mature pincer grasp

101. Which of the following is physiological in a term neonate?

(a) Hypotonia
(b) Erythema toxicum
(c) Jaundice at 20 hours of life
(d) Direct serum bilirubin level = 3.0mg/dL

EXPLANATION

Erythema Toxicum. Erythema toxicum — also called erythema toxicum neonatorum (ETN) or toxic erythema of the newborn — is a common rash seen in full term newborns. It usually appears in the first few days after birth and fades within a week

Ans. (B) i.e., Erythema toxicum

102. A preterm neonate undergoes the initial steps of resuscitation. The clinician observes that the baby is breathing, has a heart rate of 80/minute and the baby is pink. What will be the next immediate step in management?

(a) Administering intravenous epinephrine
(b) Chest compressions
(c) Positive pressure ventilation
(d) Supplemental oxygen

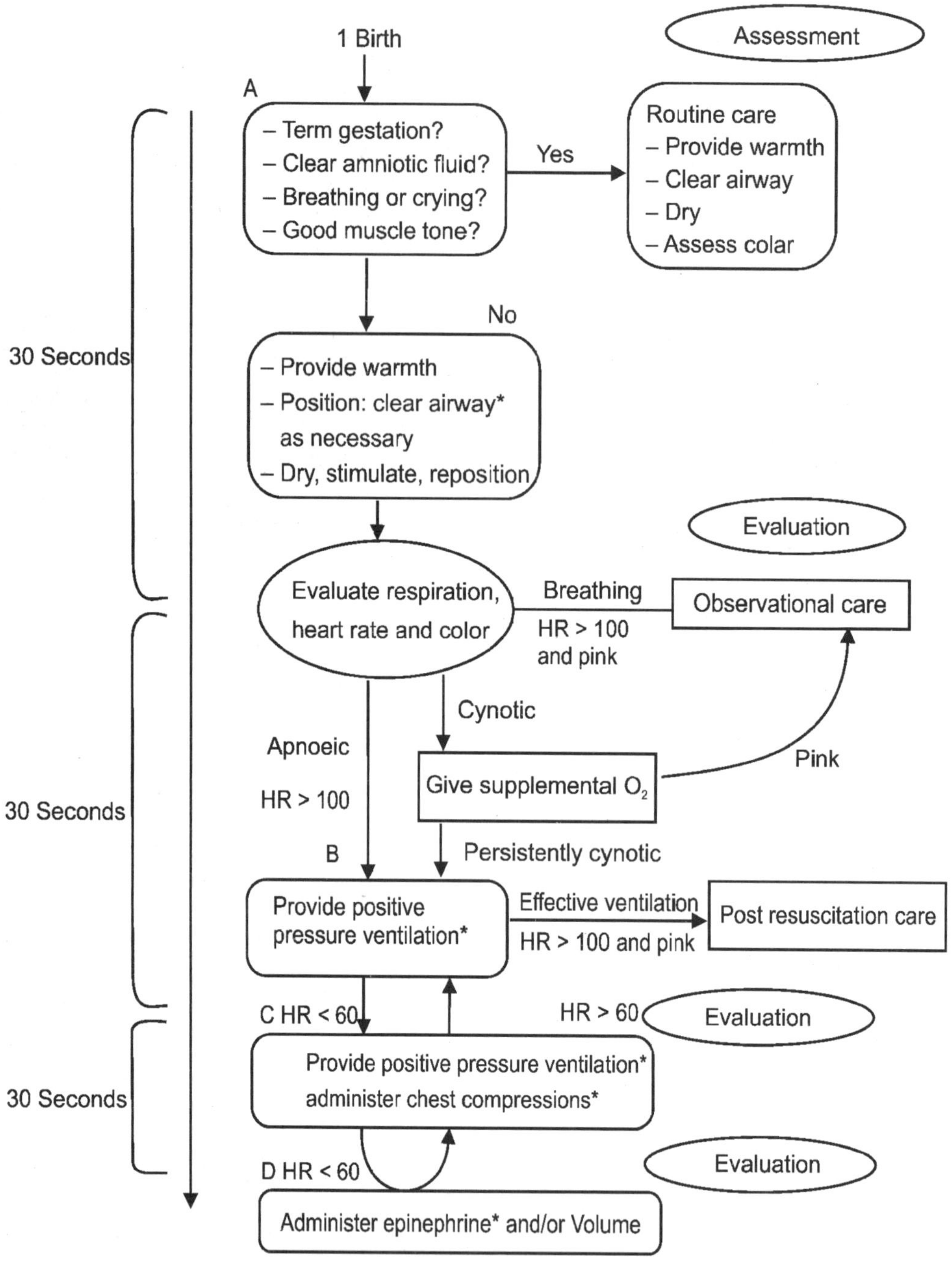

*endotracheal intubation may be considered at several steps.

Ans. (D) i.e., Supplemental oxygen

103. A child is able to copy a triangle, names 4 colours, dresses and undresses easily and is able to skip. What is the likely age of this child?

(a) 30 months (b) 36 months (c) 48 months (d) 60 months

EXPLANATION

Activity of a Five Year old child:

Social and Emotional

- Likes to sing, dance, and act
- Shows concern and sympathy for others
- Is aware of gender

- Shows more independence (for example, may visit a next door neighbour by himself [adult supervision is still needed])

Language/Communication

- Speaks very clearly
- Tells a simple story using full sentences
- Uses future tense; for example, "Grandma will be here."
- Says name and address

Cognitive (learning, thinking, problem solving)

- Counts 10 or more things
- Can draw a person with at least 6 body parts
- Can print some letters or numbers
- Copies a triangle and other geometric shapes
- Knows about things used every day, like money and food

Movement/Physical Development

- Stands on one foot for 10 seconds or longer
- Hops; may be able to skip
- Uses a fork and spoon and sometimes a table knife
- Can use the toilet on her own
- Swings and climbs

Ans. (D) i.e., 60 months

104. Which of the following will be considered to be a 'RED FLAG' in child development?

(a) No vocalization by 4 months
(b) Unable to sit without support by 10 months
(c) Unable to walk independently by 15 months
(d) Unable to speak a single word with meaning by 15 months

EXPLANATION

Developmental red flags (12–24 months)

- Cannot walk by 18 months.
- Fails to develop a mature heel toe walking pattern after several months of walking, or walks exclusively on toes.
- Does not speak at least 15 words by 18 months.
- Does not use two word sentences by age 2.
- By 15 months does not seem to know the function of common houschold objects (brush, telephone, bell, fork, spoon).
- Does not imitate actions or words by 24 months.
- Does not follow simple one step instructions by 24 months.

Ans. (D) i.e., Unable to speak a single word with meaning by 15 months

105. Gastric lavage is contraindicated in which of the following?

1. Corrosive poisoning
2. Organophosphorus poisoning
3. Iron intoxication
4. Turpentine oil ingestion

Select the correct answer using the codes given below:

(a) 1 and 2 (b) 2 and 3 (c) 3 and 4 (d) 4 and 1

EXPLANATION

Contraindications to gastric lavage

- Relative contraindications to gastric lavage include when the poisoning is due to a corrosive substance (strong acids or strong bases)
- *Gastric lavage* must not be practiced because removing *turpentine* can provoke its' aspiration with a consequent pulmonary disease in the majority of occassions.

Ans. (D) i.e., 4 and 1

106. A 10-year old girl is brought to the emergency following a road traffic accident. The child is comatose with GCS score of 4. She is hypertensive, has bradycardia and extensor posturing. CT imaging reveals comminuted skull fractures and intraparenchymal hemorrhage. The initial management should include all of the following measures except:

(a) Head of bed elevation
(b) Mechanical ventilation
(c) Intravenous dexamethasone
(d) Hypertonic saline administration

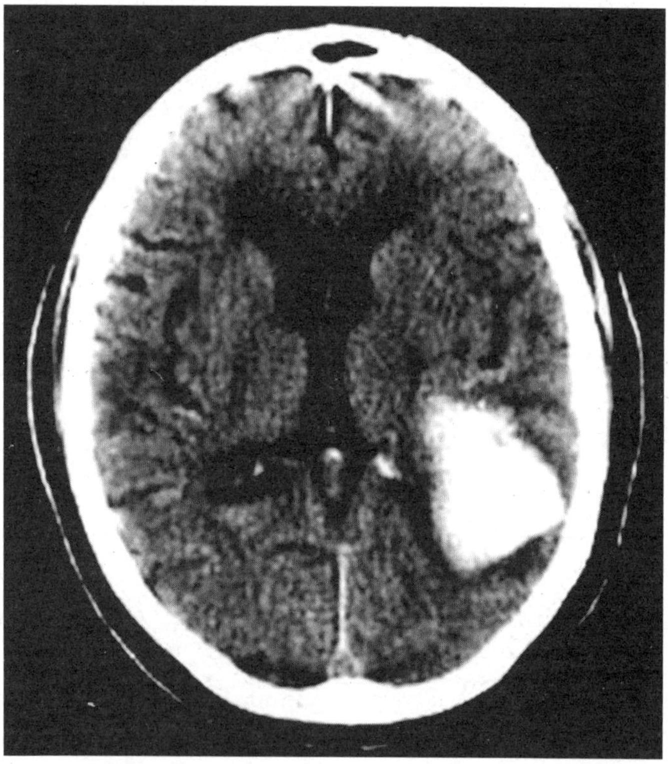

EXPLANATION

In a patient with intraparenchymal hemorrhage, the head should be elevated to 30 degrees, 1.0–1.5g/kg of 20% mannitol should be given by a rapid infusion, and the patient should be hyperventilated to a pCO_2 of 30–35mmHg. These measures are designed to lower ICP as quickly as possible prior to a definitive neurosurgical procedure (craniotomy, ventriculostomy, or placement of an ICP monitor) can be done. Corticosteroids are not recommended in the management of IPH because they have been proven to offer no benefit in randomized trials.

Ans. (C) i.e., Intravenous dexamethasone

107. A 3-year old boy is brought with complaints of staying aloof. He also has delayed speech. Rest of the developmental milestones were attained normally. The most likely diagnosis is:

(a) Selective mutism (b) Attention deficit hyperactivity disorder
(c) Autism (d) Phonological disorder

EXPLANATION

Autism is a developmental disorder characterized by troubles with social interaction and communication, and by restricted and repetitive behavior. Parents usually notice signs during the first two or three years of their child's life.

Ans. (D) i.e., Phonological disorder

2018

108. Which of the following statements regarding HPV (Human Papilloma Virus) vaccine is NOT true?

(a) It can be safely administered in pregnancy
(b) The recommended age for initiation of vaccination is 10–12 years
(c) Catch up vaccination may be permitted up to 26 years of age, provided the woman is not sexually active
(d) The vaccine is administered intramuscularly in deltoid region

EXPLANATION

Currently, the HPV vaccine is not recommended for pregnant women.

Ans. (A) i.e., It can be safely administered in pregnancy

109. A 6-year old boy comes to the immunization clinic having received all vaccines as per schedule till 18 months of age. Which vaccine should be administered now?

(a) DTPw booster (b) TdaP booster (c) DT booster (d) TT booster

EXPLANATION

The primary series of three doses of DTP (DTwP or DTaP) should be given in infancy, with a *booster* dose of a *tetanus* toxoid containing *vaccine* ideally at age 4–7 *years (DTPw)* and another *booster* in adolescence, e.g. at age 12–15 *years (TdaP).*

Ans. (A) i.e., DTPw booster

110. "Time out" strategy is used for management of children having:

(a) Tics (b) Temper tantrums (c) Stuttering (d) Breath holding spells

EXPLANATION

Time out is a form of behavioral modification that involves temporarily separating a person from an environment where unacceptable behavior has occurred. Time out should be used as a last resort for temper tantrums. It should only be used when the child has hurt someone intentionally such as biting or hitting and when he is not flooded with emotions. And it should be **non punitively** and done in a kind and firm way.

Ans. (B) i.e., Temper tantrums

111. All of the following are included in the 'Mission Indradhanush' except:

(a) Japanese Encephalitis vaccine
(b) Measles vaccine
(c) Hepatitis A vaccine
(d) Haemophilus influenza type B vaccine

EXPLANATION

Mission Indradhanush is a health mission of the government of India. It was launched by Union Health Minister J. P. Nadda on 25 December 2014. It aims to immunize all children under the age of 2 years, as well as all pregnant women, against seven vaccine preventable diseases. The diseases being targeted are diphtheria, whooping cough, tetanus, poliomyelitis, tuberculosis, measles and Hepatitis B. In addition to these, vaccines for Japanese encephalitis and Haemophilus influenzae type B are also being provided in selected states.

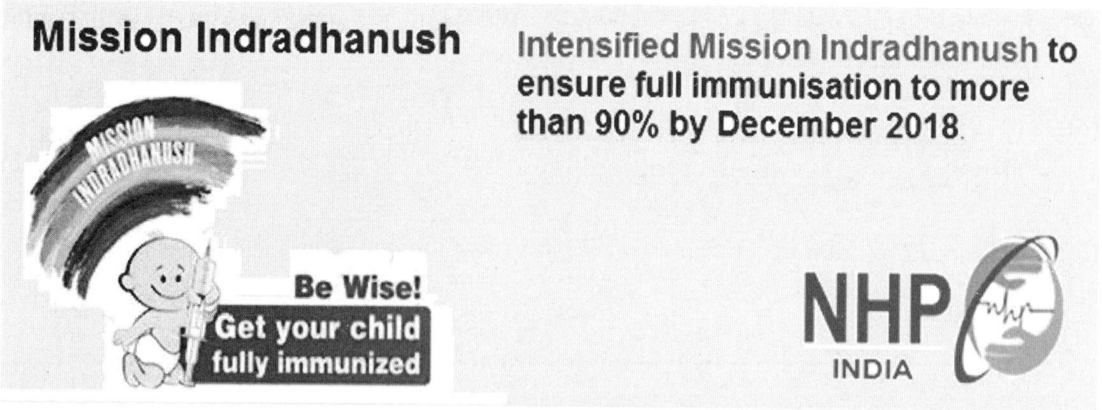

Ans. (C) i.e., Hepatitis A vaccine

112. Which of the following is the best mode of management of a newborn born to a mother with Hepatitis B infection?

(a) Hepatitis B Immunoglobulin (HBIG) and Hepatitis B vaccine at birth

(b) 1 and monotherapy with Infection

(c) 1 and monotherapy with Lamivudine

(d) 1 and monotherapy with Adefovir

EXPLANATION

Newborn born to a mother with HBV infection should receive both active (HBV vaccine) and passive immunization (HBIG).

Ans. (A) i.e., Hepatitis B Immunoglobulin (HBIG) and Hepatitis B vaccine at birth

113. At what age should a lateral neck radiograph be done for a child with Downs syndrome to rule out atlanto occipital subluxation?

(a) At birth (b) At 1 year (c) At 2 years (d) At 3 years

EXPLANATION

A screening X-ray of the upper spine is recommended:

- For children 3 years and over who will be having a procedure that will involve general anesthesia (if they have not already had a cervical spine X-ray that was read as normal)
- Every 3 years if general anesthesia is planned again
- Before taking part in sports where there is significant risk of head or neck injury

Ans. (D) i.e., At 3 years

114. Which X-ray will be used to evaluate the bone age (skeletal age) of a term newborn at birth?

(a) Wrist (b) Shoulder (c) Knee (d) Elbow

EXPLANATION

In newborns and infants skeletal age is usually determined from a lateral X-ray of the left lower leg, including knee and foot; after three month of age, an X-ray of the left hand is used.

Ans. (C) i.e., Knee

115. Which of the following permanent tooth eruption event has close correlation with menarche?

(a) First premolar (b) First molar (c) Second premolar (d) Second molar

EXPLANATION

Menarche, the onset of menstruation, is one of the most significant milestones in a woman's life. Unlike other pubertal changes that are gradual and continuous, menarche is a distinct event with a sudden onset. For most females, it occurs between the ages of 10 to 16 years. Eruption of teeth is related to chronological age, gender and ethnic origin. The permanent second molars erupt between the ages of 10 to 13 years.

Ans. (D) i.e., Second molar

116. Which one of the following is NOT a component of the '4 Ds' that are the focus of the Rashtriya Bal Suraksha Karyakram' (RBSK)?

(a) Deficit (b) Disease (c) Deficiency (d) Developmental delay

EXPLANATION

Rashtriya Bal Swasthya Karyakram (RBSK) is a new initiative aiming at early identification and early intervention for children from birth to 18 years to cover 4 'D's viz. Defects at birth, Deficiencies, Diseases, Development delays including disability.

RBSK

RASHTRIYA BAL SWASTHYA KARYAKRAM

राष्ट्रीय बाल स्वास्थ्य कार्यक्रम

FROM SURVIVAL TO HEALTHY SURVIVAL

Ans. (A) i.e., Deficit

117. In which one of the following age groups is the highest rate of drowning observed, worldwide?

(a) Less than 1 year (b) 1–4 years (c) 4–10 years (d) 10–15 years

EXPLANATION

In 2014, among children 1 to 4 years old who died from an unintentional injury, one third died from *drowning*. Among children *ages* 1 to 4, *most drowning* occur in home swimming pools.

Ans. (B) i.e., 1–4 years

118. Which of the following is the recommended initial intravenous therapy in a 2-year old child with Severe Acute Malnutrition with Severe Dehydration and Shock?

(a) Ringer Lactate (R) at the rate of 30mL/kg over first 30 minutes

(b) Half normal saline (N/2) in 5% dextrose at the rate of 15mL/kg over first 60 minutes

(c) Normal saline (NS) at the rate of 20 mL/kg over the first 30 minutes

(d) N/5 saline with 5% dextrose at the rate of 30mL/kg over first 60 minutes

EXPLANATION

For the shocked child (or child with severe dehydration who is unable to tolerate oral fluids), WHO guidelines recommends 15mls/Kg of intravenous fluid over 1 hour (repeated once if necessary) and a 10ml/Kg blood transfusion over 3 hours if there is no subsequent improvement.

Ans. (B) i.e., Half normal saline (N/2) in 5% dextrose at the rate of 15 mL/kg over first 60 minutes

119. A female carrier for hemophilia A gene gets married to a genetically normal male. What are the chances of her delivering a male offspring with hemophilia?

(a) 0% (b) 25% (c) 50% (d) 100%

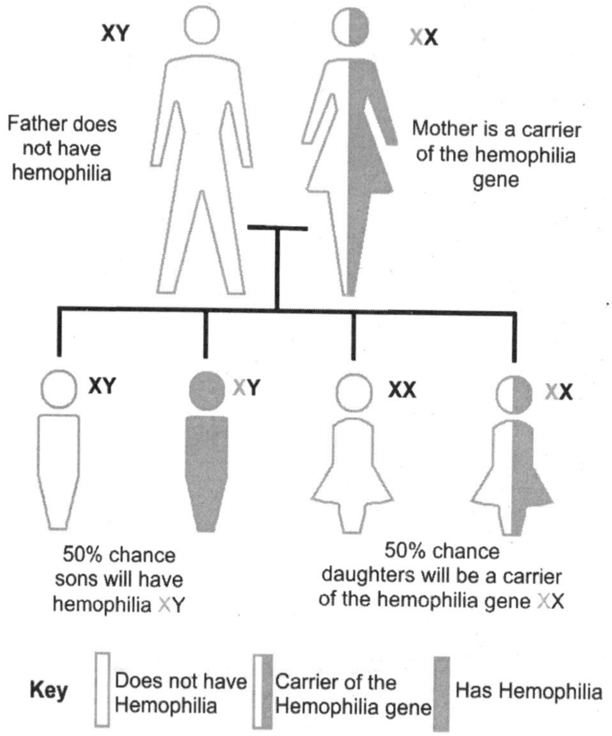

Ans. (C) i.e., **50%**

120. What is the definition of 'Cold stress' in a newborn as measured by the axillary temperature?

(a) 35.0 – 35.5 °C (b) 35.0 – 36.0 °C (c) 35.5 – 36.5 °C (d) 36.0 – 36.4 °C

EXPLANATION

Hypothermia occurs when the body temperature drops below 36.5°C (97.7°F), the lower limit of the normal range of 36.5–37.5°C (97.7–99.5°F). The *newborn infant* with a body temperature of between 36.0–36.4°C (96.8–97.5°F) may be under *cold stress* which gives rise to concern.

Ans. (D) i.e., **36.0–36.4°C**

CHAPTER

3 CMS EXAMINATION 2017

PAPER - 2

1. **The external opening of branchial fistula is present in:**

   (a) Lower third of the neck

   (b) Middle third of the neck

   (c) Upper third of the neck

   (d) Suprasternal notch

   EXPLANATION:

   Second branchial cleft fistulae typically open onto the skin at the anterior border of sternocleidomastoid at the junction of middle and lower 1/3rd.

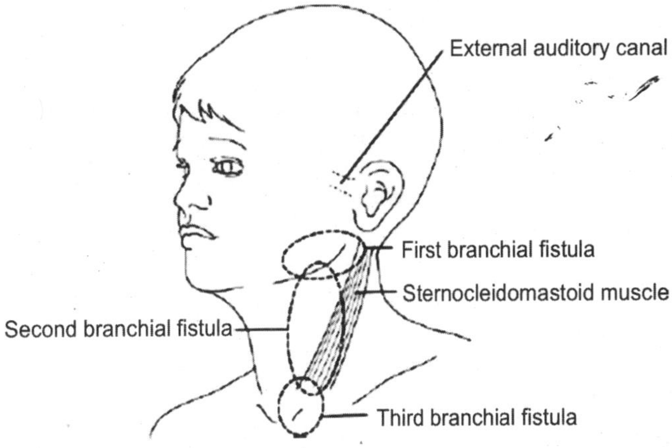

Ans. (A) i.e., Lower third of the neck

2. **A eight year old male child complains of severe pain in right testes. The most probable diagnosis is:**

   (a) Torsion of right testis

   (b) Strangulated Inguinal hernia

   (c) Acute epididym orchitis

   (d) Undescended testis

   EXPLANATION:

   Testicular torsion occurs when the spermatic cord (from which the testicle is suspended) twists, cutting off the testicle's blood supply. The most common symptom in children is rapid onset of severe testicular pain. The testicle may also be higher than usual and vomiting may occur. In newborns pain is often absent and instead the scrotum may become discolored or a testicle may disappear from its usual place.

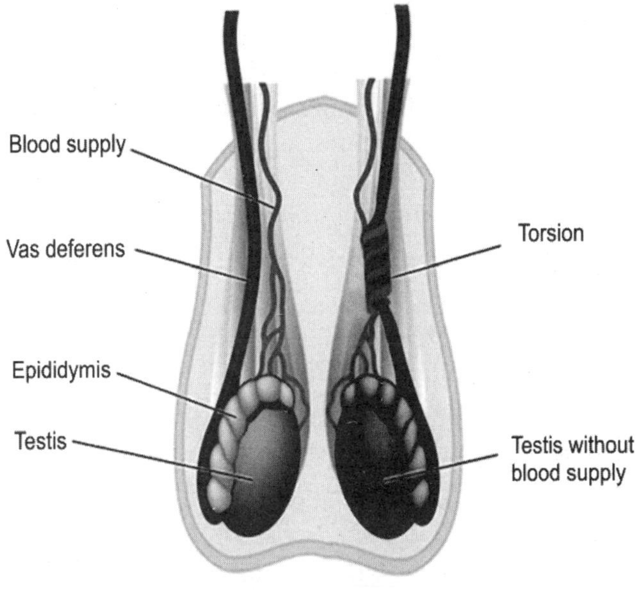

Torsion of Testis

Ans. (A) i.e., Torsion of right testis

3. **Which one of the following statements is NOT correct regarding Gastroschisis?**
   (a) It is a ruptured exomphalos
   (b) Gut has herniated through a defect to right of umbilicus
   (c) Normally limited to midgut
   (d) There is no covering membrane

EXPLANATION:

Omphalocele, also called **exomphalos**, is a rare abdominal wall defect in which the intestines, liver and occasionally other organs remain outside of the abdomen in a sac because of failure of the normal return of intestines and other contents back to the abdominal cavity during around the ninth week of intrauterine development.

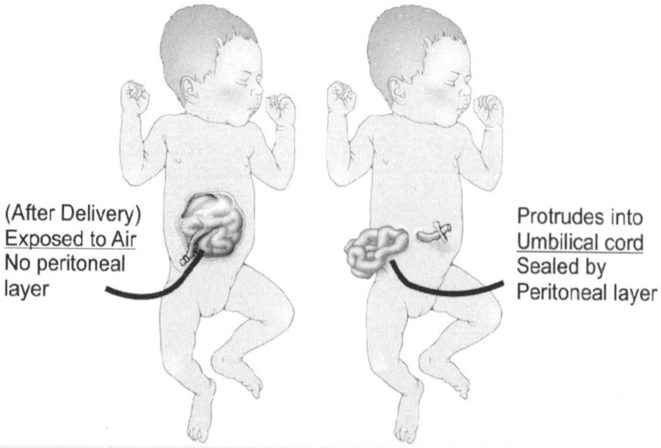

Ans. (A) i.e., It is a ruptured exomphalos

4. **Heineke Mikulicz operation is done for:**
   (a) Ureteric stricture
   (b) Urethral stricture
   (c) Pyloric stenosis
   (d) Stricture common bile duct

EXPLANATION:

The most commonly performed **pyloroplasty** is known as Heineke-Mikulicz **pyloroplasty**. This type consists of a transversely closed longitudinal **incision** across the pylorus.

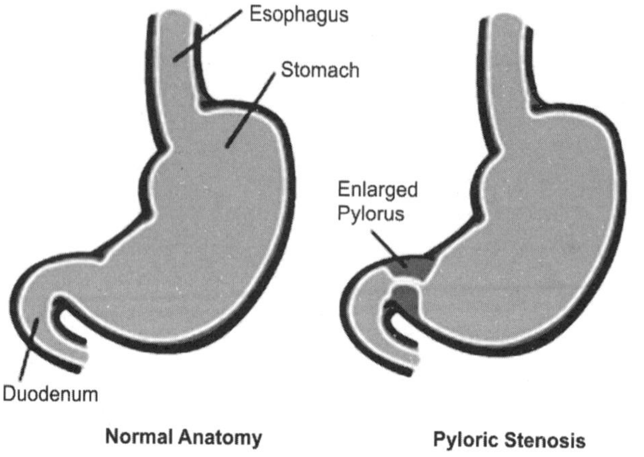

Ans. (C) i.e., Pyloric stenosis

5. **A 32 year old female underwent laparoscopic cholecystectomy which was difficult. On her second post operative day, she develops jaundice. Her LFT parameters show serum bilirubin 6.8mg/dL; direct bilirubin 5.6 and indirect bilirubin 1.2mg/dL; and serum alkaline phosphatase 1226IU/L. She is most likely suffering from obstructive jaundice due to:**
   (a) Bile duct injury
   (b) Carcinoma gallbladder
   (c) Hepatocellular carcinoma
   (d) Carcinoma head of pancreas

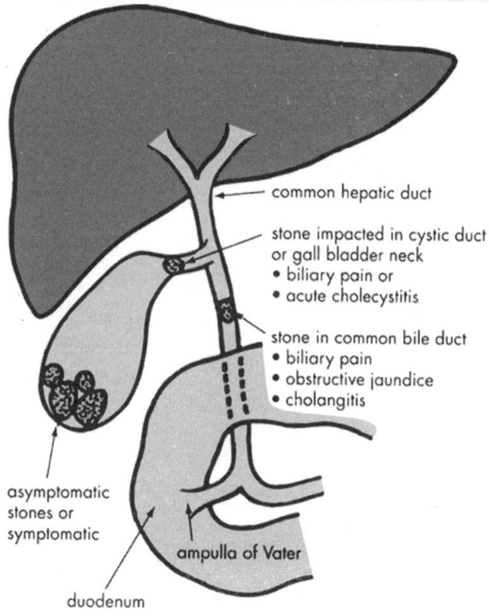

EXPLANATION:

Biliary injury (bile duct injury) is the traumatic damage of the bile ducts. It is most commonly an iatrogenic complication of cholecystectomy—surgical removal of gall bladder, but can also be caused by other operations or by

2017

major trauma. The risk of biliary injury is more during laparoscopic cholecystectomy than during open cholecystectomy.

Ans. (A) i.e., Bile duct injury

6. **A 60 year old man presents with painless progressive jaundice for two months. He has a history of weight loss. On examination, his gallbladder is palpable which is smooth, non tender and globular. His serum bilirubin is 18.2 mg/dL. He is most likely suffering from:**

(a) Carcinoma head of pancreas
(b) Carcinoma stomach
(c) Choledocholithiasis
(d) Klatskin tumour

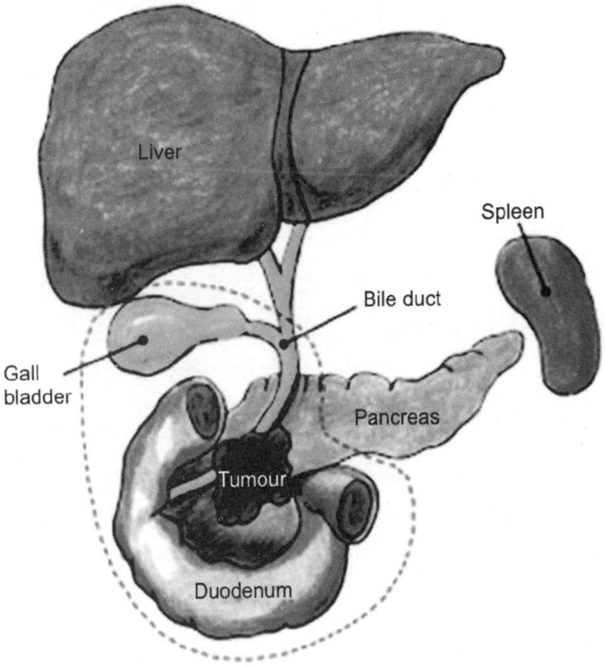

EXPLANATION:

Signs and symptoms of the most common form of pancreatic cancer may include jaundice, abdominal or back pain, unexplained weight loss, light colored stools, dark urine and loss of appetite. There are usually no symptoms in the disease's early stages, and symptoms that are specific enough to suggest pancreatic cancer typically do not develop until the disease has reached an advanced stage. By the time of diagnosis, pancreatic cancer has often spread to other parts of the body.

Ans. (A) i.e., Carcinoma head of pancreas

7. **A young 23 year old male riding his motorcycle meets with a road accident. He is tachypnoeic with HR 110/m and BP 112/74mmHg. On examination, he has tenderness over left side of chest with decreased air entry. His trachea is pushed to opposite side. Abdominal examination is unremarkable. Most probably he is suffering from:**

(a) Haemothorax
(b) Consolidation
(c) Subcutaneous emphysema
(d) Tracheal rupture

EXPLANATION:

Hemothorax tends to occur following blunt or penetrating trauma to the thorax or thoracoabdominal area. It may also follow thoracic surgery, or may be spontaneous. Chest pain, dyspnea, and tachypnea are common presenting features. Other symptoms of hemothorax are dependent on the mechanism of injury, but may include:

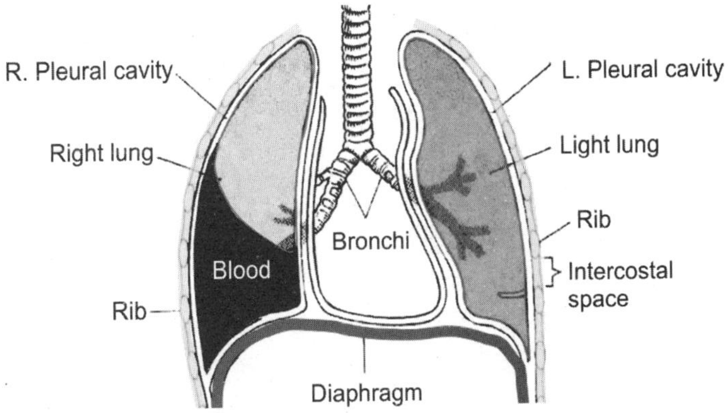

- Cyanosis
- Decreased or absent breath sounds on affected side
- Tracheal deviation to unaffected side

- Dull resonance on percussion
- Unequal chest rise
- Tachycardia
- Hypotension
- Pale, cool, clammy skin
- Possible subcutaneous emphysema
- Narrowing pulse pressure

Ans. (A) i.e., Haemothorax

8. **Mondor's disease is:**

(a) Lymphangitis of mammary lymphatics
(b) Multiple breast cysts
(c) Eczema by nipple and areola
(d) Thrombophlebitis of superficial veins of breast

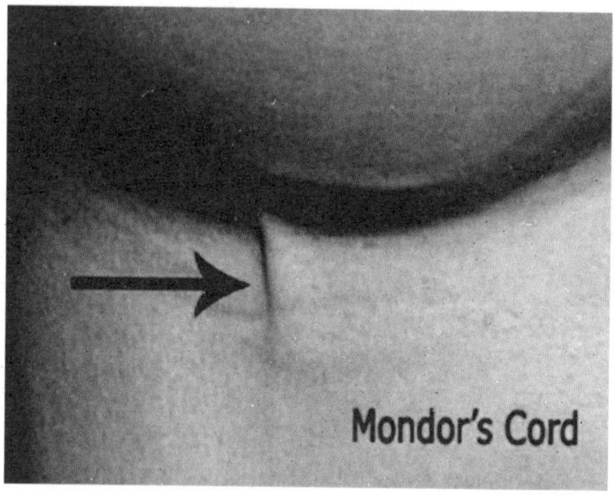

EXPLANATION:

Mondor's disease (also known as "Mondor's syndrome of superficial thrombophlebitis") is a rare condition which involves thrombophlebitis of the superficial veins of the breast and anterior chest wall. It sometimes occurs in the arm or penis. In axilla, this condition is known as axillary web syndrome.

Ans. (D) i.e., Thrombophlebitis of superficial veins of breast

2017

9. **Which of the following is NOT true regarding 'Renal Carbuncle'?**

(a) It is an abscess in renal parenchyma
(b) It occurs in diabetic patient
(c) It is a type of renal tuberculosis
(d) It occurs in intravenous drug abusers

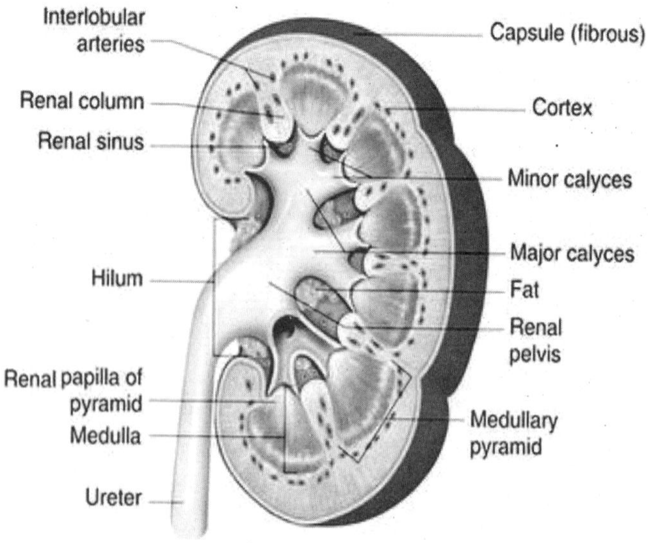

EXPLANATION:

Carbuncle of the kidney may be defined as a metastatic, circumscribed, conglomerate suppurative process, usually caused by *Staphylococcus aureus*, having its origin in some superficial focus, such as a furuncle, paronychia or carbuncle.

Ans. (C) i.e., It is a type of renal tuberculosis

10. **Anderson Hynes operation is performed for:**

(a) Achalasia cardia
(b) Pyloric stenosis
(c) Pseudo-pancreatic cyst
(d) Pelvi-ureteric junction obstruction

EXPLANATION:

Dismembered pyeloplasty (technique by Anderson and Hynes) is indicated as surgical therapy for ureteropelvic obstruction in cases:

- With scintigraphic evidence of obstruction
- With decreasing (but sufficient) renal function of the affected kidney
- With clinical symptoms (flank pain, nephrolithiasis or recurrent infections)

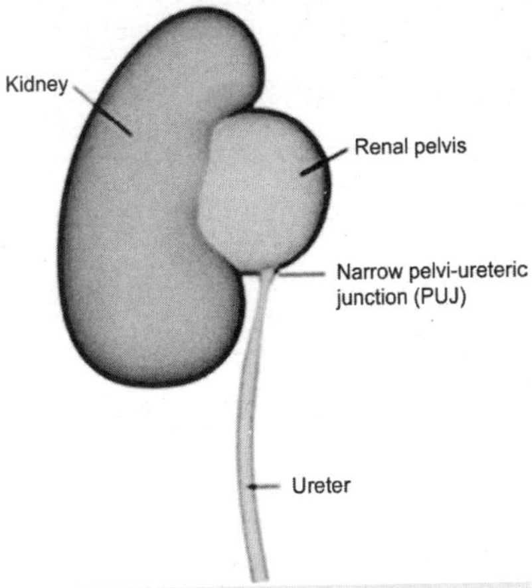

Ans. (D) i.e., Pelvi ureteric junction obstruction

11. Which of the following is NOT correct for 'strawberry gall bladder'?

(a) It is a malignant condition of gall bladder
(b) It has sub mucous aggregation of cholesterol crystals
(c) It may be associated with cholesterol Stones
(d) Simple cholecystectomy is the treatment of choice

EXPLANATION:

The name *strawberry gallbladder* comes from the typically stippled appearance of the mucosal surface on gross examination, which resembles a strawberry. Cholesterolosis results from abnormal deposits of cholesterol esters in macrophages within the lamina propria (foam cells) and in mucosal epithelium. The gallbladder may be affected in a patchy localized form or in a diffuse form. The diffuse form macroscopically appears as a bright red mucosa with yellow mottling (due to lipid), hence the term *strawberry* gallbladder.

Gallbladder and Extrahepatic Bile Ducts Sections

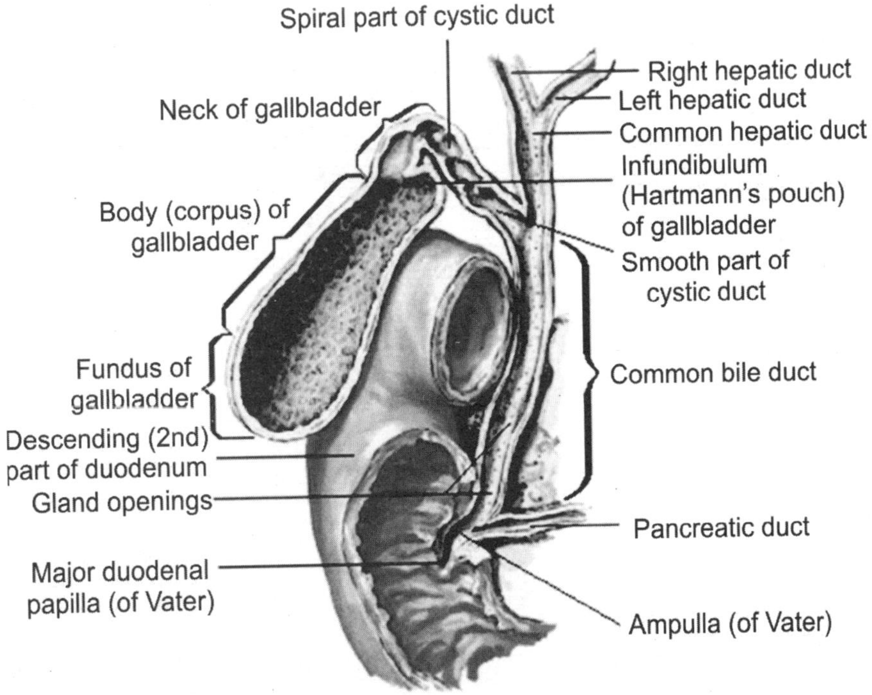

Ans. (A) i.e., It is a malignant condition of gall bladder

2017

2017

12. **Treatment of choice for Recurrent Thyrotoxicosis after surgery is:**
   (a) Further surgery
   (b) Radio iodine followed by surgery
   (c) Radio iodine
   (d) Observe/follow up

EXPLANATION:

Radioiodine (^{131}I) therapy for thyrotoxicosis has the advantages of simplicity, effectiveness and safety in patients over 40 years of age and especially in the frail and elderly when there is often associated cardiac disease. ^{131}I should not be used in children except in unusual circumstances such as drug sensitivity and refusal to have an operation. There is, however, only a relative contraindication to its use in adults less than 40 years of age and it is the best treatment for a post operative recurrence irrespective of the age of the patient. The physician must be sure the patient is not in early pregnancy and she should avoid this state for several months.

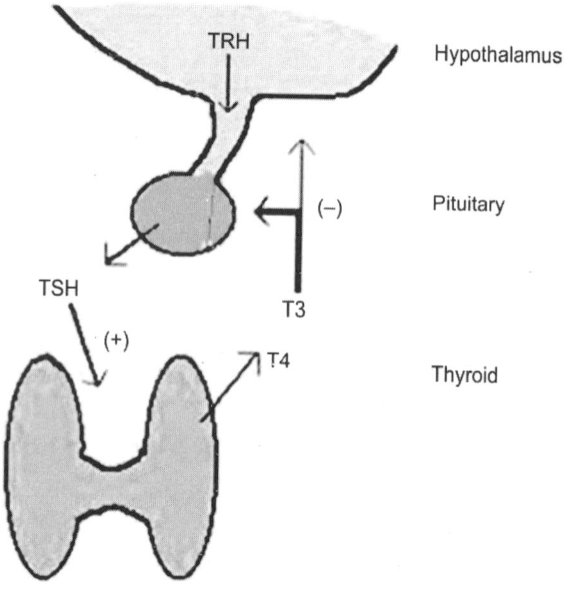

Diagram of the negative feedback loop for thyroid hormone (T3 & T4) homeostasis

Ans. (C) i.e., Radio iodine

13. **All the following are features of Polycystic disease of kidneys except:**
   (a) Haematuria (b) Hypertension
   (c) Renal failure (d) Erythrocytosis

EXPLANATION:

PCKD

- Cysts in PCKD are non functioning tubules filled with fluid pumped into them, which range in size from microscopic to enormous, crushing adjacent normal tubules and eventually rendering them non functional as well.
- Signs and symptoms of PCKD include hypertension, headaches, abdominal pain, hematuria, and excessive urination. Other symptoms include pain in the back, and cyst formation (renal and other organs).

Polycystic Kidney Disease

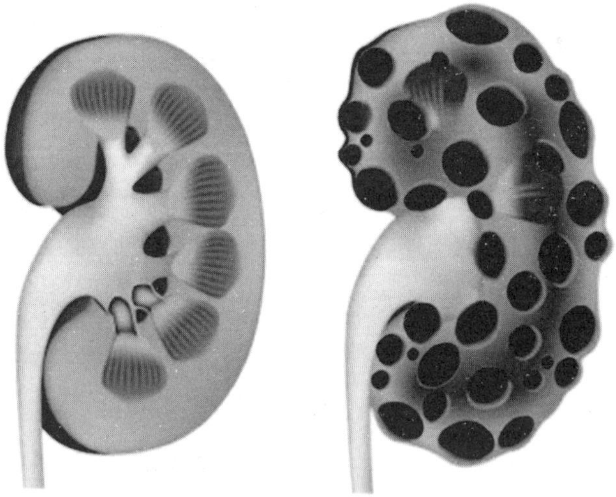

Ans. (D) i.e., Erythrocytosis

14. **Which one of the following is the most important selection criteria for obesity surgery?**
   (a) BMI > 40
   (b) BMI 30
   (c) BMI 30 with co-morbid disease
   (d) BMI 35 without any co-morbid disease

EXPLANATION:

The U.S. National Institutes of Health recommends bariatric surgery for obese people with a body mass index (BMI) of at least 40, and for people with BMI of at least 35 and serious coexisting medical conditions such as diabetes.

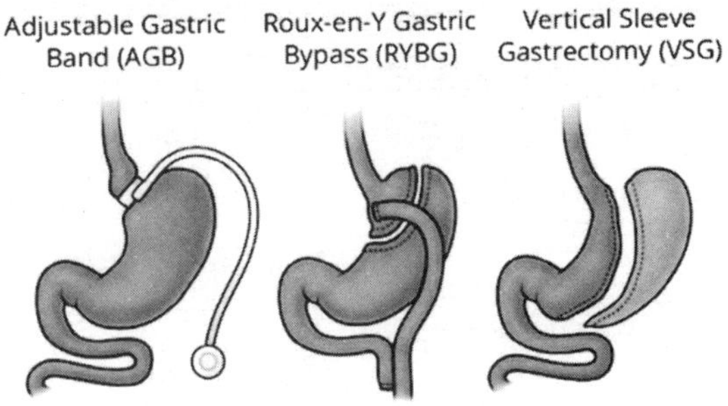

Ans. (A) i.e., BMI > 40

15. **A 45 year old underwent abdominal rectal prolapse surgery. At present, he complains of sexual dysfunction which is probably due to the injury of:**

(a) Pelvic autonomic nerves
(b) Inferior mesenteric artery
(c) Rectum
(d) Urinary bladder

EXPLANATION:

In **pelvic surgery** there is a risk of damage to the **pelvic autonomic nerves** with consequent urinary **dysfunction**, **impotence** and orgasmic failure.

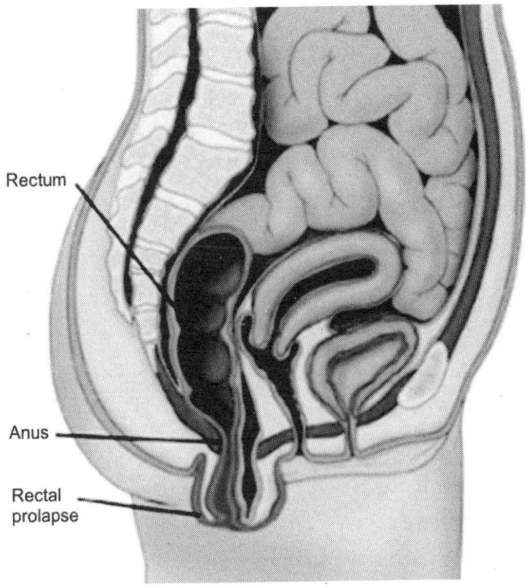

Ans. (A) i.e., Pelvic autonomic nerves

16. **In endoscopic retrograde cholangiopancreatography, endoscope used is:**

(a) End viewing
(b) Side viewing
(c) Rigid
(d) Front viewing

EXPLANATION:

ERCP has been used for the diagnosis and treatment of pancreatic diseases for over 20 years. This procedure is performed on an outpatient basis under sedation (rarely under general anesthesia). Using a "side viewing" endoscope, called a duodenoscope, the duodenal "papilla" (a mound like structure that houses the opening of the common bile duct and the pancreatic duct) is identified and manipulated. The scope contains a working channel through which flexible instruments are passed into the bile and/or pancreatic ducts to diagnose and treat pancreatic diseases.

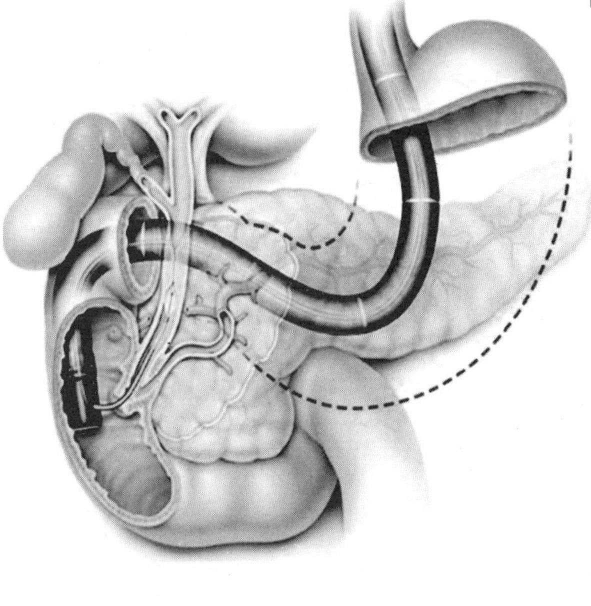

Ans. (B) i.e., Side viewing

2017

2017

17. **Oliguria is defined as:**
   (a) Absence of urine production
   (b) More than 900ml of urine excreted in a day
   (c) 600 ml to 700ml of urine excreted in a day
   (d) Less than 300ml of urine excreted in a day

EXPLANATION:

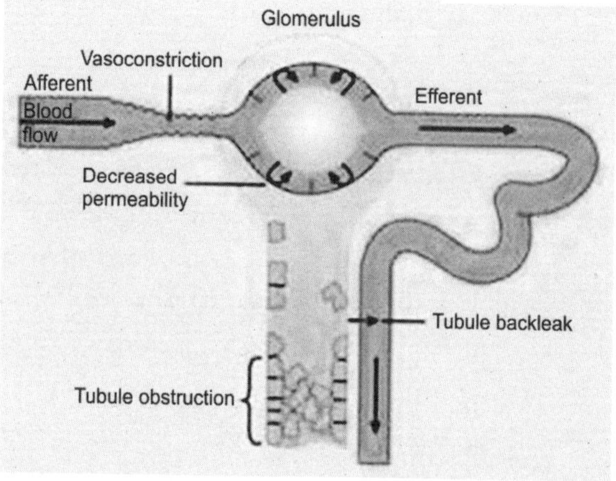

Oliguria or **hypouresis** (both names from roots meaning "not enough urine") is the low output of urine. In humans, it is clinically classified as an output more than 80ml/day but less than 400ml/day. The decreased output of urine may be a sign of dehydration, kidney failure, hypovolemic shock, HHNS (hyperosmolar Hyperglycemic Nonketotic Syndrome), multiple organ dysfunction syndrome, urinary obstruction/urinary retention, DKA, preeclampsia, and urinary tract infections, among other conditions.

Ans. (D) i.e., Less than 300ml of urine excreted in a day

18. **A 40 year old man, with a history of a reducible left groin swelling of two years, comes with severe pain over left groin. The swelling is now non reducible and is very tender to touch. The most probable treatment plan for this patient would be:**
   (a) Continue conservative management
   (b) Hot fomentation of groin area
   (c) Oral antibiotics
   (d) Prepare for emergency surgery

EXPLANATION:

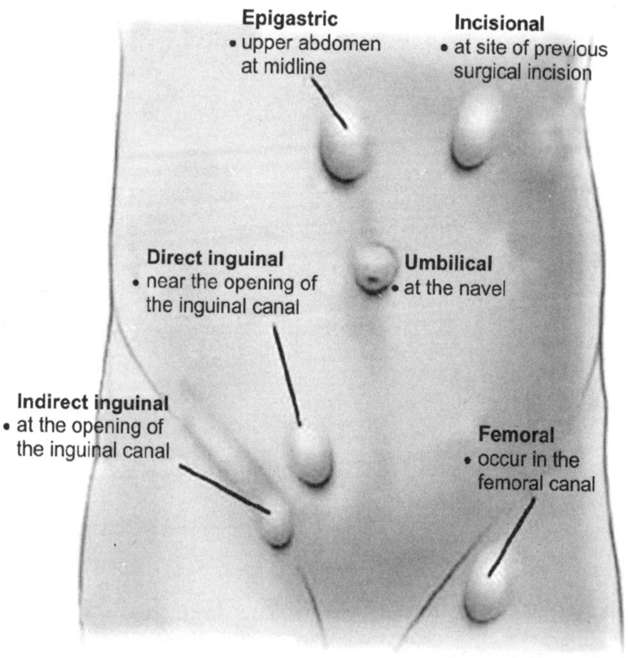

Irreducibility or Incarceration is a complication, in which hernia cannot be reduced, or pushed back into place, at least not without very much external effort. In intestinal hernias, this also substantially increases the risk of bowel obstruction and strangulation.

Ans. (D) i.e., Prepare for emergency surgery

19. **During laparoscopic inguinal hernia repair, in the 'triangle of doom', the following are true except:**
   (a) Vas deferens on medial side
   (b) Cord structures on lateral side
   (c) Base by iliac vessels
   (d) Dangerous area for dissection

EXPLANATION:

The **Triangle of Doom** is an anatomical triangle defined by the vas deferens medially, spermatic vessels laterally and peritoneal fold inferiorly. This triangle contains external iliac artery and vein, the deep circumflex iliac vein, the genital branch of genitofemoral nerve and hidden by fascia, the femoral nerve. It bears significance in laparoscopic repair of groin hernia. Surgical staples are avoided here.

Quadrangle of Pain and Doom

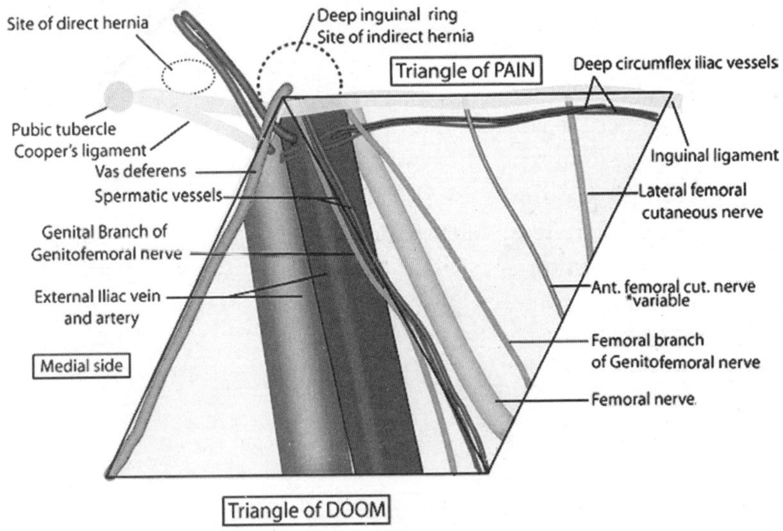

Preperitoneal view of the right inguinal space

Ans. (C) i.e., Base by iliac vessels

20. **All are rare type of lateral Hernia of abdominal wall, except:**
    (a) Spigelian
    (b) Obturator
    (c) Superior lumbar
    (d) Inferior lumbar

EXPLANATION:

An **obturator hernia** is a rare type of hernia of the pelvic floor in which pelvic or abdominal contents protrudes through the obturator foramen. Because of differences in anatomy, it is much more common in women, especially multiparous and older women who have recently lost a lot of weight. The diagnosis is often made intraoperatively after presenting with bowel obstruction.

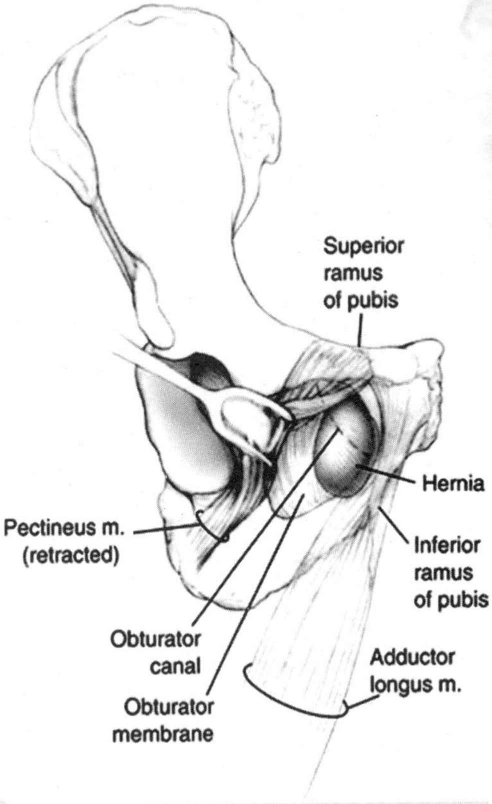

Ans. (B) i.e., Obturator

21. A 35 year old female had laparoscopic ventral hernia repair using polypropylene mesh in January 2015. In June 2015, she is again admitted with features of subacute intestinal obstruction and is managed conservatively. She continues to have recurrent colicky pain after that. Most probably she is suffering from:

(a) Recurrence of hernia
(b) New hernia
(c) Acute appendicitis
(d) Bowel adhesion to mesh

EXPLANATION:

Ventral hernia mesh repair is a common surgical procedure and may be performed by open or laparoscopic technique. Most patients have favorable outcome after surgery, but some patients experience problems such as pain, discomfort, and hernia recurrences. Intra abdominal adhesions may have deleterious effects, like intestinal obstruction followed by chronic pain and reduced quality of life. Adhesion seems to be associated with abdominal pain and discomfort.

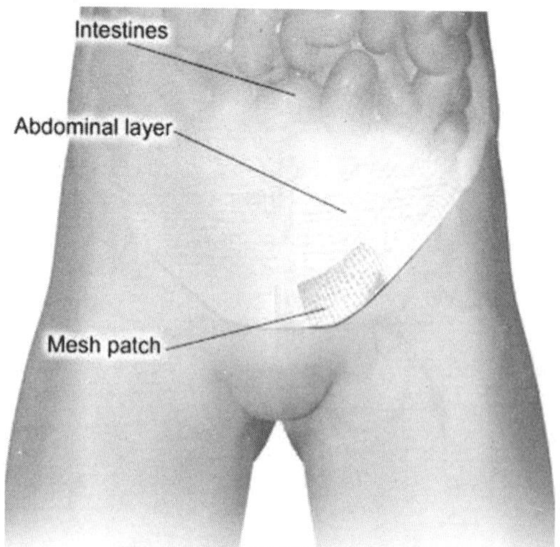

Post-Inguinal Hernia Repair

Ans. (D) i.e., Bowel adhesion to mesh

22. **Which of the following is NOT correct for breast abscess?**
(a) Drainage of abscess by a radial incision
(b) Antibiotic is given if pus is already present
(c) A counter incision is made in the dependant part
(d) Dressings are changed frequently

EXPLANATION:

A breast abscess is a collection of pus that develops into the breast with different causes. During lactation, breast abscess develops only rarely, most sources cite about 0.4–0.5% of breastfeeding women. Known risk factors are age over 30, primiparous and late delivery. Antibiotics were not shown effective in prevention of lactation abscess but are useful to treat a secondary infection.

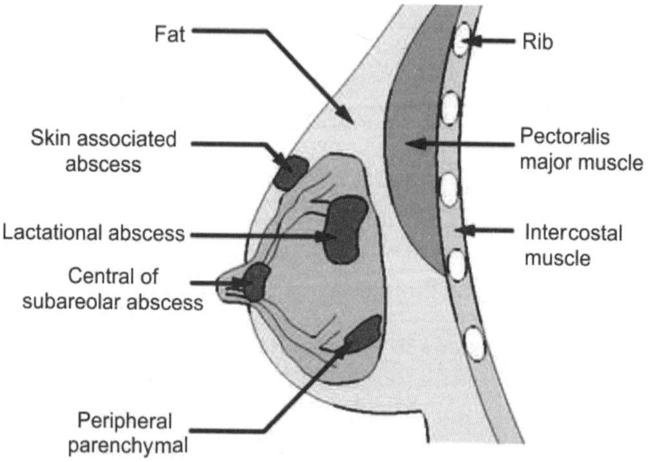

Ans. (B) i.e., Antibiotic is given if pus is already present

23. **Important landmark in submandibular gland dissection is:**
(a) Posterior border of mylohyoid muscle
(b) Posterior belly of digastrics muscle
(c) Anterior belly of digastrics muscle
(d) Facial artery

EXPLANATION:

Surgical excision of the submandibular gland (SMG) is commonly indicated in patients with neoplasms, and non neoplastic conditions such as chronic sialadenitis, sialolithiasis, ranula and drooling. Each submandibular gland has a larger,

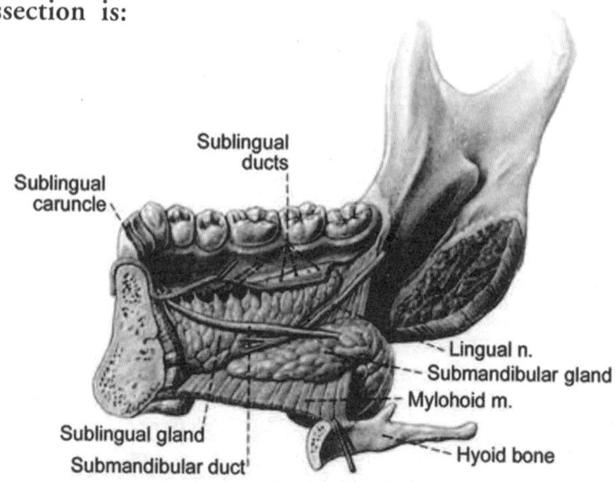

2017

superficial part and a smaller deep part. The two are separated by the mylohyoid muscle. The two parts however are continuous with each other posteriorly and the concavity thus formed is occupied by the free posterior border of the mylohyoid muscle.

Ans. (A) i.e., Posterior border of mylohyoid muscle

24. **Which of the following is NOT a feature of Systemic Inflammatory Response Syndrome?**

(a) Hyperthermia (more than 38°C)
(b) Hypothermia (less than 36°C)
(c) Leucocytosis
(d) Bradycardia

EXPLANATION:

Systemic inflammatory response syndrome (SIRS) is an inflammatory state affecting the whole body. It is the body's response to an infectious or noninfectious insult. Although the definition of SIRS refers to it as an "inflammatory" response, it actually has pro and anti inflammatory components.

Systematic Inflammatory Response Syndrome
Temperature > 38.3°C, or < 36°C
Heat Rate > 90 bmp
Respiratory rate > 20 breaths/min
White cell count < 4 or > 12g/L
Blood glucose > 7.7 mmol/L not diabetic
New altered mental state

Ans. (D) i.e., Bradycardia

25. **A 35 year old man presents to Emergency with acute onset pain abdomen radiating to whole abdomen and abdominal distension for one day. On examination, he has tenderness and guarding all over abdomen with pulse rate of 100/m and BP 116/84 mmHg. Chest X-ray erect position shows gas under bilateral domes of diaphragm. Probably he is suffering from:**

(a) Acute pancreatitis
(b) Ruptured liver abscess
(c) Appendicular perforation
(d) Colonic perforation

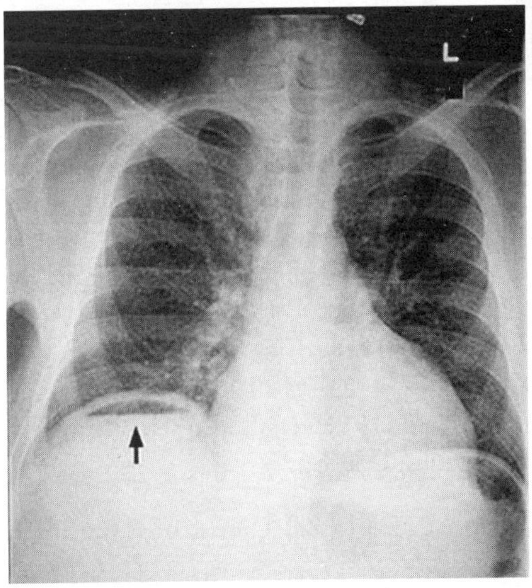

EXPLANATION:

The most common cause of air under diaphragm (pneumoperitoneum) is a perforated abdominal viscus, generally a perforated peptic ulcer, although any part of the bowel may perforate from a benign ulcer, tumor or abdominal trauma. A perforated appendix seldom causes a pneumoperitoneum.

Ans. (D) i.e., Colonic perforation

26. **A 70-year old man comes to Emergency with pain lower abdomen and not passing urine for eight hours. He has a past history of urgency, hesitancy and frequency of urine. On examination, he has a lump up to the umbilicus which is slightly tender.**

What is the next step of management?

(a) Get an urgent USG
(b) Per rectal examination
(c) Per urethral catheterise the patient
(d) Start antibiotics

EXPLANATION:

Urinary retention is characterised by poor urinary stream with intermittent flow, straining, a sense of incomplete voiding, and hesitancy (a delay between trying to urinate and the flow actually beginning). As the bladder remains full, it may lead to incontinence, nocturia (need to urinate at night), and high frequency. Acute retention, causing complete anuria, is a medical emergency, as the bladder can stretch to an enormous size, and possibly tear if not dealt with quickly. If the bladder distends enough, it becomes painful. In such a case, there may be suprapubic constant, dull, pain. In acute urinary retention, urinary catheterization, placement of a prostatic stent, or suprapubic cystostomy relieves the retention.

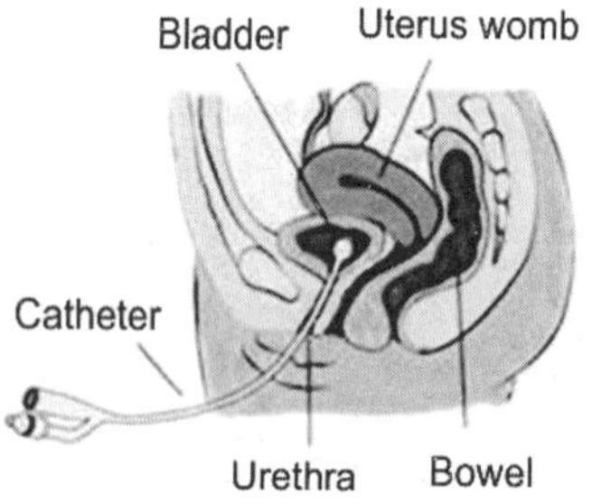

Figure 1 - Female catheter

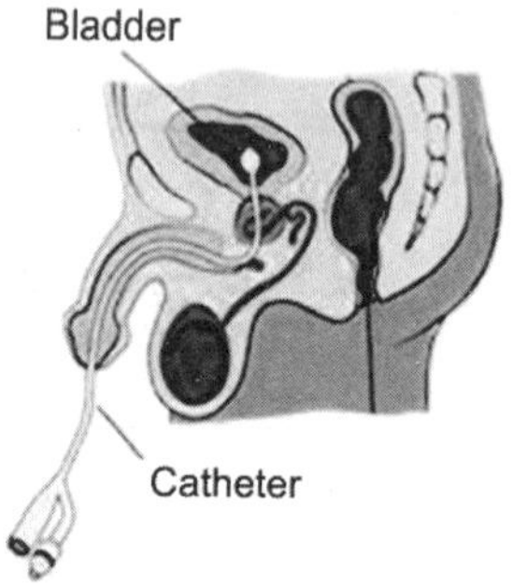

Figure 2 - Male catheter

Ans. (C) i.e., Per urethral catheterise the patient

2017

27. **'Swiss cheese defects' of anterior abdominal wall after exploratory laparotomy is best seen while doing:**

(a) Open ventral hernia repair
(b) Open inguinal hernia repair
(c) Laparoscopic ventral hernia repair
(d) Laparoscopic inguinal hernia repair

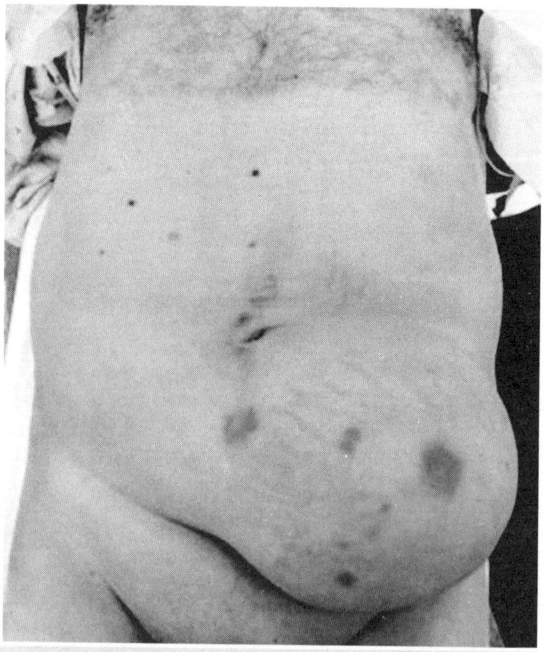

EXPLANATION:

Incisional hernias can be a significant problem after open abdominal surgery. Laparoscopic incisional hernia repair (LIHR) is conceptually appealing: a large, abdominal wall reincision with potential wound related ill effects is avoided and an intraperitoneal onlay mesh is expected to provide security that is equivalent to open, retromuscular mesh repair. Complete division of adhesions to the anterior abdominal wall may identify subclinical "Swiss cheese" defects but incurs some risk of additional complications.

Ans. (C) i.e., Laparoscopic ventral hernia repair

28. **A 35 year old male patient comes to casualty with acute pain abdomen; and on examination found to have cold, clammy extremities, sunken eyes, dry tongue, thready pulse, drawn and anxious face with abdominal guarding and rigidity. This clinical picture indicates:**

(a) Local peritonitis
(b) Diffuse early peritonitis
(c) Diffuse late peritonitis
(d) Acute cholecystitis

EXPLANATION:

Diffuse late peritonitis features:

- Abdomen becomes rigid
- Distension
- Bowel sounds absent
- Shock
  - o Cold clammy extremities
  - o Sunken eyes
  - o Dry tongue
  - o Rapid thread pulse
  - o Anxious facies

Peritonitis

Type	Definition	Microbiology
Primary	Due to bacterial translocation or hematogenous seeding. No break in integrity of GI tract	**Monomicrobial;** coliforms or streptococci
Secondary	Microscopic or macroscopic perforation	**Polymicrobial;** coliforms gram positive cocci and enteric anaerobes
Tertiary	Persistent or recurrent peritoneal infection developing after treatment of secondary peritonitis	**Nosocomial** organisms; enterococci, staphylococci resistant gram negative bacilli and yeast
Dialysis associated	Seeding of peritoneum due to dialysis catheter or breaks in sterility	Usually **monomicrobial;** skin flora, yeast

2017

Ans. (C) i.e., Diffuse late peritonitis

29. **All of the following statements are true for keloids except:**
   (a) It is rarely seen in white skinned persons and is more common over the sternum
   (b) True keloid continues to become worse even after one year
   (c) True keloid does not spread into surrounding tissue
   (d) The maturation and stabilization of the collagen fibrils is inhibited

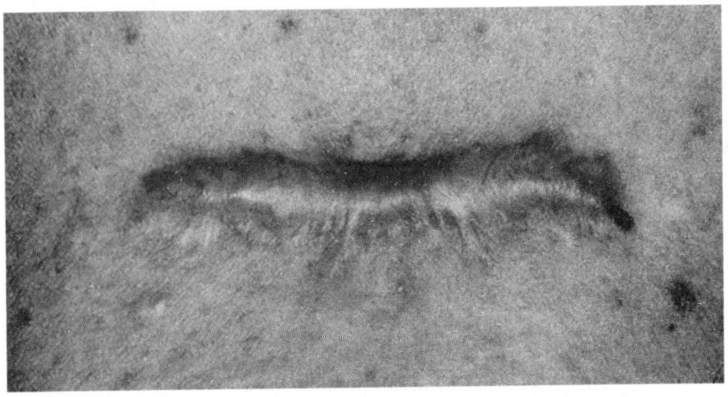

EXPLANATION:

Keloids should not be confused with hypertrophic scars, which are raised scars that do not grow beyond the boundaries of the original wound.

Ans. (C) i.e., True keloid does not spread into surrounding tissue

30. **Which of these is a palliative shunt procedure created between the left subclavian artery and pulmonary artery to treat cyanotic congenital heart disease?**
   (a) Gott's shunt
   (b) Lieno renal shunt
   (c) Blalock Taussig shunt
   (d) Waterstons shunt

EXPLANATION:

The **Blalock–Thomas–Taussig shunt** (commonly called the **Blalock–Taussig shunt**) is a surgical procedure used to increase pulmonary blood flow for palliation in duct dependent cyanotic heart defects like pulmonary atresia, which are common causes of blue baby syndrome. In modern surgery, this procedure is temporarily used to direct blood flow to the lungs and relieve cyanosis while the infant is waiting for corrective or definitive surgery. One branch of the subclavian artery or carotid artery is separated and connected with the pulmonary artery. The first area of application was tetralogy of Fallot.

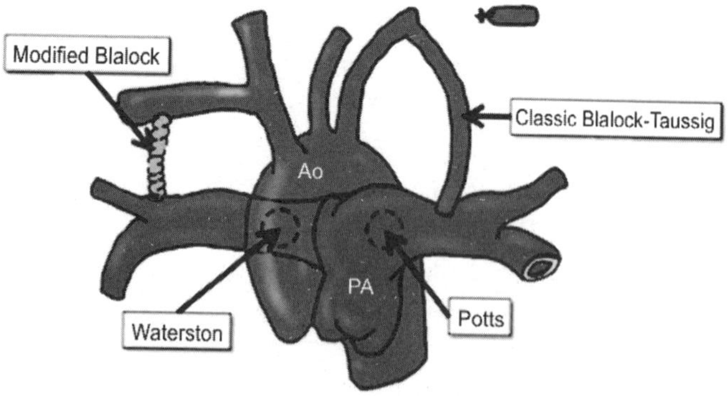

Ans. (C) i.e., Blalock Taussig shunt

31. A young male is undergoing emergency surgery for a clinical diagnosis of acute appendicitis. Intraoperatively minimal pus was found but the appendix was normal.
What is the next step of management?

(a) Appendectomy
(b) Right hemicolectomy
(c) Close the abdomen without doing anything
(d) Search for perforated Meckel's diverticulum

EXPLANATION:

Meckel's diverticulum (MD) occurs when the omphalomesenteric duct fails to obliterate completely during fetal life. It is the most common congenital abnormality of the gastrointestinal tract, classically thought to represent about 2% of the population. Despite the fact that this condition is relatively common, only about 4–16% of cases will lead to complications, which include hemorrhage, intussusception, inflammation and, occasionally, perforation. Many of the other presenting symptoms, such as abdominal pain and nausea, are non specific and may mimic appendicitis.

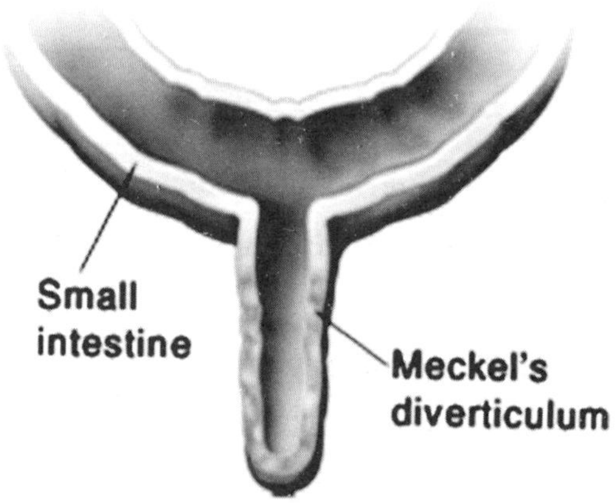

Ans. (D) i.e., Search for perforated Meckel's diverticulum

32. Which of the following is NOT considered as an indicator of adequate fluid resuscitation?

(a) Urine output
(b) Respiratory rate
(c) Pulse
(d) Blood pressure

EXPLANATION:

Volume depletion takes place when fluid is lost from the extracellular space at a rate exceeding net intake. Acute hemorrhage is the leading cause of acute life threatening intravascular volume loss requiring aggressive fluid resuscitation to maintain tissue perfusion until the underlying cause can be corrected. Intravascular volume depletions may also result from gastrointestinal disorders (e.g., vomiting, diarrhea, or ascites), burns, environmental exposure, or renal salt wasting. Volume depletion may result from

2017

acute sequestration in the body in a "third space" that is not in equilibrium with the intracellular fluid, as seen in septic shock.

Fluid Management in the Severely Burned Patient

Criteria for adequate fluid resuscitation
Normalization of blood pressure
Urine output (1–2mL/Kg/hr)
Blood lactate (<2mM/L)
Base deficit (<–5)
Gastric intramucosal pH (>7.23)
Central venous pressure and pulmonary occlusion pressure
Intrathoracic blood volume index
Cardiac index (4.5L/min/m^2)
Oxygen delivery index (600mL/min/m^2)

Ans. (B) i.e., Respiratory rate

33. **In a 65-year old, double contrast barium enema shows cancer of colon with an apple core appearance. Colonoscopic biopsy shows adenocarcinoma. What will be the next step of management?**

(a) Surgery
(b) Chemotherapy
(c) CECT to stage disease
(d) Radiotherapy

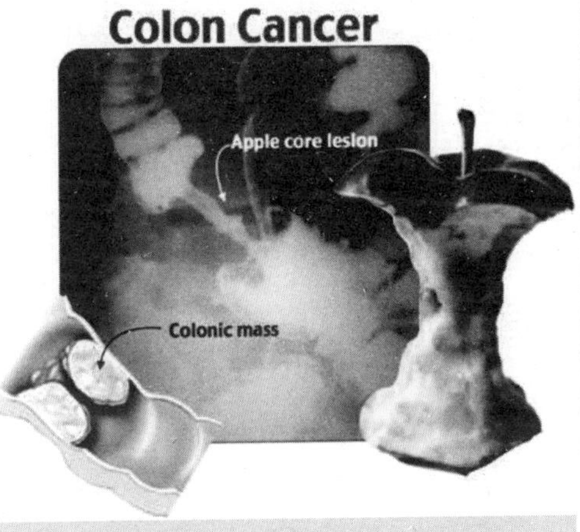

EXPLANATION:

Colorectal cancer diagnosis is performed by sampling of areas of the colon suspicious for possible tumor development, typically during colonoscopy or sigmoidoscopy, depending on the location of the lesion. It is confirmed by microscopical examination of a tissue sample.

Disease extent is usually determined by a CT scan of the chest, abdomen and pelvis. Other potential imaging tests such as PET and MRI may be used in certain cases.

Ans. (C) i.e., CECT to stage disease

34. **A 35-year old woman presented with a lump in her upper abdomen for two months which was slightly increasing. She also complained of early satiety. She gave a history of acute severe pain in upper abdomen for which she was admitted in hospital for 10 days, about three months ago. On examination, the mass was firm, smooth surfaced and not moving with respiration. She was most likely suffering from:**

(a) Cancer stomach
(b) Cancer colon
(c) Pseudocyst pancreas
(d) Splenic cyst

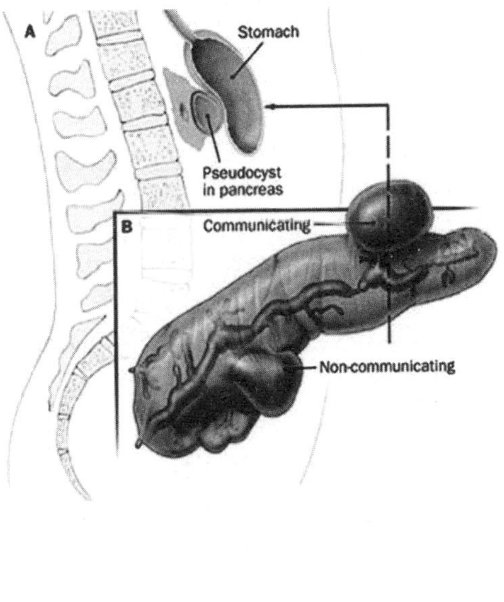

EXPLANATION:

A **pancreatic pseudocyst** is a circumscribed collection of fluid rich in pancreatic enzymes, blood, and necrotic tissue, typically located in the lesser sac of the abdomen. Pancreatic pseudocysts are usually complications of pancreatitis, although in children they frequently occur following abdominal trauma. Pancreatic pseudocysts account for approximately 75% of all pancreatic masses.

Ans. (C) i.e., Pseudocyst pancreas

35. **While working in a primary health centre, an elderly patient presents with a history of sudden loss of vision and curtain falling sensation in one eye. This symptom is highly suggestive that the patient has the following condition:**

(a) Retinal detachment

(b) Vitreous haemorrhage

(c) Acute onset ptosis

(d) Intracranial haemorrhage

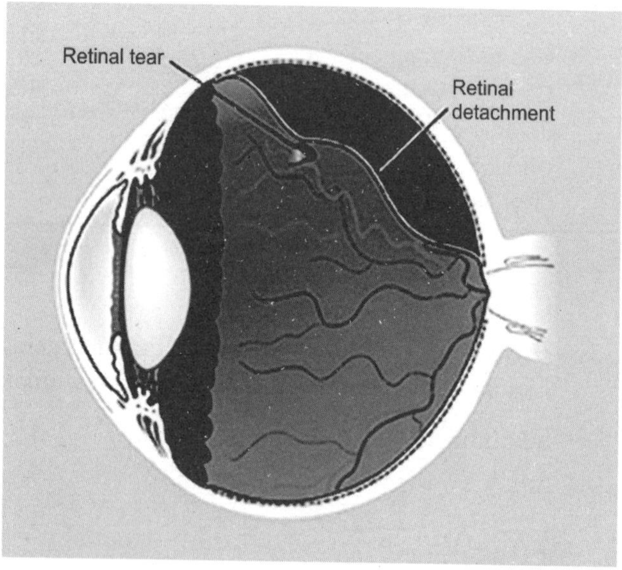

EXPLANATION:

Retinal detachment is a disorder of the eye in which the retina separates from the layer underneath. Symptoms include an increase in the number of floaters, flashes of light, and worsening of the outer part of the visual field. This may be described as a curtain over part of the field of vision. In about 7% of cases both eyes are affected. Without treatment permanent loss of vision may occur

Ans. (A) i.e., Retinal detachment

36. **Pringle's manoeuvre is done to stop bleeding at:**

(a) Left gastric artery

(b) Splenic artery

(c) Renal artery

(d) Hepatoduodenal ligament

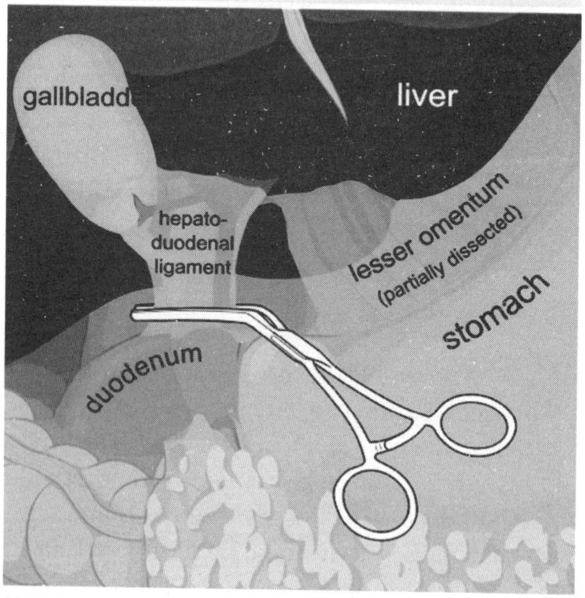

EXPLANATION:

The **Pringle maneuver** is a surgical **maneuver** used in some abdominal operations. A large atraumatic haemostat is used to clamp the hepatoduodenal ligament (free border of the lesser omentum) interrupting the flow of blood through the hepatic artery and the portal vein and thus helping to control bleeding from the liver.

Ans. (D) i.e., Hepatoduodenal ligament

37. **What is the most common malignant tumour of eyelid?**

(a) Neurofibroma

(b) Meibomian cancer

(c) Basal cell cancer

(d) Pseudotumour

EXPLANATION:

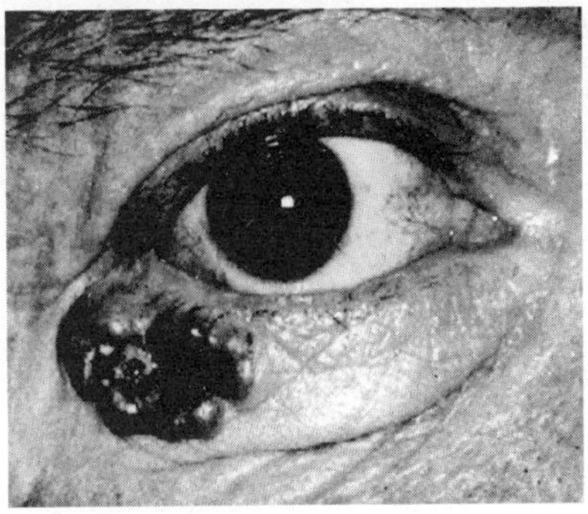

Basal cell carcinoma (BCC), also known as **basal cell cancer,** is the most common type of skin cancer. It often appears as a painless raised area of skin, which may be shiny with small blood vessels running over it; or it may present as a raised area with ulceration. Basal cell cancer grows slowly and can damage the tissue around it but is unlikely to spread to distant areas or to result in death.

Ans. (C) i.e., Basal cell cancer

38. Which of the following is NOT a symptom of atherosclerotic occlusive disease at the bifurcation of aorta (Leriche syndrome)?

(a) Claudication of the buttock and thigh
(b) Claudication of the calf
(c) Sexual impotence
(d) Gangrene localised to the feet

EXPLANATION:

Aortoiliac occlusive disease, also known as **Leriche's syndrome** and **Leriche syndrome,** is a form of central artery disease involving the blockage of the abdominal aorta as it transitions into the common iliac arteries.

Symptoms according to the Area of Arterial Lesion

Area of lesion	Clinical picture
Aortoiliac	Buttock-thigh-calf claudication
	Impotency in a man (if bilateral involvement is present): Leriche syndrome
Femoropopliteal	Calf claudication with/without plantar claudication
Infrapopliteal	Plantar claudication

Ans. (D) i.e., Gangrene localised to the feet

39. Which of the following factors is labelled as cytokine in the pathogenesis of Systemic Inflammatory Response Syndrome (SIRS)?

(a) Nitric oxide
(b) Complements
(c) Leukotrienes
(d) Tumor necrosis factor

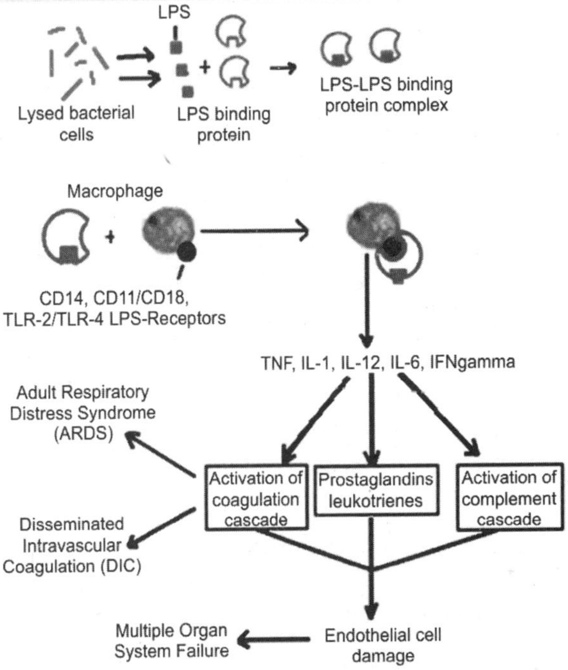

EXPLANATION:

SIRS is a serious condition related to systemic inflammation, organ dysfunction, and organ failure. It is a subset of cytokine storm, in which there is abnormal regulation of various cytokines. SIRS is also closely related to sepsis, in which patients satisfy criteria for SIRS and have a suspected or proven infection.

Ans. (D) i.e., Tumor necrosis factor

40. **Vocal cord palsy after thyroid surgery is due to injury to:**

(a) Superficial laryngeal nerve
(b) Recurrent laryngeal nerve
(c) Ansa cervicalis
(d) Vagus nerve

EXPLANATION:

The **recurrent laryngeal nerve** (RLN) is a branch of the vagus nerve (cranial nerve X) that supplies all the intrinsic muscles of the larynx, with the exception of the cricothyroid muscles. There are two recurrent laryngeal nerves, right and left, in the human body. The right and left nerves are not symmetrical, with the left nerve looping under the aortic arch, and the right nerve looping under the right subclavian artery then traveling upwards. They both travel alongside of the trachea. Additionally, the nerves are one of few nerves that follow a *recurrent* course, moving in the opposite direction to the nerve they branch from, a fact from which they gain their name.

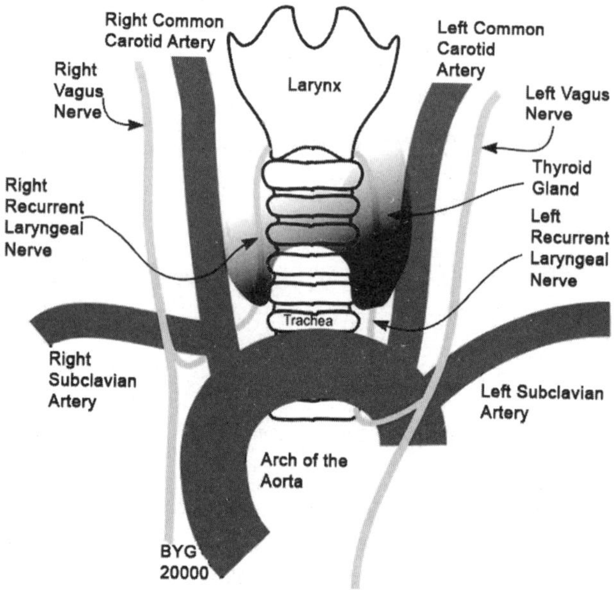

Ans. (B) i.e., Recurrent laryngeal nerve

2017

41. **A infertile woman presents with yellow or green vaginal discharge, bartholin cyst and proctitis. What is the most probable diagnosis?**

(a) Syphilis
(b) Trichomomiasis
(c) Gonorrhoea
(d) Candidiasis

EXPLANATION:

Symptoms of gonorrhea in women include vaginal discharge, dysuria, intermenstrual bleeding, ***dyspareunia*** and abdominal pain. In men, gonorrhea causes anterior urethritis. Many people with gonococcal ***proctitis*** don't have any symptoms. In a small fraction of men, ascending ***urethritis*** progresses to epididymitis. Discharge is usually described as thin, purulent, and mildly odorous; however, many patients have minimal or no symptoms from gonococcal cervicitis.

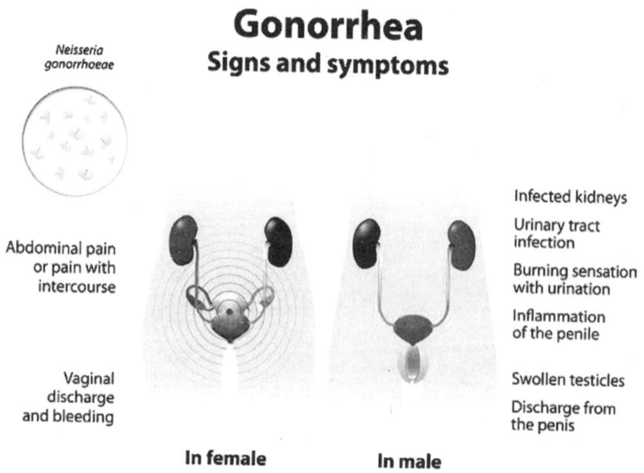

Ans. (C) i.e., Gonorrhoea

42. **Absolute contraindication to combined oral contraceptive is:**

(a) History of GDM
(b) History of thrombo embolism
(c) History of previous two caesarean section
(d) History of gallbladder disease

EXPLANATION:

Contraindications of OCP use (ABBCCCD)

- Acute or chronic liver disease (e.g. Wilson's disease).
- Bad migraines (with focal neurological signs).
- Bleed per vagina undiagnosed.
- Cancer (endometrial, breast).
- Cardiovascular disease.
- Cardiovascular disease risk factors.
  - Smoking >35 years.
  - Uncontrolled BP.
- DVT.

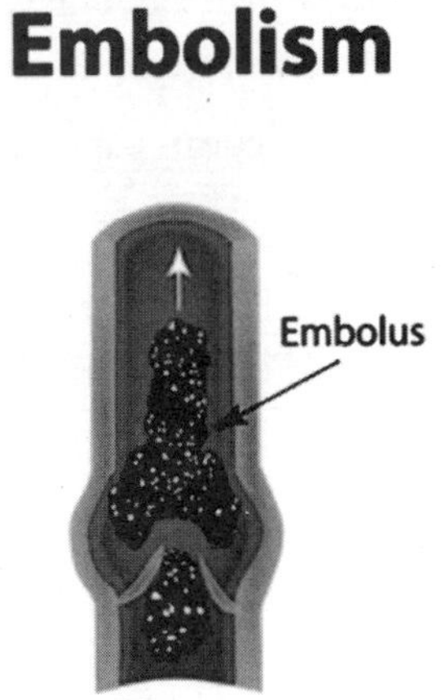

Ans. (B) i.e., History of thrombo embolism

43. A 28 year old P1L1 presents with severe pain in her abdomen and is taken for laparotomy. On opening the abdomen pseudomyxoma of the peritoneum is present. What should be the probable reason?

(a) Mucinous cystadenoma of ovary
(b) Serous cystadenoma of ovary
(c) Rupture of dermoid tumor
(d) Endometriosis

EXPLANATION:

Pseudomyxoma peritonei (PMP) is a clinical condition caused by cancerous cells (mucinous adenocarcinoma) that produce abundant mucin or gelatinous ascites. The tumors cause fibrosis of tissues and impede digestion or organ function, and if left untreated, the tumors and mucin they produce will fill the abdominal cavity. This will result in compression of organs and will destroy the function of colon, small intestine, stomach, or other organs. Prognosis with treatment in many cases is optimistic, but the disease is lethal if untreated, with death by cachexia, bowel obstruction, or other types of complications.

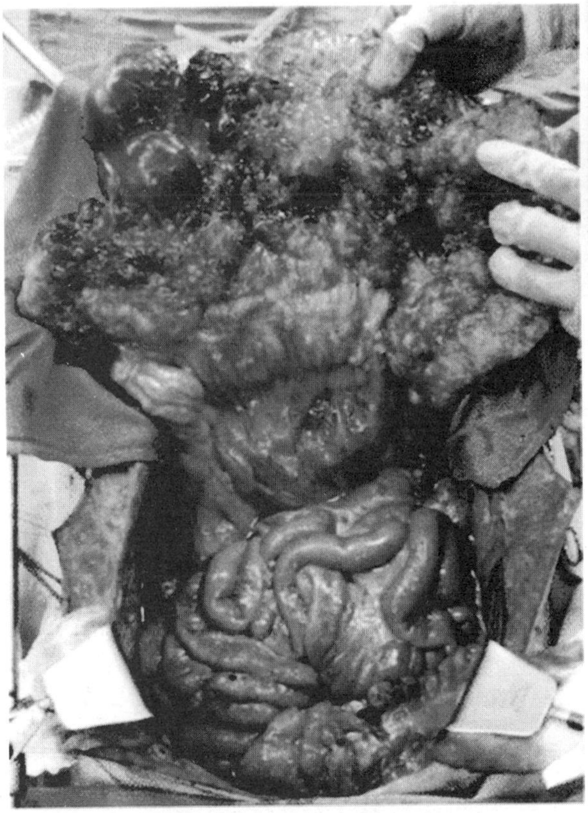

This disease is most commonly caused by an appendiceal primary cancer (cancer of the appendix); mucinous tumors of the ovary have also been implicated, although in most cases ovarian involvement is favored to be a metastasis from an appendiceal or other gastrointestinal source. Disease is typically classified as low or high grade (with signet ring cells). When disease presents with low grade histologic features the cancer rarely spreads through the lymphatic system or through the bloodstream.

Ans. (A) i.e., Mucinous cystadenoma of ovary

44. In a 40 year old woman, pap smear shows atypical glandular cells. The next step of management should be:

(a) Repeat pap smear after three months

(b) Colposcopic directed cervical biopsy

(c) Colposcopy, cervical biopsy, endocervical curettage and endometrial biopsy

(d) Hysteroscopy and directed endometrial biopsy

EXPLANATION:

The **Papanicolaou test** (abbreviated as **Pap test**, also known as **Pap smear, cervical smear**, or **smear test**) is a method of cervical screening used to detect potentially precancerous and cancerous processes in the cervix. Abnormal findings are often followed up by more sensitive diagnostic procedures, and, if warranted, interventions that aim to prevent progression to cervical cancer. The test was invented by, and named for, doctor Aurel Babe' and doctor Georgios Papanikolaou.

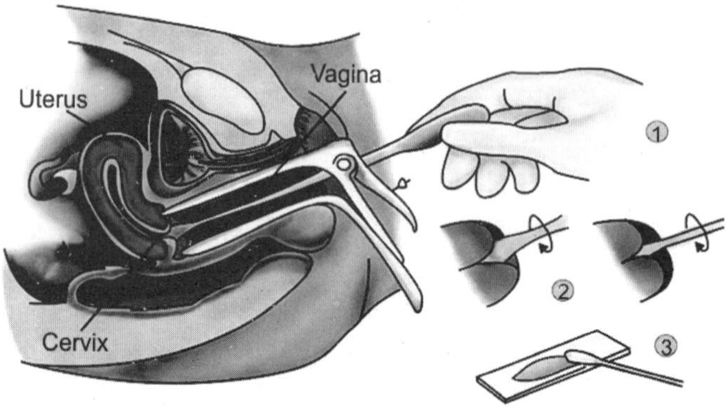

Ans. (C) i.e., Colposcopy, cervical biopsy, endocervical curettage and endometrial biopsy

45. A 50 year old P4L4 has a simple left ovarian cyst of 10cm. Ca 125 is 30U/mL. Treatment of choice would be:

(a) TAH + BSO (Total abdominal hysterectomy + Bilateral salpingo oopherectomy)

(b) Laparoscopic cystectomy

(c) Laparoscopic oophorectomy

(d) Medical management with oral contraceptives

EXPLANATION:

CA-125 is useful in differential diagnosis and in follow up of the disease of ovarian tumours, but it by itself has not been shown to be an effective method to screen for early stage ovarian cancer due to its unacceptable low sensitivity and specificity. CA-125 levels in premenopausal people over 200 U/mL may indicate ovarian cancer, as may any elevation in CA-125 above 35 U/mL in post menopausal people. CA-125 levels are not accurate in early stage ovarian cancer, as fully half of stage I ovarian cancer patients have a normal CA-125 level.

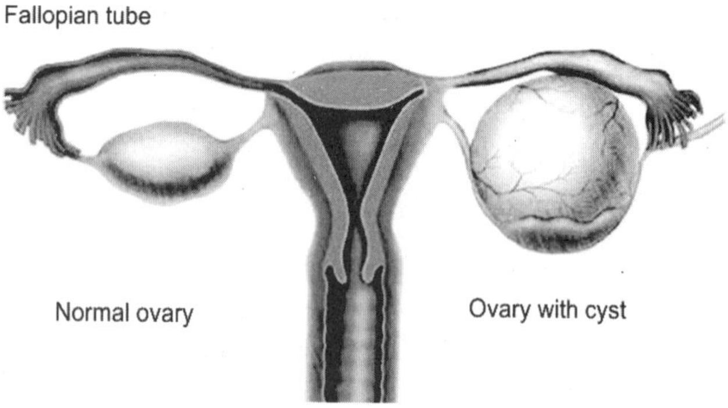

If a tumor in a premenopausal woman is determined to be a low malignant potential tumor during surgery, and it is clearly stage I cancer, only the affected ovary is removed. For postmenopausal women with low malignant potential tumors, hysterectomy with bilateral salpingo-oophorectomy is still the preferred option.

Ans. (A) i.e., TAH + BSO (Total abdominal hysterectomy + Bilateral salpingo oopherectomy)

46. **A seven year old girl with precocious puberty is found to be having a 10cm. ovarian cyst on USG. The most likely etiology is:**

(a) Benign cystic teratoma
(b) Brenner tumour
(c) Choriocarcinoma
(d) Granulosa cell tumour

EXPLANATION:

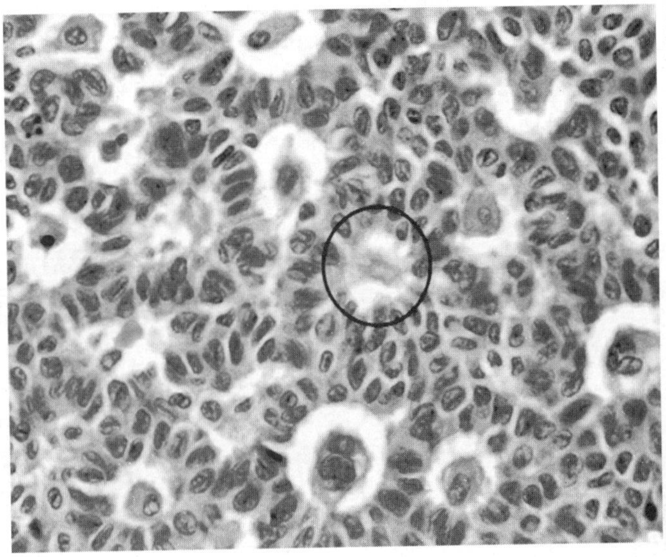

Granulosa cell tumours (or **granulosatheca cell tumoursor folliculoma**) are tumours that arise from granulosa cells. These tumours are part of the sex cord gonadal stromal tumour or non epithelial group of tumours. Although granulosa cells normally occur only in the ovary, granulosa cell tumours occur in both ovaries and testicles. These tumours should be considered malignant and treated in the same way as other malignant tumours of ovary. The ovarian disease has two forms, juvenile and adult, both characterized by indolent growth, and therefore has high recovery rates. The staging system for these tumours is the same as for epithelial tumours and most present as stage I. The peak age at which they occur is 50–55 years, but they may occur at any age. Histology shows Call Exner bodies.

Ans. (D) i.e., Granulosa cell tumour

2017

47. **A 17-year old girl presents with an ovarian cyst of 5cm. The cyst is echo free, unilocular and CA 125 of 8U/ml. What is most appropriate management?**

(a) Laproscopy for cyst removal
(b) Laparotomy for cyst removal
(c) Conservative with follow up ultrasound
(d) Medical treatment

EXPLANATION:

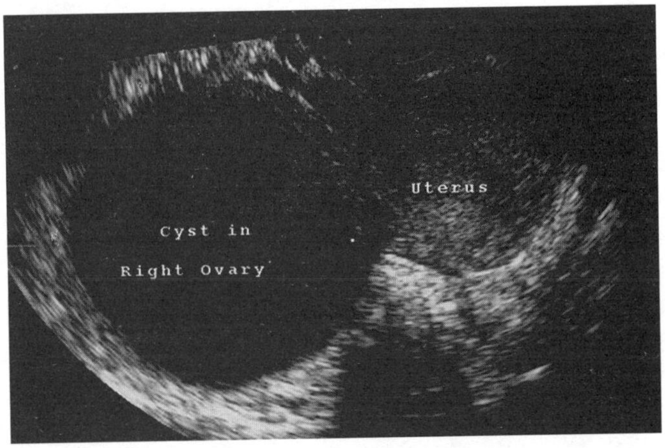

Follow up imaging in women of reproductive age for incidentally discovered simple cysts on ultrasound is not needed until 5 cm, as these are usually normal ovarian follicles. Simple cysts 5 to 7 cm in premenopausal females should be followed yearly. Simple cysts larger than 7 cm require further imaging with MRI or surgical assessment. Because they are large, they cannot be reliably assessed by ultrasound alone because it may be difficult to see the soft tissue nodularity or thickened septation at their posterior wall due to limited penetrance of the ultrasound beam.

Ans. (C) i.e., Conservative with follow up ultrasound

48. **The contraceptive choice for a 38 year old P1L1 woman having chronic hypertension, dysmenorrhoea and menorrhagia is:**
   (a) Copper intrauterine device
   (b) Sterilization
   (c) Levenorgestrel intrauterine device
   (d) Combined oral contraceptive pills

EXPLANATION:

Intrauterine device (IUD) with progestogen, sold under the brand name **Mirena** among others, is a intrauterine device that releases the hormone levonorgestrel. It is used for birth control, heavy menstrual periods, and to prevent excessive build of the lining of the uterus in those on estrogen replacement therapy. It is one of the most effective forms of birth control with a one year failure rate around 0.2%. The device is placed in the uterus and lasts three to five years. Following removal fertility returns quickly.

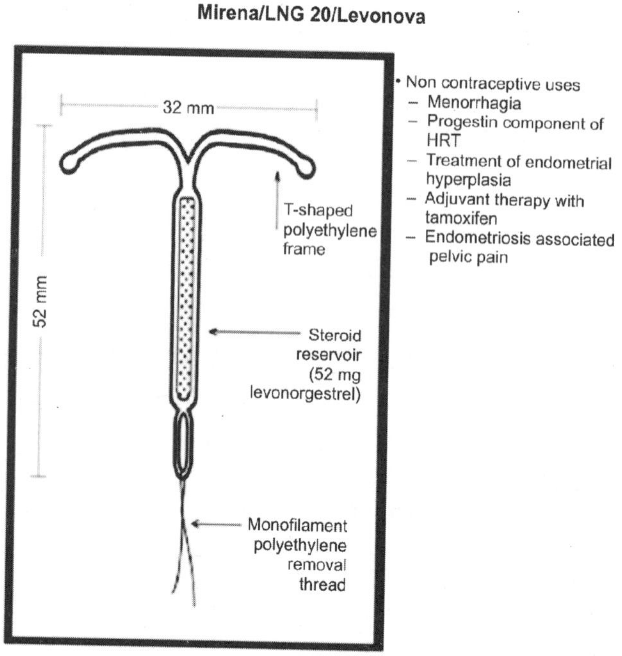

Ans. (C) i.e., Levenorgestrel intrauterine device

49. **Most probable cause of heavy bleeding in a P2L2 during tenth day post partum is:**
   (a) Retained bits of cotyledons and membranes
   (b) Subinvolution of placental site
   (c) Resumption of menstruation
   (d) Infected episiotomy wound

EXPLANATION:

Cause of PPH	Incidence
Uterine atony	70%
Trauma	20%
Retained tissue	10%
Coagulopathy	1%

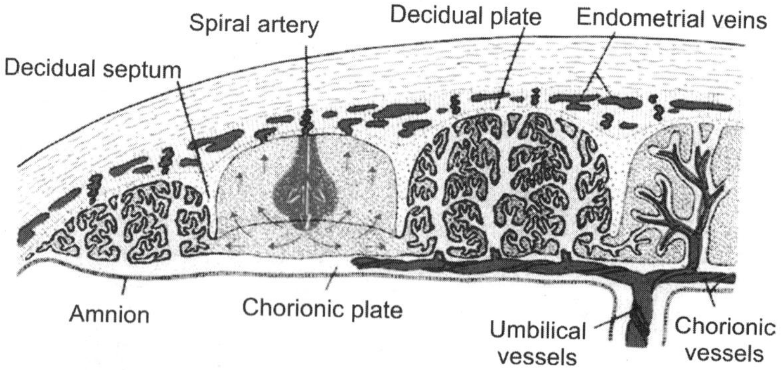

Ans. (A) i.e., Retained bits of cotyledons and membranes

50. **A woman with which of the following health problems should avoid centchromen?**
   (a) Polycystic ovarian syndrome
   (b) Woman with dysfunctional uterine bleeding
   (c) Endometrial hyperplasia
   (d) Endometriosis

EXPLANATION:

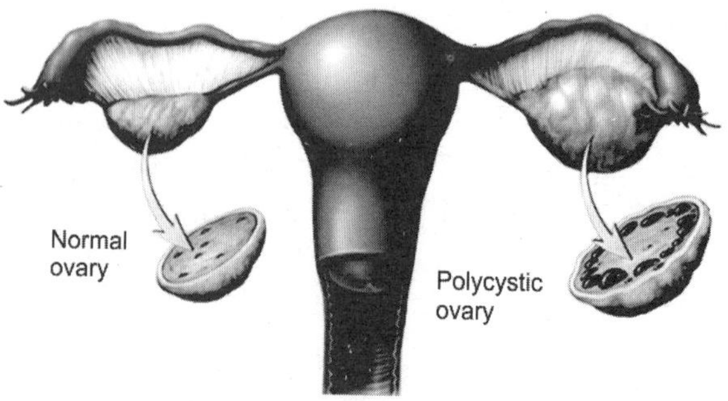

Saheli/ Centchroman does not have the short term side effects like nausea, vomiting, weight gain etc. which are commonly reported with the other oral contraceptive pills. The only side effects reported with Saheli (Centchroman) is the delay in the menstrual cycles in around 8% of the cases.

Ans. (A) i.e., Polycystic ovarian syndrome

51. Combined contraceptive pills give protection from the following except:

(a) Cancer of ovary
(b) Cancer of endometrium
(c) Cancer of cervix
(d) Ectopic pregnancy

EXPLANATION:

The use of oral contraceptives (birth control pills) for five years or more decreases the risk of ovarian cancer in later life by 50%. Combined oral contraceptive use reduces the risk of ovarian cancer by 40% and the risk of endometrial cancer by 50% compared with never users. The risk reduction increases with duration of use, with an 80% reduction in risk for both ovarian and endometrial cancer with use for more than 10 years. The risk reduction for both ovarian and endometrial cancer persists for at least 20 years.

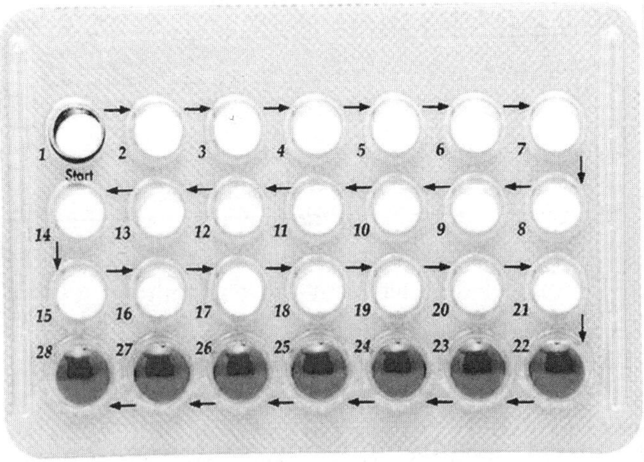

Ans. (C) i.e., Cancer of cervix

52. A woman presents with heavy foul smelling discharge with sharply demarcated ulcers without induration on the perineum and the labia majora. Inguinal lymphadenopathy is also present. What is the most probable diagnosis?

(a) Gonorrhoea
(b) Tuberculosis
(c) Chancroid
(d) Trichomoniasis

EXPLANATION:

The ulcer of chancroid characteristically:

- Ranges in size dramatically from 3 to 50mm (1/8 inch to two inches) across
- Is painful
- Has sharply defined, undermined borders
- Has irregular or ragged borders
- Has a base that is covered with a gray or yellowish gray material
- Has a base that bleeds easily if traumatized or scraped
- Painful swollen lymph nodes occurs in 30 to 60% of patients.
- Dysuria (pain with urination) and dyspareunia (pain with intercourse) in females

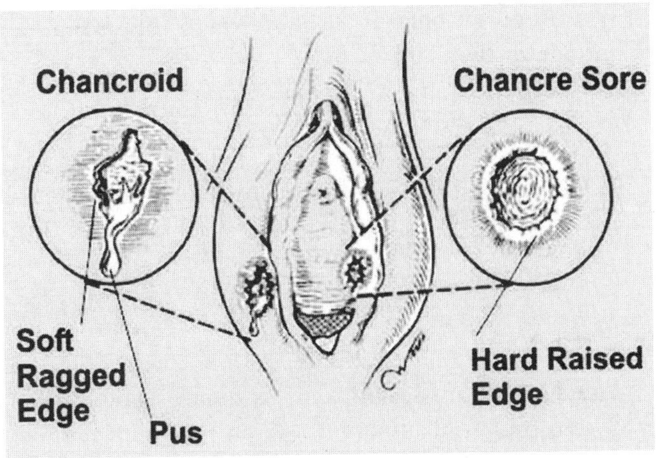

Ans. (C) i.e., Chancroid

53. **A 28 year old woman develops amenorrhoea after having dilatation and curettage. The most likely diagnosis is:**

(a) Kallman syndrome
(b) Asherman syndrome
(c) Anorexia nervosa
(d) Turner syndrome

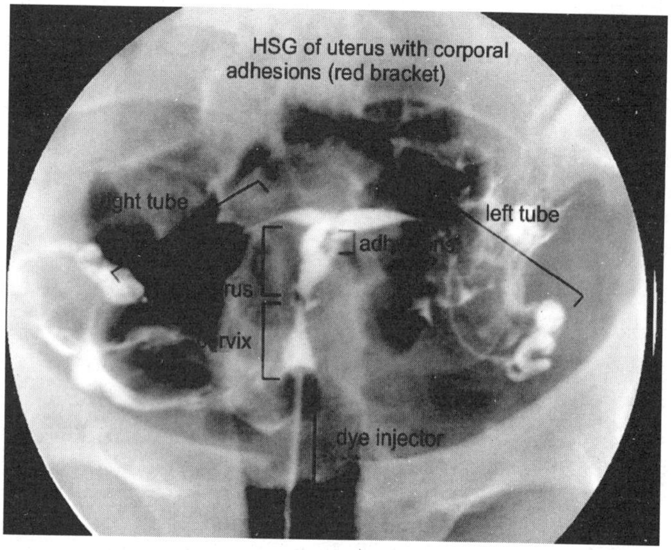

EXPLANATION:

"**Asherman's Syndrome**", which is also referred to as intrauterine adhesions (IUA) or intrauterine synechiae, is an acquired uterine condition that occurs when scar tissue (adhesions) form inside the uterus and/or the cervix. It is characterized by variable scarring inside the uterine cavity, where in many cases the front and back walls of the uterus stick to one another. AS can be the cause of menstrual disturbances, infertility, and placental abnormalities etc.

Ans. (B) i.e., Asherman syndrome

54. **Which of the following tests is NOT used for diagnosing syphilis?**

(a) Frie's test
(b) Direct fluorescent antibody test
(c) FTA – ABS test
(d) TPHA

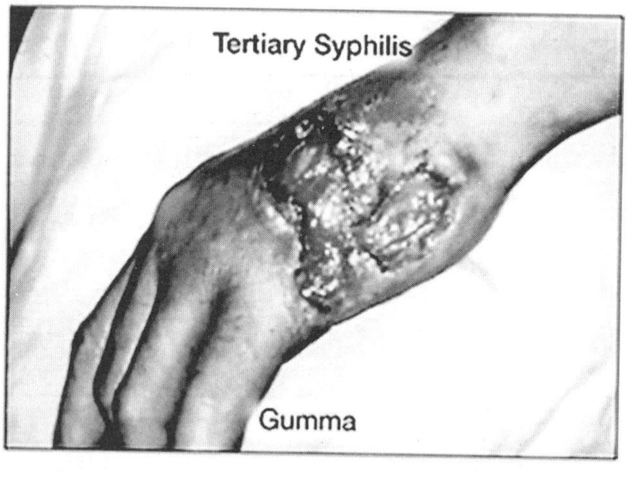

EXPLANATION:

The **Frei test** was developed in 1925 by Wilhelm Siegmund Frei, a German dermatologist, to identify lymphogranuloma inguinale. Antigen made from sterile pus aspirated from previously unruptured abscesses, produced a reaction in patients with lymphogranuloma inguinale when injected intradermally.

Ans. (A) i.e., Frie's test

55. **Fitz Hugh Curtis syndrome involving perihepatitis is present in the following:**

(a) Moniliasis
(b) Syphilis
(c) Tuberculosis
(d) Gonorrhoea

EXPLANATION:

Fitz Hugh–Curtis syndrome is a rare complication of pelvic inflammatory disease (PID) involving liver capsule inflammation leading to the creation of adhesions. The condition is named after the two physicians, Thomas **Fitz Hugh**, Jr and Arthur Hale **Curtis** who first reported this condition in 1934 and 1930 respectively. Fitz Hugh–Curtis syndrome occurs almost exclusively in women. It is usually caused by Chlamydia trachomatis (Chlamydia) or Neisseria gonorrhoeae (Gonorrhea) though other bacteria such as Bacteroides, Gardnerella, E. coli and Streptococcus have also been found to cause Fitz Hugh Curtis syndrome on occasion.

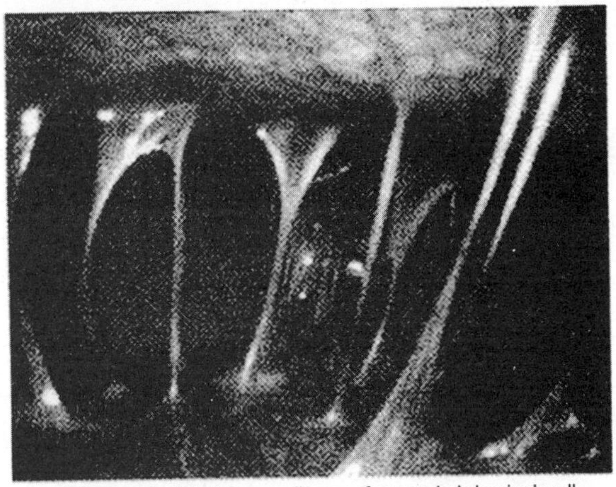
Fibrinous exudate between liver surface and abdominal wall

Ans. (D) i.e., Gonorrhoea

56. Which of the following cause/causes bacterial vaginosis?

1. Gardnerella 2. Mycoplasma 3. Ureaplasma urealyticum

Select the correct answer using the code given below:

(a) 1 only (b) 2 and 3 only (c) 1 and 3 only (d) 1, 2 and 3

EXPLANATION:

Bacterial vaginosis (BV) is a disease of the vagina caused by excessive growth of bacteria. Common symptoms include increased vaginal discharge that often smells like fish. The discharge is usually white or gray in color. Burning with urination may occur. Itching is uncommon. Occasionally, there may be no symptoms. Having BV approximately doubles the risk of infection by a number of other sexually transmitted infections, including HIV/AIDS. It also increases the risk of early delivery among pregnant women.

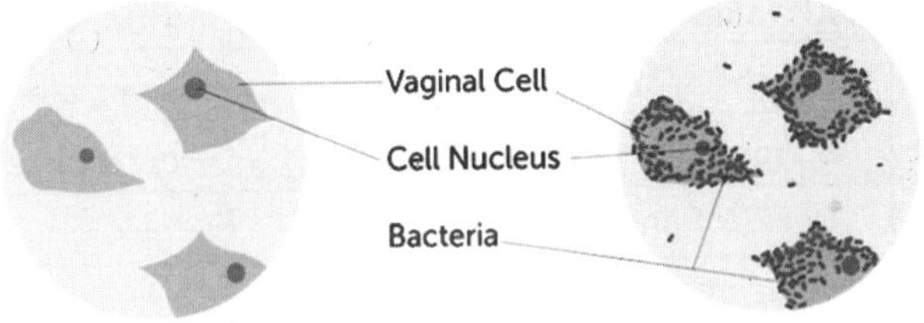

Normal vaginal cells seen under a microscope.
"Clue Cells", vaginal cells with bacteria stuck to them.

Ans. (D) i.e., 1, 2 and 3

57. Where are antisperm antibodies usually present?

(a) Uterus (b) Vagina
(c) Fallopian tube (d) Cervix

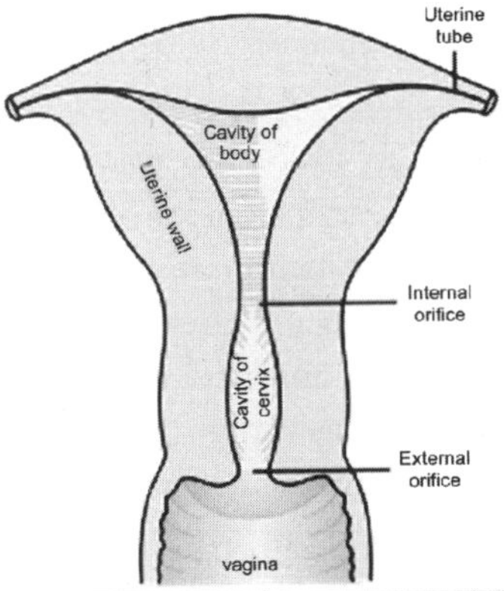

EXPLANATION:

Antisperm antibodies (ASA) are immunoglobulins of IgG, IgA, and/or IgM, which are directed against sperm antigens. ASA can be detected in ejaculate, cervical mucus, follicular fluid, and blood serum.

Ans. (D) i.e., Cervix

2017

58. **Modified Bishop's score includes all except:**

(a) Cervical length and dilatation
(b) Consistency of cervix
(c) Position of os
(d) Position of occiput

EXPLANATION:

According to the Modified Bishop's preinduction cervical scoring system, effacement has been replaced by cervical length in cm, with scores as follows: 0 for >3cm, 1 for >2cm, 2 for >1 m, 3 for >0cm. Cervical length may be easier and more accurate to measure and have less interexaminer variability.

Score	0	1	2
Cervical dilatation (cm)	<1	1–2	3–4
Length of cervix (cm)	>2	1–2	<1
Station of presenting part (cm)	Spines-3	Spines-2	Spines-1
Consistency	Firm	Medium	Soft
Position	Posterior	Central	Anterior

Ans. (D) i.e., Position of occiput

59. **The engaging diameter of brow presentation is:**

(a) Mento vertical
(b) Submento vertical
(c) Suboccipito bregmatic
(d) Submento bregmatic

EXPLANATION:

AP diameter	Attitude	Presenting part
Suboccipitobregmatic 9.4 cm	Complete flexion	Vertex occipitoanterior
Suboccipitofrontal 10.5 cm	Incomplete flexion	Vertex occipitoposterior
Occipitofrontal 11 cm	Deflexion	Vertex occipitoposterior
Verticomental 13.5 cm	Extension	Brow
Submentobregmatic 9.4 cm	Complete extension	Face

Ans. (A) i.e., Mento vertical

60. **Intramuscular injection of iron dextran is given by 'Z' technique to:**

(a) Alleviate the pain
(b) Decrease the incidence of infection
(c) Reduce the staining
(d) Increase the iron absorption

EXPLANATION:

The **Z-track method** is a type of IM **injection technique** used to prevent tracking (leakage) of the medication into the subcutaneous tissue (underneath the skin). During the procedure, skin and tissue are pulled and held firmly while a long needle is inserted into the muscle.

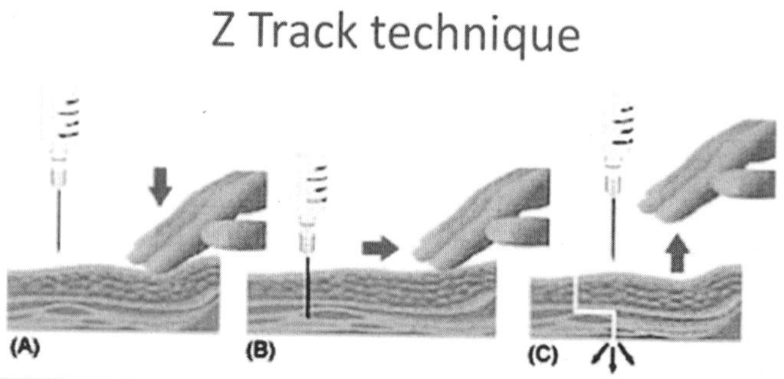

Ans. (C) i.e., Reduce the staining

61. Which of the following is/are the risk factors for acute pelvic inflammatory disease in women?

1. Intercourse during menstruation
2. Multiple sex partners

Select the correct answer using the code given below:

(a) 1 only (b) 2 only
(c) Both 1 and 2 (d) Neither 1 nor 2

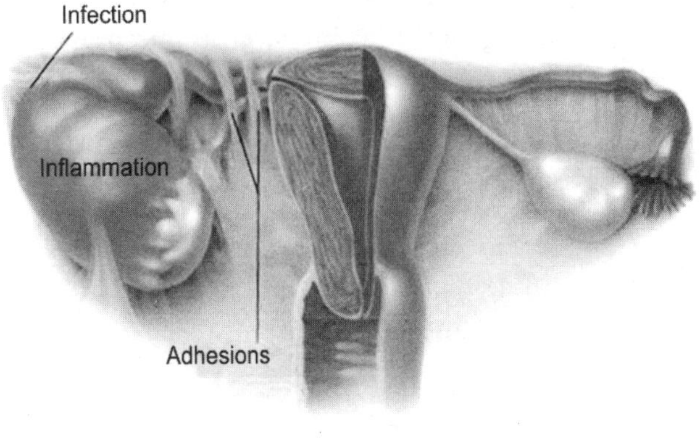

EXPLANATION:

Risk factors for PID

- A high number of sexual partners.
- Vaginal douching may also increase the risk.
- Pelvic inflammatory disease (PID) is the most threatening risk of having coitus during menses.

Ans. (C) i.e., Both 1 and 2

62. The umbilical cord normally contains:

(a) Two arteries and two veins (b) One artery and one vein
(c) Two arteries and one vein (d) One artery and two veins

EXPLANATION:

During prenatal development, the umbilical cord is physiologically and genetically part of the fetus and (in humans) normally contains two arteries (the umbilical arteries) and one vein (the umbilical vein), buried within Wharton's jelly. The umbilical vein supplies the fetus with oxygenated, nutrient rich blood from the placenta. Conversely, the fetal heart pumps deoxygenated, nutrient depleted blood through the umbilical arteries back to the placenta.

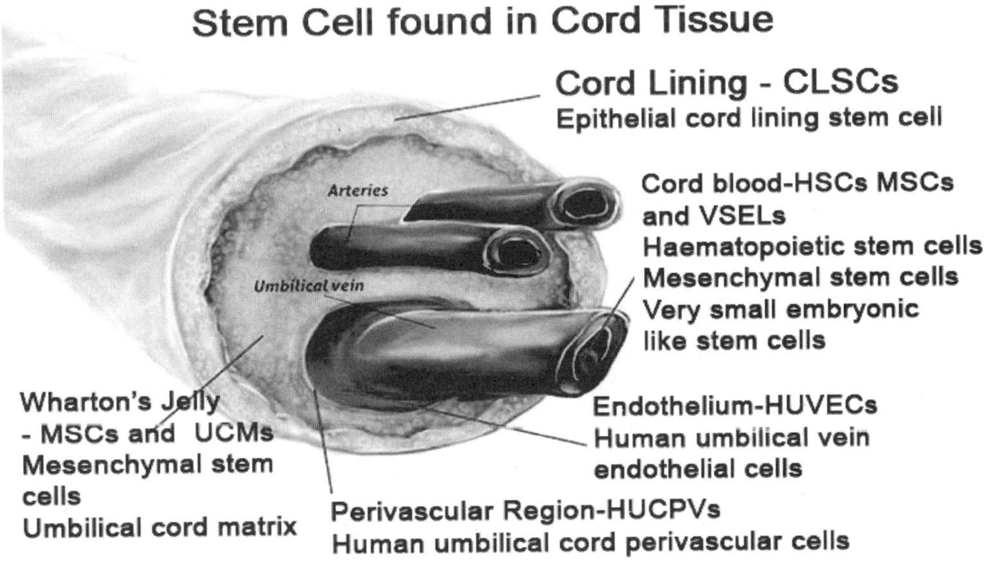

Ans. (C) i.e., Two arteries and one vein

63. Painless genital ulcer is found in which one of the following genital infections?

(a) Grannloma inguinale (b) Chancroid
(c) Lymphogranuloma venerum (d) Herpes simplex

EXPLANATION:

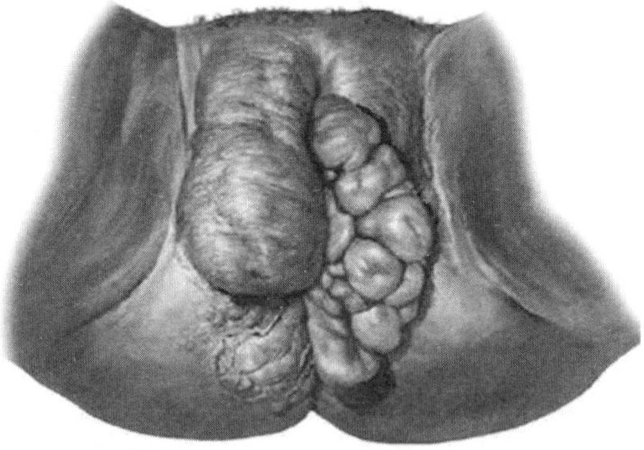

LGV may begin as a self limited painless genital ulcer that occurs at the contact site 3–12 days after infection. Women rarely notice a primary infection because the initial ulceration where the organism penetrates the mucosal layer is often located out of sight, in the vaginal wall. In men fewer than 1/3 of those infected notice the first signs of LGV. This primary stage heals in a few days.

Ans. (C) i.e., Lymphogranuloma venerum

64. Medical management of tubular ectopic pregnancy can be done in the following except:

(a) Period of gestation 5 weeks

(b) β HCG level more than 10,000 IU

(c) Absent foetal cardiac activity

(d) Gestational sac diameter 3 cm

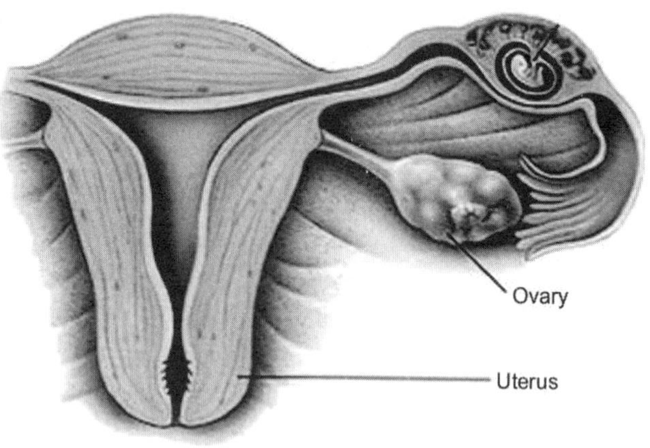

EXPLANATION:

The use of the medication methotrexate works well in some cases of ectopic pregnancy. Specifically it works well when the β HCG is low and the size of the ectopic is small. Surgery is still typically recommended if the tube has ruptured, there is a fetal heartbeat, or the person's vital signs are unstable.

Ans. (B) i.e., β HCG level more than 10,000 IU

65. Cholestasis may lead to the following complications except:

(a) Intrauterine foetal death

(b) Meconium stained liquor

(c) Preterm labour

(d) Neonatal jaundice

EXPLANATION:

Intrahepatic Cholestasis of Pregnancy (ICP) is a condition in which the normal flow of bile is affected by the increased amounts of pregnancy hormones. Cholestasis is more common in the last trimester of pregnancy when hormones are at their peak, but it usually goes away within a few days after delivery. Cholestasis may increase the risks for fetal distress, preterm birth, or stillbirth.

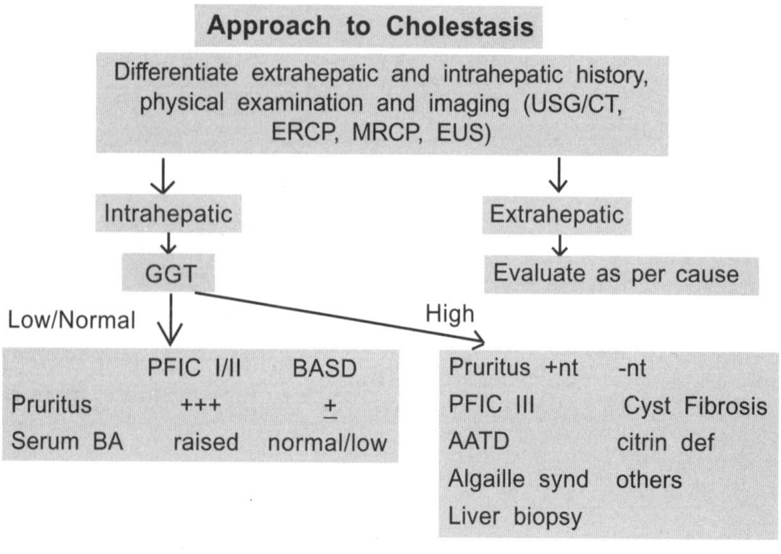

Ans. (D) i.e., Neonatal jaundice

66. **Which of the following genital infections is associated with preterm labour?**

(a) Human Papilloma Virus
(b) Trichomonas vaginalis
(c) Monilial vaginitis
(d) Bacterial vaginosis

EXPLANATION:

Risk factor for preterm labor
Black ethnicity/race
Filipino ancestry
High or low BMI
Large or small pregnancy weight gain
Short maternal height
History of spontaneous preterm birth
Being single/unmarried
Bacterial vaginosis
Asymptomatic bacteriuria
Periodontitis
Low socioeconomic status
Short cervical length
Fetal fibronectin
Chlamydia
Celiac disease

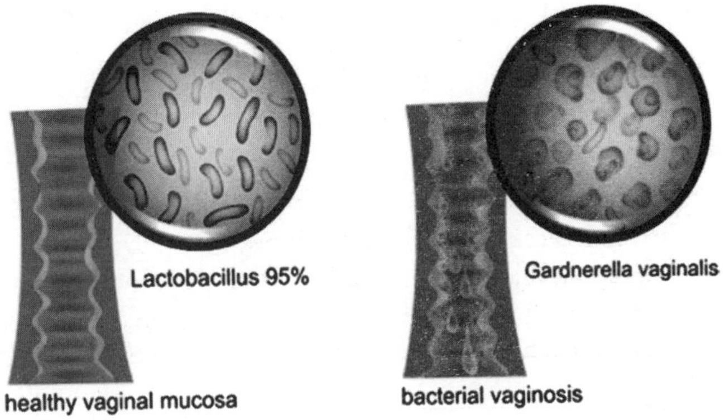

2017

Ans. (D) i.e., Bacterial vaginosis

67. **Multiple pregnancy is associated with an increased incidence of the following except:**

(a) Hyperemesis gravidarum
(b) Congenital malformations
(c) Pregnancy induced hypertension
(d) Post date pregnancy

EXPLANATION:

Risk factors for preterm birth include diabetes, high blood pressure, multiple pregnancy, being either obese or underweight, a number of vaginal infections, tobacco smoking and psychological stress, among others.

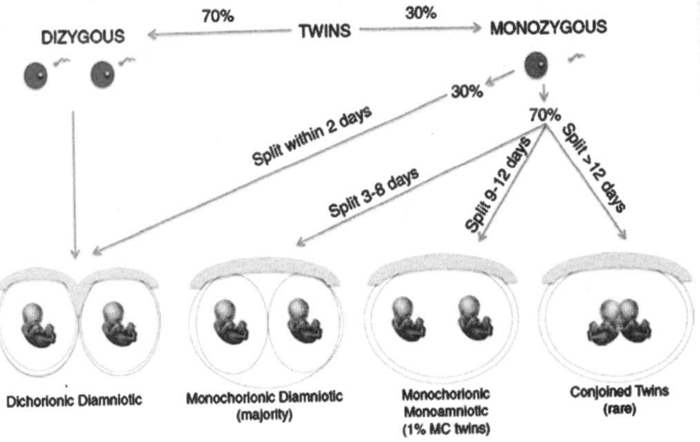

Ans. (D) i.e., Post date pregnancy

68. **Which of the following conditions of the endometrium is associated with a significantly increased risk of development of cancer?**

(a) Simple hyperplasia
(b) Complex hyperplasia with atypia
(c) Simple atypical hyperplasia
(d) Complex hyperplasia

EXPLANATION:

Many women who have symptoms of **endometrial** cancer (vaginal bleeding after menopause or abnormal menstrual bleeding) may have a biopsy that shows precancerous changes of the endometrium, called **complex hyperplasia with atypia.**

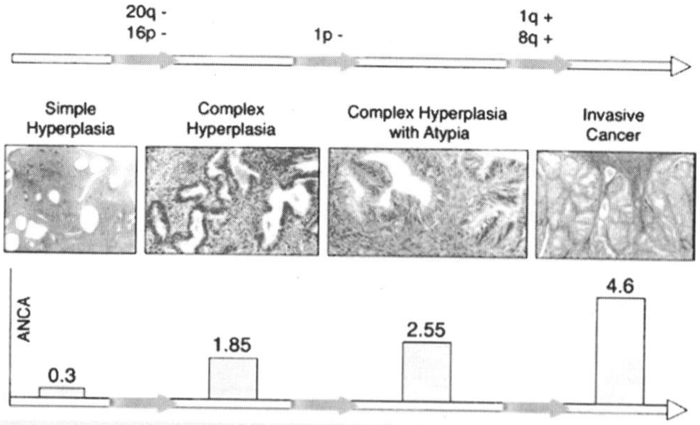

Ans. (B) i.e., Complex hyperplasia with atypia

69. **Surgical staging is done for all the genital malignancies except:**

(a) Ovarian malignancy
(b) Gestational trophoblastic neoplasia
(c) Endometrial carcinoma
(d) Fallopian tube malignancy

EXPLANATION:

There are several different types of GTD. Hydatidiform moles are benign in most cases, but sometimes may develop into invasive moles, or, in rare cases, into choriocarcinoma, which is likely to spread quickly, but which is very sensitive to chemotherapy, and has a very good prognosis.

Feature	Complete mole	Partial mole
Synonyms	Classic, true	Incomplete
Fetal or embryonic tissue or membranes	Absent	Usually present
Villous capillaries	Usually absent; when present, no fetal blood cells	Usually present; may contain fetal blood cells
Hydatidiform swelling of chorionic villi	Diffuse	Focal
Trophoblastic hyperplasia	Usually present	Mild and focal
Malignant potential (%)	15–25	5–10
Karyotype	46, XX; 46, XY	69, XXX; 69, XXY

Ans. (B) i.e., Gestational trophoblastic neoplasia

70. **B-Lynch suture for atonic postpartum haemorrhage:**

(a) compresses the uterus
(b) ligates the uterine arteries
(c) ligates the utero ovarian anastomosis
(d) ligates the ovarian vessels

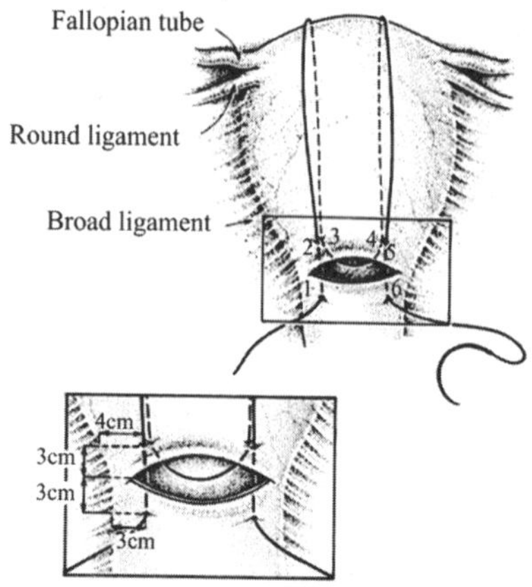

EXPLANATION:

The **B-Lynch suture** or **B-Lynch procedure** is a form of compression suture. It is used to mechanically compress an atonic uterus in the face of severe postpartum hemorrhage. It was developed by Christopher B-Lynch, a consultant obstetrician and gynaecological surgeon based at Milton Keynes General Hospital, Milton Keynes, Buckinghamshire, England. B-Lynch was born in 1947 in Sierra Leone with the birth name of Christopher Balogun-Lynch.

Ans. (A) i.e., compresses the uterus

71. Regarding 'Delancy's levels of vaginal support', consider the following pairs:

1. Level I .... Supports distal urethra perineal body
2. Level II .... Supports mid vagina
3. Level III .... Supports apical defect

Which of the pairs given above is/are correctly matched?

(a) 1 and 3 only
(b) 2 only
(c) 2 and 3 only
(d) 1, 2 and 3

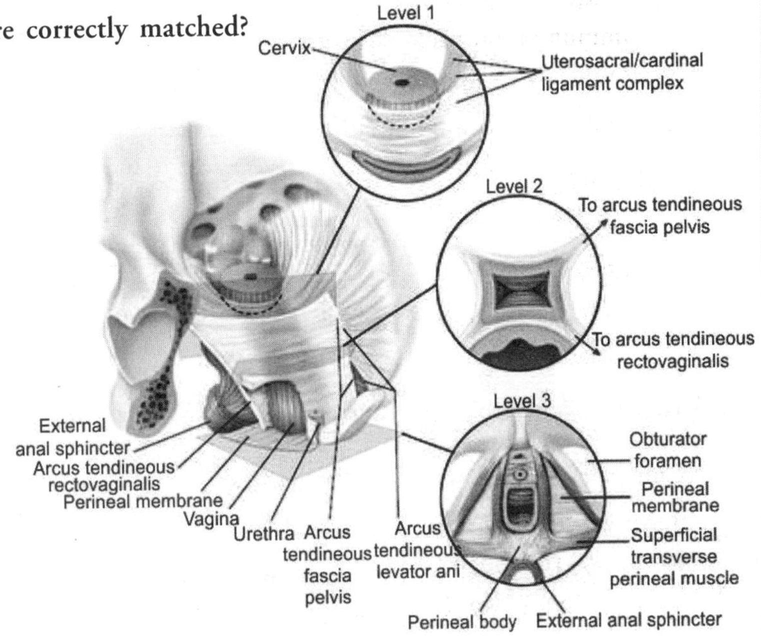

EXPLANATION:

Delancy's levels of vaginal support

- Level 1: Uterosacral and cardinal ligaments
- Level 2: Pelvic fascia and paracolpos connects the vagina to the lateral pelvic wall through the arcus tendineus
- Level three: Levator ani muscle supports lower one third of the vagina.

Ans. (B) i.e., 2 only

72. Regarding "conjoined twins", which of the following statements is/are true?

1. These are always monozygotic
2. These result when division occurs before the embryonic disc is formed
3. Most common variety is thoracopagus

Select the correct answer using the code given below:

(a) 1 and 2 only (b) 2 and 3 only
(c) 1 and 3 only (d) 1, 2 and 3

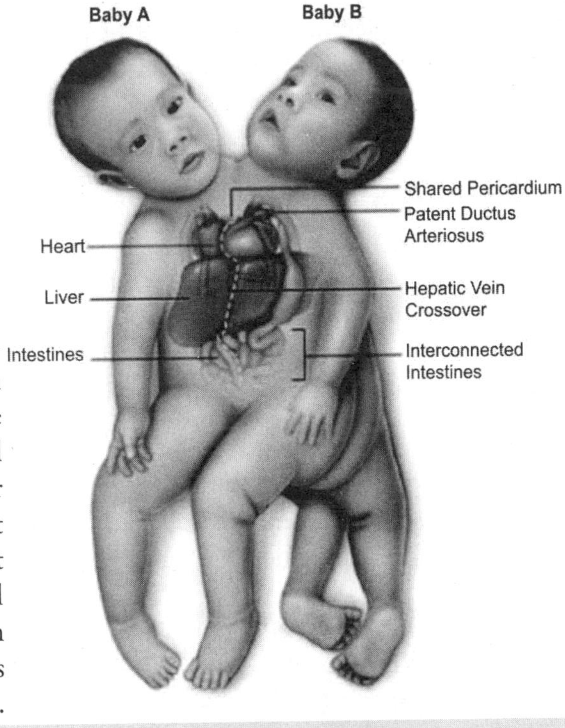

EXPLANATION:

Conjoined twins are always identical and **mono-amniotic-monochorionic** (sharing the same amnion and chorion). Identical twins happen when one fertalized egg spontaneously splits into two identical halves. So, this type of twinning is thought to occur because of an extremely late split, one that does not completely separate into individual fetuses. The result is a set of twins who will have skin and even internal organs that are fused together. The most common type is known as thoracopagus twins. These twins are connected at the upper portion of thier torsos.

Ans. (C) i.e., 1 and 3 only

73. **The appropriate treatment for the baby of a woman who is HBsAg positive but HBeAg negative is:**

(a) Both active and passive immunisation soon after birth

(b) Passive immunisation soon after birth but active immunisation after one year of age

(c) Only active immunisation soon after birth

(d) Only passive immunisation soon after birth

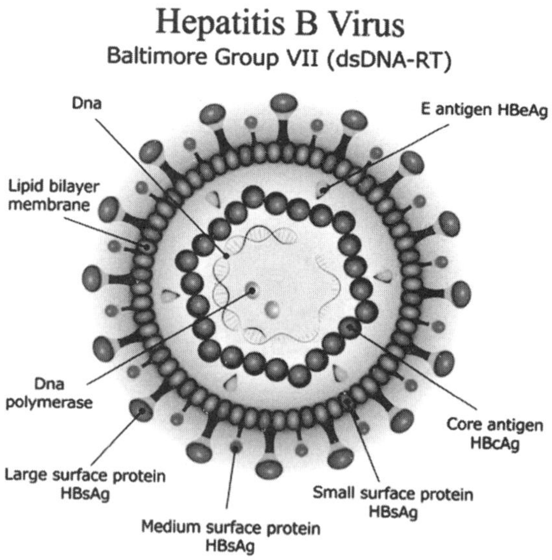

EXPLANATION:

HBeAg negativity denotes that mother is least infectious as the virus is not replicating actively. Child born to HBsAg positive mothers should be offered both active as well as passive immunization.

Ans. (A) i.e., Both active and passive immunisation soon after birth

74. **Consider the following pairs regarding foetal heart during labour:**

Term .... Description

1. **Early decelerations ....** Most common during labour and are due to cord compression
2. **Late decelerations ....** Result due to any process leading to maternal hypotension, placental insufficiency or excessive uterine activity
3. **Variable decelerations ....** Are due to head compression leading to vagal stimulation

Which of the pairs given above is/are correctly matched?

(a) 1 and 2 (b) 2 and 3

(c) 1 and 3 (d) 2 only

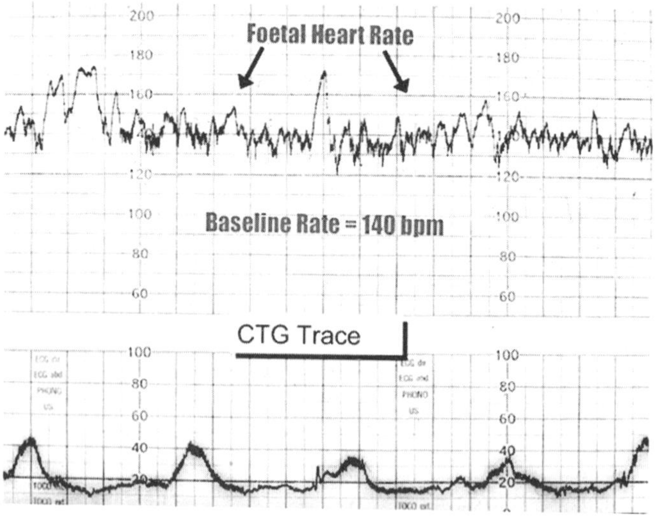

EXPLANATION:

Late Decelerations are a result of placental insufficiency, which can result in fetal distress. Monitoring usually shows symmetrical gradual decrease and return to baseline of the fetal heart rate in association with a uterine contraction. A 'gradual' deceleration has onset to nadir of 30 seconds or more. In contrast to early deceleration, the low point of fetal heart rate occurs after the peak of the contraction, and returns to baseline after the contraction is complete.

Ans. (D) i.e., 2 only

75. **A 26 year old woman P_1L_1 reports with High Grade Squamous Intraepithelial Lesion (HGSIL) on Pap smear (Papanicolaou smear). Further management for her is:**

(a) VIA, VILI

(b) Colposcopy and directed biopsy

(c) LEEP

(d) Conisation

2017

EXPLANATION:

Colposcopy is a medical diagnostic procedure to examine an illuminated, magnified view of the cervix and the tissues of the vagina and vulva. Many premalignant lesions and malignant lesions in these areas have discernible characteristics which can be detected through the examination. It is done using a colposcope, which provides an enlarged view of the areas, allowing the colposcopist to visually distinguish normal from abnormal appearing tissue and take directed biopsies for further pathological examination. The main goal of colposcopy is to prevent cervical cancer by detecting precancerous lesions early and treating them. The procedure was developed by the German physician Hans Hinselmann, with help from Eduard Wirths. The development of colposcopy involved experimentation on Jewish inmates from Auschwitz.

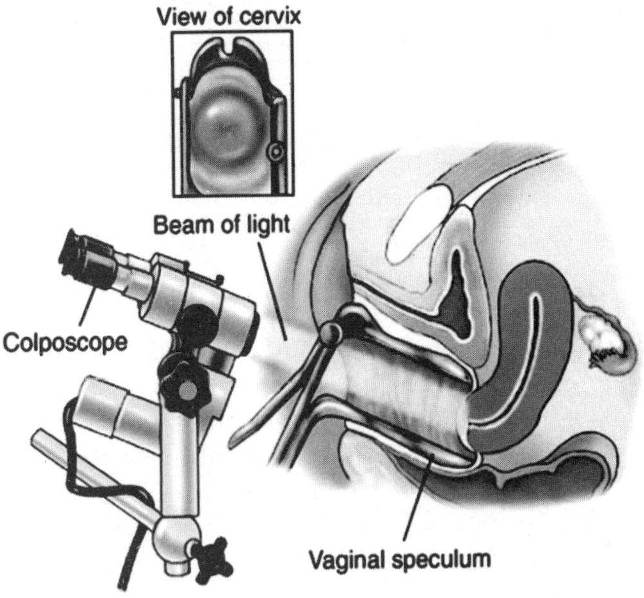

Ans. (B) i.e., Colposcopy and directed biopsy

76. **With reference to the displacement of uterus, the treatment of choice for genuine stress urinary incontinence is:**
   (a) Kegel's perineal exercises
   (b) Kelly's placation
   (c) TVT O mid urethral tape
   (d) Periurethral injection of bulking agents

EXPLANATION:

The transobturator tape (TOT or Monarc) sling procedure aims to eliminate stress urinary incontinence by providing support under the urethra. The minimally invasive procedure eliminates retropubic needle passage and involves inserting a mesh tape under the urethra through three small incisions in the groin area.

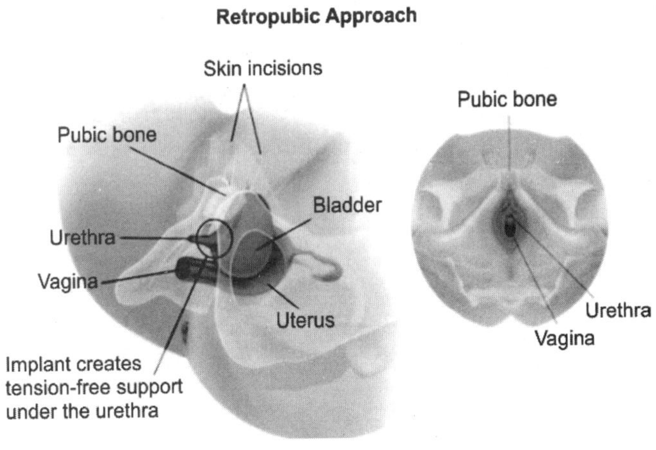

Ans. (C) i.e., TVT O mid urethral tape

77. **Regarding placental separation in III stage of labour, consider the following statements:**
   1. **Separation of placenta occurs at deciduas spongiosa**
   2. **In Shultz method, separation of placenta starts at centre**
   3. **In Mathew Duncan's method, separation begins at margin**

   Which of the statements given above is/are correct?
   (a) 1 only
   (b) 1 and 2 only
   (c) 2 and 3 only
   (d) 1, 2 and 3

2017

EXPLANATION:

Placental separation

- Decidua basalis, where the implantation takes place and the basal plate is formed. This can be subdivided into a zona compacta and a zona spongiosa (where the detachment of the placenta takes place following birth).
- There are two methods by which the placenta separates from the uterine wall:
  - o Schultze method — in the majority of cases separation starts in the centre of the placenta and this part descends first. The foetal surface therefore appears at the vulva with the membranes trailing behind. The retroplacental clot is contained within the inverted sac, thus there is minimal blood loss.
  - o Mathew Duncan method — less commonly separation starts at the lower edge of the placenta. The placenta slips down sideways and maternal surface appears first at the vulva. This method of separation is usually accompanied by some bleeding per vaginum, since blood from placental site escapes immediately, thus a retroplacental clot does not form. This method results in slower separation of the placenta and bleeding is likely to be profuse.

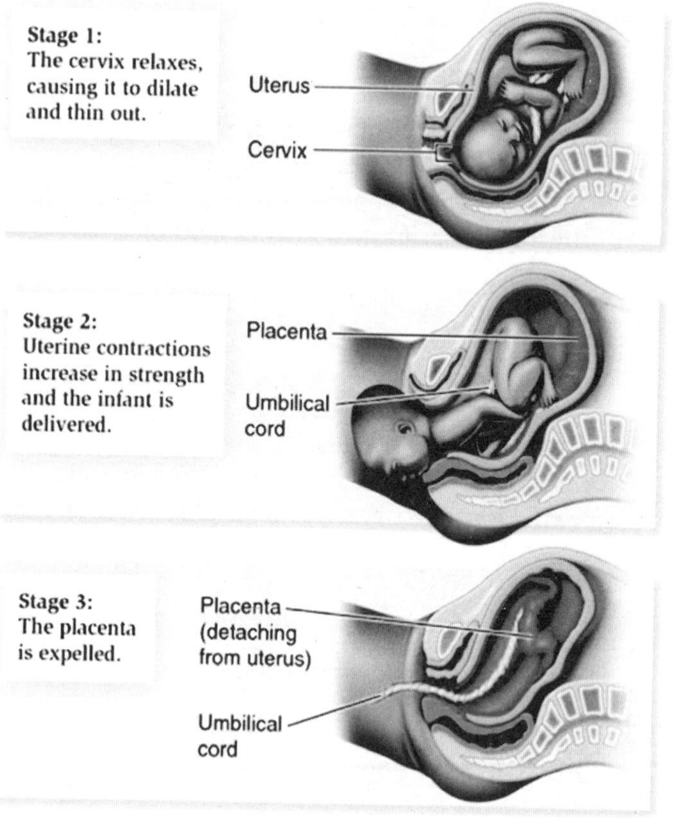

Ans. (D) i.e., 1, 2 and 3

78. **A 16 year old girl presents with primary amenorrhea with absent vagina, cervix and uterus in the presence of normal secondary sexual characteristics. Ovaries are present on USG. The most probable diagnosis is:**

(a) Kleinfelter's syndrome

(b) Androgen Insensitivity syndrome

(c) Mayer Rockitansky Kuster Hauser syndrome

(d) Prader Willi syndrome

EXPLANATION:

Müllerian agenesis, also known as **Mayer–Rokitansky–Küster–Hauser syndrome** (MRKH) or **vaginal agenesis**, is a congenital malformation characterized by a failure of the Müllerian duct to develop, resulting in a missing uterus and variable degrees of vaginal hypoplasia of its upper portion. Müllerian agenesis (including absence of the uterus, cervix and/or vagina) is the cause in 15% of cases of primary amenorrhoea. Because most of the vagina does not develop from the Müllerian duct, instead developing from the urogenital sinus, along with the bladder and urethra, it is present even when the Müllerian duct is completely absent. Because ovaries do not develop from the Müllerian ducts, affected women might have normal secondary sexual characteristics but are infertile due to the lack of a functional uterus. However, motherhood is possible through use of gestational surrogates.

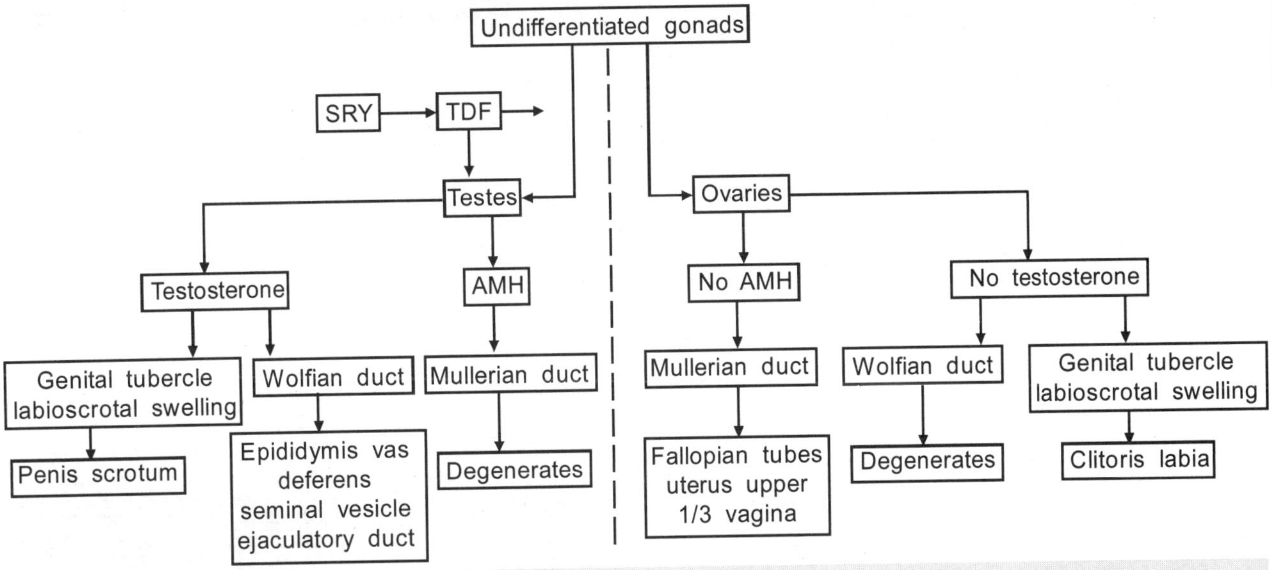

Ans. (C) i.e., Mayer Rockitansky Kuster Hauser syndrome

79. A 32-year old woman is noted to have 1200cc of blood loss following a spontaneous vaginal delivery and delivery of placenta. The uterine fundus is palpated and noted to be firm. Which of the following is the most likely treatment for this patient?

(a) B-lynch suture

(b) Surgical repair of cervical tear

(c) Intramuscular prostaglandin

(d) Replacement of inverted uterus

EXPLANATION:

Injury to the birth canal, which includes the uterus, cervix, vagina and the perineum, which can happen, even if the delivery is monitored properly. The bleeding is substantial as all these organs become more vascular during pregnancy.

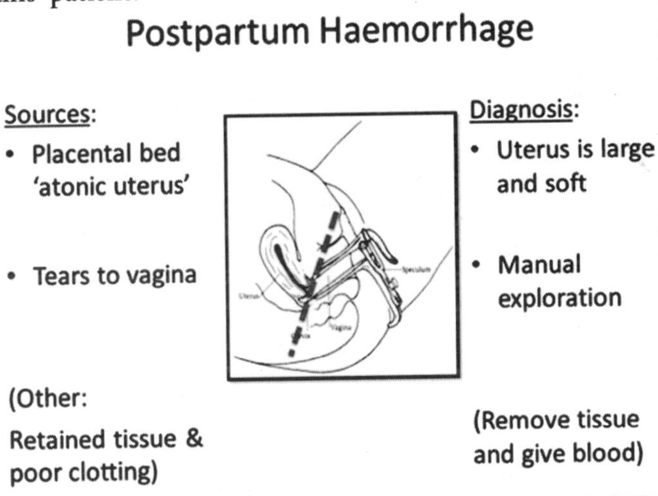

Ans. (B) i.e., Surgical repair of cervical tear

80. Which of the following statements is/are correct regarding physiology of menstruation?

1. LH surge precedes ovulation
2. There are two peaks in serum estradiol levels, first in follicular and second in luteal phase
3. Serum progesterone has only one peak i.e., in luteal phase

Select the correct answer using the code given below:

(a) 1 only (b) 1 and 2 only (c) 2 and 3 only (d) 1, 2 and 3

EXPLANATION:

Physiology of menstruation

- Since the **LH surge** always **precedes ovulation**, detecting this hormone is critical in predicting two peak fertility days.

- In the normal menstrual cycle, estradiol levels measure typically <50pg/ml at menstruation, rise with follicular development (peak: 200pg/ml), drop briefly at ovulation, and rise again during the luteal phase for a second peak. At the end of the luteal phase, estradiol levels drop to their menstrual levels unless there is a pregnancy.
- Progesterone levels are relatively low during the preovulatory phase of the menstrual cycle, rise after ovulation, and are elevated during the luteal phase.

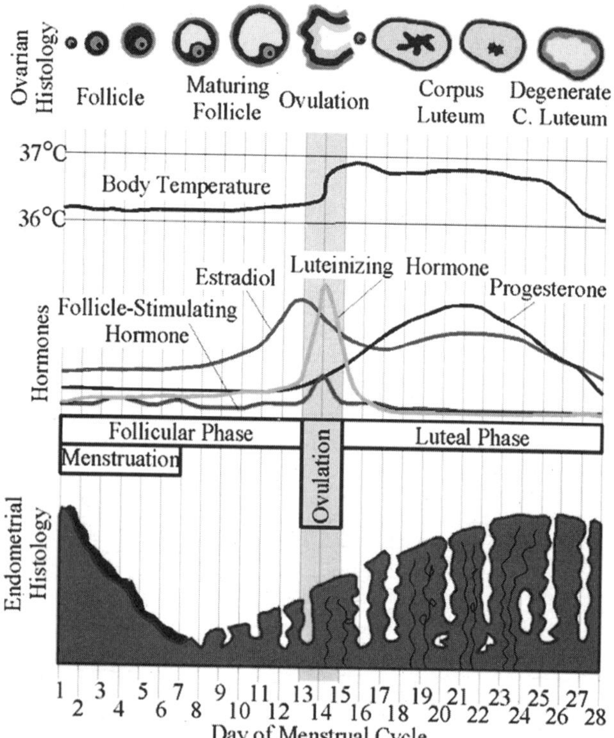

(Average values. Durations and values may differ between different females or different cycles.)

Ans. (D) i.e., 1, 2 and 3

81. **Which of the following is/are the measure(s) of dispersion?**

   1. Mode **2. Median** **3. Standard Deviation**

   Select the correct answer using the code given below:

   (a) 1 and 2 only (b) 3 only (c) 2 and 3 only (d) 1, 2 and 3

EXPLANATION:

Most measures of dispersion have the same units as the quantity being measured. In other words, if the measurements are in metres or seconds, so is the measure of dispersion. Examples of dispersion measures include:

- Standard deviation
- Interquartile range (IQR)
- Range
- Average absolute deviation (or simply called average deviation)
- Mean absolute difference (also known as Gini mean absolute difference)
- Median absolute deviation (MAD)
- Distance standard deviation

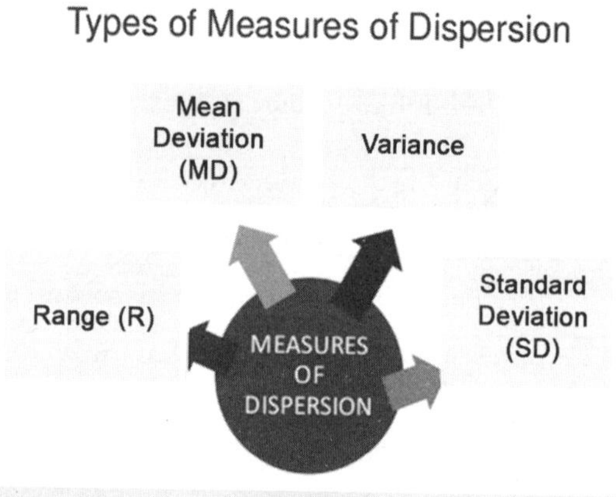

Ans. (B) i.e., 3 only

82. **Which among the following is/are the examples of primordial prevention?**

   1. **Adopting healthy lifestyles from childhood**
   2. **Immunization of infants**

3. Screening of cervical cancer

Select the correct answer using the code given below:

(a) 1 only (b) 1 and 2 only (c) 1 and 3 only (d) 1, 2 and 3

EXPLANATION:

Primordial prevention refers to all measures designed to prevent the development of risk factors in the first place, early in life.

A Classification of Preventive Strategies

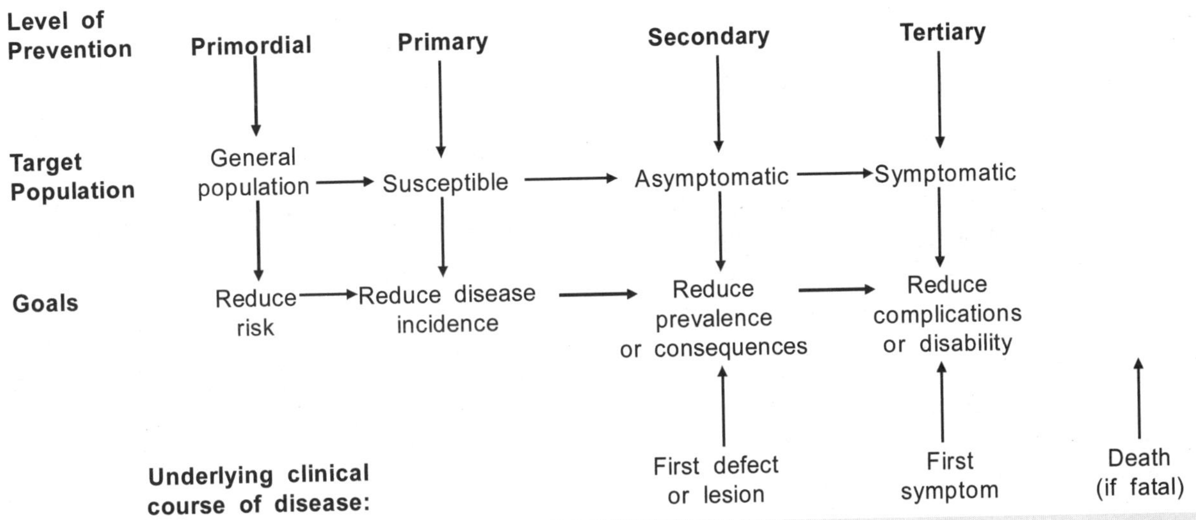

Ans. (A) i.e., 1 only

83. The appropriate statistical test to find out obesity as a significant risk factor for breast cancer is:

(a) Student's paired 't' test
(b) Student's unpaired 't' test
(c) Chi square test
(d) Wilcoxon's signed rank test

EXPLANATION:

A **chi squared test,** also written as χ^2 **test,** is any statistical hypothesis test where the sampling distribution of the test statistic is a chi squared distribution when the null hypothesis is true. Without other qualification, 'chi squared test' often is used as short for *Pearson's* chi squared test. The chi squared test is used to determine whether there is a significant difference between the expected frequencies and the observed frequencies in one or more categories.

Ans. (C) i.e., Chi square test

84. **In a case control study, confounding factors can be minimized by the following except:**

(a) Matching of variables such as age and sex
(b) Randomization during selection
(c) Stratification during analysis
(d) Increasing sample size for cases and controls

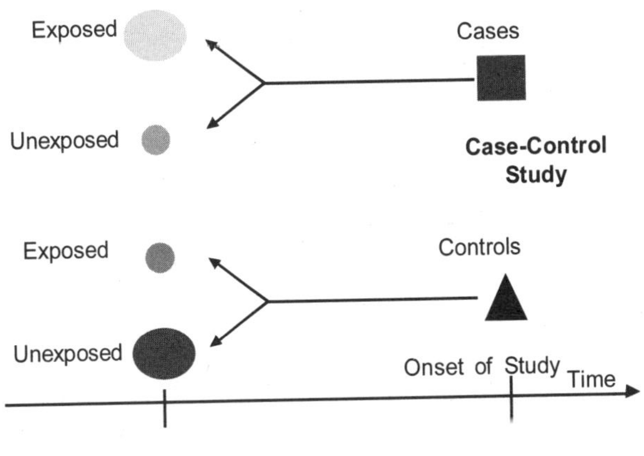

EXPLANATION:

A **case control study** is a type of observational study in which two existing groups differing in outcome are identified and compared on the basis of some supposed causal attribute. Case control studies are often used to identify factors that may contribute to a medical condition by comparing subjects who have that condition/disease (the "cases") with patients who do not have the condition/disease but are otherwise similar (the "controls"). They require fewer resources but provide less evidence for causal inference than a randomized controlled trial.

Ans. (D) i.e., Increasing sample size for cases and controls

85. Which one of the following is FALSE regarding confounding factor in epidemiological studies?

(a) Associated both with exposure and disease

(b) Distributed equally between study and control groups

(c) Independent risk factor for disease in question

(d) Source of bias is interpretation

EXPLANATION:

A **confounder** (also **confounding variable, confounding factor** or **lurking variable**) is a variable that influences both the dependent variable and independent variable causing a spurious association. Confounding is a causal concept, and as such, cannot be described in terms of correlations or associations

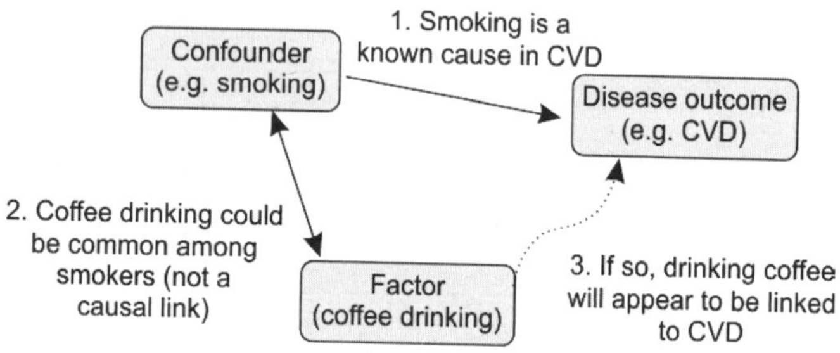

Ans. (B) i.e., Distributed equally between study and control groups

86. Denominator in calculation of case fatality rate is:

(a) Total number of deaths due to all causes

(b) Total number of hospital admissions

(c) Total number of cases due to the disease concerned

(d) Total number of deaths due to the disease concerned

EXPLANATION:

A **case fatality rate** (CFR)—or **case fatality risk, case fatality ratio** or just **fatality rate**—is the proportion of deaths within a designated population of "cases" (people with a medical condition) over the course of the disease. A CFR is conventionally expressed as a percentage and represents a measure of risk. CFRs are most often used for diseases with discrete, limited time courses, such as outbreaks of acute infections.

Types of Mortality Rates

Crude mortality rate	$\frac{\text{Deaths}}{\text{Population}}$
Cause-specific mortality rate	$\frac{\text{Deaths from cause}}{\text{Population}}$
Case-fatality rate	$\frac{\text{Deaths from cause}}{\text{Number of persons with disease/cause}}$
Proportionate mortality rate (PMR)	$\frac{\text{Deaths from cause}}{\text{All deaths}}$

Ans. (C) i.e., Total number of cases due to the disease concerned

87. A well of contaminated water resulting in an epidemic of acute watery diarrhoea is a typical example for:

(a) Common source, single exposure epidemic

(b) Common source, continuous exposure epidemic

(c) Slow epidemic

(d) Propagated epidemic

EXPLANATION:

Common source epidemic–All victims acquire the infection from the same source (e.g. a contaminated water supply).

- Continuous source – Common source outbreak where the exposure occurs over multiple incubation periods
- Point source – Common source outbreak where the exposure occurs in less than one incubation period

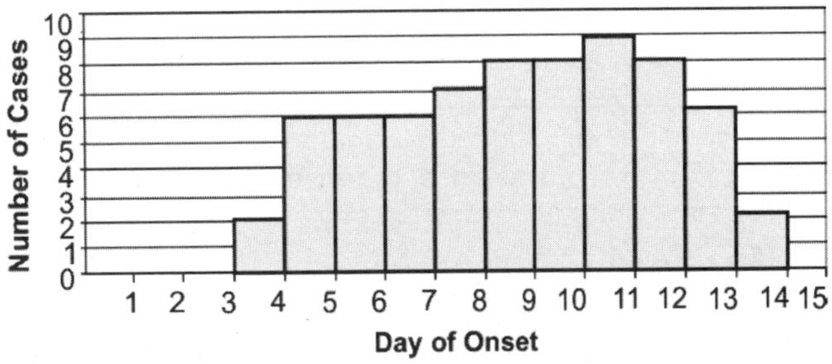

Ans. (B) i.e., Common source, continuous exposure epidemic

88. An important measure of communicability of a disease is:

(a) Incidence rate

(b) Case fatality rate

(c) Prevalence rate

(d) Secondary attack rate

EXPLANATION:

The **secondary attack rate** is defined as the probability that infection occurs among susceptible persons within a reasonable incubation period following known contact with an infectious person or an infectious source.

- **Secondary Attack Rate** : Number of exposed persons developing the diseas with the range of the incubation period folowing exposure to the primary case:

$$SAR = \frac{\text{No. of exposed persons developing the disease with the range of the IP}}{\text{Total No. of exposed/susceptible contacts}} \times 100$$

Ans. (D) i.e., Secondary attack rate

89. Which of the following statements is NOT correct regarding case fatality rate?

(a) Very useful indicator for both acute and chronic diseases

(b) One of the measures related to virulence

(c) It is the ratio of deaths to cases expressed as percentage

(d) Variation can occur for the same disease because of changes in the agent factors

EXPLANATION:

Case fatality rate, also called **case fatality ratio**, in epidemiology, the proportion of people who die from a specified disease among all individuals diagnosed with the disease over a certain period of time. Case fatality rate typically is used as a measure of disease severity and is often used for prognosis (predicting disease course or outcome), where comparatively high rates are indicative of relatively poor outcomes. It also can be used to evaluate the effect of new treatments, with measures decreasing as treatments improve. Case fatality rates are not constant; they can vary between populations and over

2017

time, depending on the interplay between the causative agent of disease, the host, and the environment as well as available treatments and quality of patient care.

Rate	Calculation	Measure of
Attack rate	(No. of individuals during an outbreak/population at risk at the beginning of the outbreak)* 10^n	Identifying risk factors for specific disease in outbreak investigation
Incidence rate	(No. of new cases of disease over a time interval/ avg. population at risk during the time interval)* 10^n	• Monitoring the course of epidemic • Cohort study—Measure of effect of suspected or known risk factors
Prevalence rate	(No. of existing cases of disease at a point of time/ population at risk during same point of time)* 10^n	• Static measure of risk of having a particular disease • Case control study—effect of suspected or known risk factors
Case fatality rate	No. of deaths from a specified cause/Total No. of cases of same disease	• Determine prognosis of disease • Severity of the disease

Ans. (A) i.e., Very useful indicator for both acute and chronic diseases

90. Farmer's lung is caused by the inhalation of:

(a) Grain dust with actinomycetes
(b) Sugarcane dust
(c) Silica dust
(d) Cotton fibre dust

EXPLANATION:

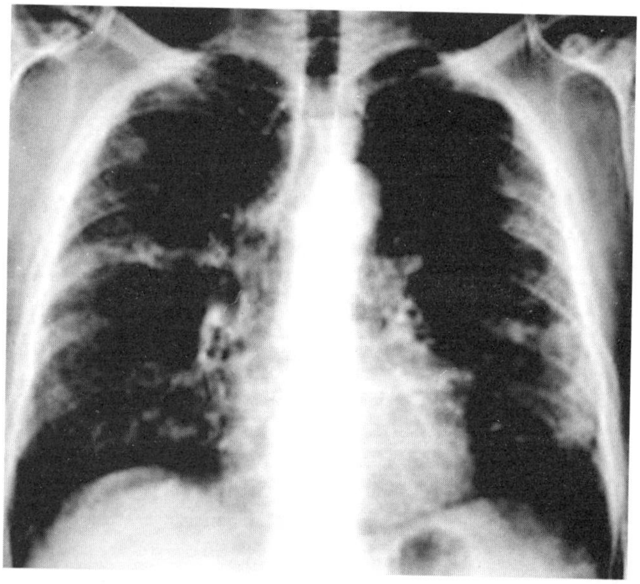

Farmer's lung occurs because repeated exposure to antigens, found in the mold spores of hay, crops, and animal feed, triggers an allergic reaction within the farmer's immune system. The defense mechanisms of the body present as cold and flu like symptoms that occur in individuals who experience either acute or chronic reactions. The mold spores are inhaled and provoke the creation of IgE antibodies that circulate in the bloodstream, these types of immune response are most often initiated by exposure to thermophilic actinomycetes (most commonly *Saccharopolyspora rectivirgula*, which generate IgG type antibodies.

Ans. (A) i.e., Grain dust with actinomycetes

91. Suraksha Clinics are conducted under the aegis of which National Health Programme?

(a) Revised National Tuberculosis Control programme
(b) Iodine Deficiency Disorders Programme
(c) National AIDS Control Programme
(d) Reproductive and Child Health Programme

EXPLANATION:

Suraksha Clinic (formerly Designated STI/RTI Clinics) are a chain of STI/RTI Clinics. These clinics are established by National AIDS Control Organisation for the better health services and for the prevention of HIV/AIDS in India.

suraksha clinic
Sexual and Reproductive Health Services

Ans. (C) i.e., National AIDS Control Programme

92. **Mean + 2 S.D. contains:**

(a) 68.3% values (b) 91.2% values
(c) 95.4% values (d) 99.7% values

EXPLANATION:

If the observations follow a Normal distribution, a range covered by one standard deviation above the mean and one standard deviation below it $(\bar{x} \pm 1SD)$ includes about 68% of the observations; a range of two standard deviations above and two below $(\bar{x} \pm 2SD)$ about 95% of the observations; and of three standard deviations above and three below $(\bar{x} \pm 3SD)$ about 99.7% of the observations.

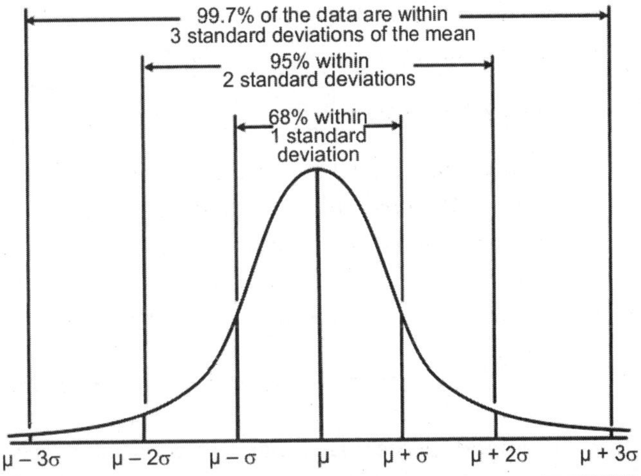

Ans. (C) i.e., 95.4% values

93. **Infant Mortality Rate is expressed per:**

(a) 1000 pregnancies (b) 1000 live births
(c) 1000 under five children (d) 100,000 live births

EXPLANATION:

Infant mortality refers to deaths of young children, typically those less than one year of age. It is measured by the **infant mortality rate** (IMR), which is the number of deaths of children under one year of age per 1000 live births.

Infant Mortality Rate

- Ratio of infant deaths registered in a given year to the total number of live births registered in the same year.
- Usually expressed as a rate per 1000 live births
- **STRICTLY SPEAKING – NOT A 'RATE', BUT A 'RATIO'**

$$\text{Infant Mortality Rate} = \frac{\text{Deaths among children} < 1 \text{ year}}{\text{Number of live births}} \times 1000$$

Ans. (B) i.e., 1000 live births

94. **Which of the following tests is NOT used for checking quality of pasteurisation of milk?**

(a) Phosphatase test
(b) Standard Plate count
(c) Coliform count
(d) Orthotoludine test

EXPLANATION:

Orthotoludine (OT) test enables total, free and combined chlorine in water to be determined with speed and accuracy.

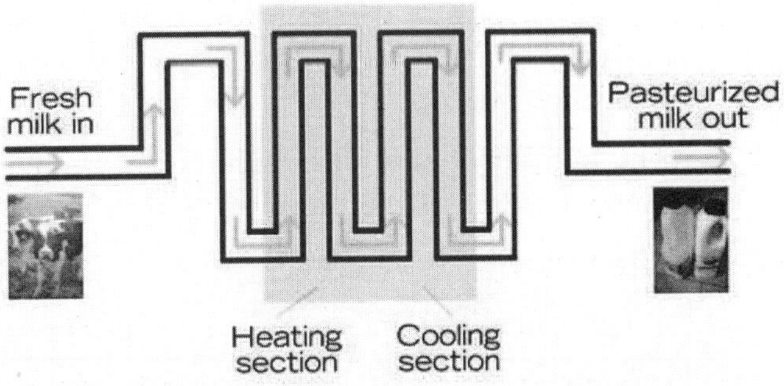

Ans. (D) i.e., Orthotoludine test

95. **Which of the following are components of epidemiological triad?**

(a) Sensitivity, specificity and predictive value
(b) Time, place and person distribution
(c) Agent, host and environmental factors
(d) Prevalence, incidence and attack rate

The 'epidemiological triad' of causal factors

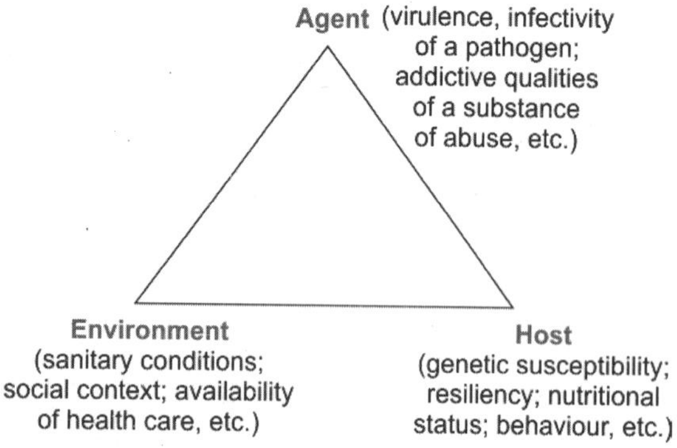

EXPLANATION:

A traditional model of infectious disease causation, known as the **Epidemiologic Triad** is depicted in Figure. The **triad** consists of an external agent, a host and an environment in which host and agent are brought together, causing the disease to occur in the host.

Ans. (C) i.e., Agent, host and environmental factors

96. **By applying the principles of ergonomics which of the following can be improved?**

1. **Designing of equipment and tools**
2. **Human efficiency**
3. **Layout of place of work**
4. **Reduction in industrial accidents**

Select the correct answer using the code given below:

(a) 1, 2 and 3 only (b) 1, 2, 3 and 4
(c) 2, 3 and 4 only (d) 1, 3 and 4 only

EXPLANATION:

Human factors and ergonomics (commonly referred to as **Human Factors**), is the application of psychological and physiological principles to the (engineering and) design of products, processes, and systems. The goal of human factors is to reduce human error, increase productivity, and enhance safety and comfort with a specific focus on the interaction between the human and the thing of interest.

Ergonomics

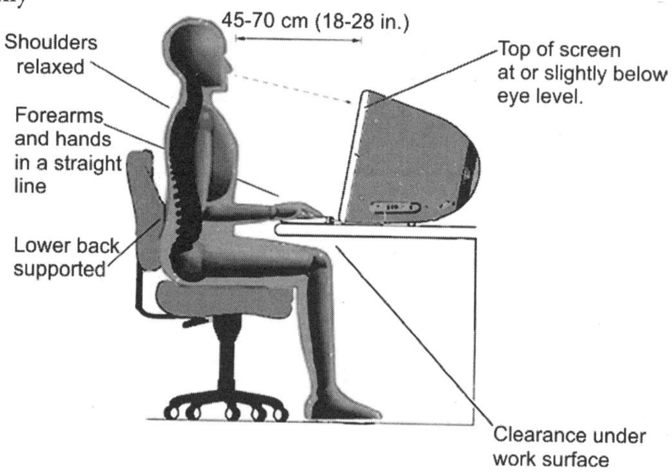

Ans. (B) i.e., 1, 2, 3 and 4

97. **The risk of disease is measured by:**

(a) Prevalence Rate (b) Incidence Rate (c) Attrition Rate (d) Fatality Rate

EXPLANATION:

- **Incidence rate**

  The number of new cases occuring in the population during a specified time/number of persons exposed to the risk of developing the disease during that time.

- **Attack rate**

  o The cumulative incidence rate of infection in a group over a period of an epidemic

  o Number of people at risk who are infected / Total number of people at risk

Ans. (B) i.e., Incidence Rate

98. **Tetanus spores can only be killed by:**

(a) Large doses of penicillin
(b) Anti tetanus Serum
(c) Tetanus toxoid
(d) Gamma irradiation

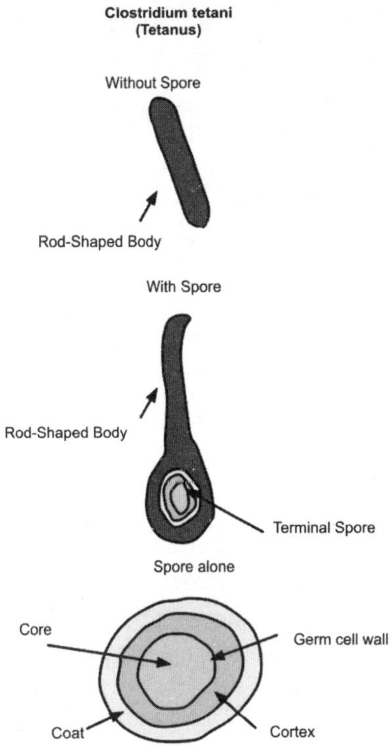

EXPLANATION:

Endospores are resistant to most agents that would normally kill the vegetative cells they formed from. Prolonged exposure to ionising radiation, such as X rays and gamma rays, will also kill most endospores.

Ans. (D) i.e., Gamma irradiation

99. **Which is/are the correct statements regarding the cut off points for the diagnosis of anaemia?**

1. **Haemoglobin for adult males is 13g/dL**
2. **Haemoglobin for adult non pregnant female is 12g/dL**
3. **Haemoglobin for adult pregnant female is 11g/dL**
4. **Haemoglobin for children six months to six years of age is 11g/dL**

Select the correct answer using the code given below:

(a) 1 only (b) 1, 2, 3 and 4
(c) 2 and 4 only (d) 1 and 3 only

EXPLANATION:

Normal levels of hemoglobin are:

- Men: 13.8 to 18.0g/dL (138 to 180g/L, or 8.56 to 11.17mmol/L)
- Women: 12.1 to 15.1g/dL (121 to 151g/L, or 7.51 to 9.37mmol/L)
- Children: 11 to 16g/dL (110 to 160g/L, or 6.83 to 9.93mmol/L)
- Pregnant women: 11 to 14 g/dL (110 to 140g/L, or 6.83 to 8.69mmol/L) (9.5 to 15 usual value during pregnancy)
- Normal values of hemoglobin in the 1st and 3rd trimesters of pregnant women must be at least 11g/dL and at least 10.5g/dL during the 2nd trimester.

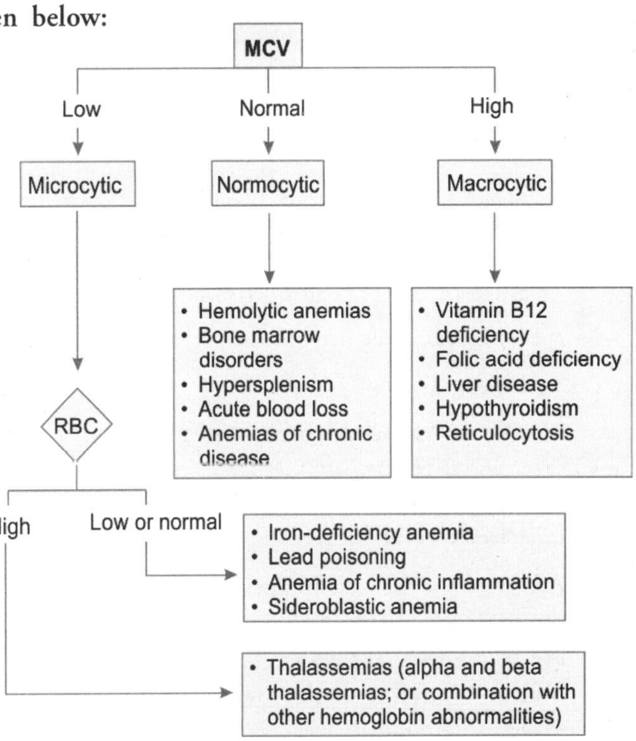

Ans. (B) i.e., 1, 2, 3 and 4

100. Health functionary at PHC level is:

(a) ASHA
(b) Anganwadi Worker
(c) Health Assistant (Female)
(d) Health Worker (Female)

EXPLANATION:

Staff for New Primary Health Centre

1. Medical Officer	1
2. Pharmacist	1
3. Nurse Midwife (Staff Nurse)	1
4. Health Worker (Female)/ANM	1
5. Health Educator	1
6. Health Assistant (Male)	1
7. Health Assistant (Female)/LHV	1
8. Upper Division Clerk	1
9. Lower Division Clerk	1
10. Laboratory Technician	1
11. Driver (Subject to Vehicle availability)	1
12. Class IV	4
Total	15

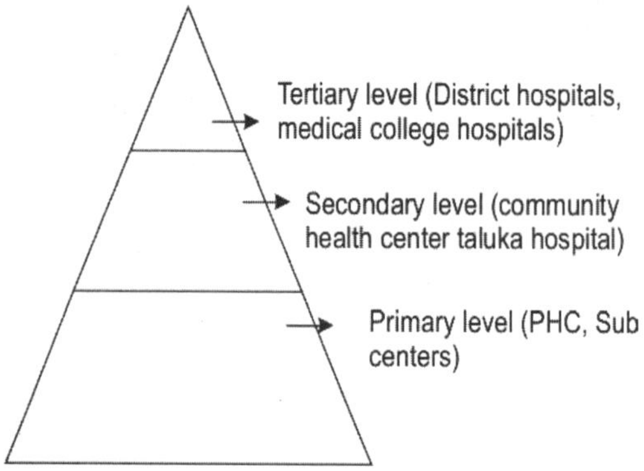

Ans. (C) i.e., Health Assistant (Female)

101. Due to a measles **outbreak in a community, a medical officer decided to immunize a child aged seven months with measles vaccine. When should the next measles vaccine be administered?**

(a) Not required
(b) After four weeks
(c) When the child completes nine months of age
(d) When the child completes fifteen months of age

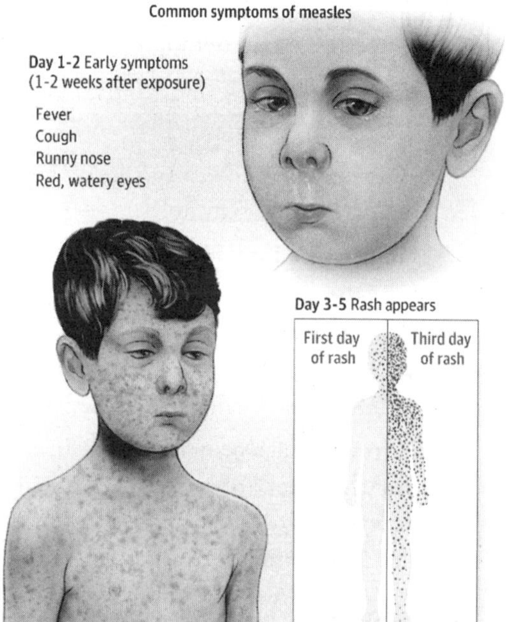

EXPLANATION:

After one dose of measles, 85% of children nine months of age and 95% over twelve months of age are immune. Nearly all of those who do not develop immunity after a single dose develop it after a second dose. When rates of vaccination within a population are greater than ~92% outbreaks of measles typically no longer occur; however, they may occur again if rates of vaccination decrease. The vaccine's effectiveness lasts many years. The vaccine may also protect against measles if given within a couple of days of exposure to measles.

Ans. (C) i.e., When the child completes nine months of age

102. Which of the following is/are the methods of assessment of nutritional status?

1. Clinical examination
2. Anthropometry
3. Biochemical evaluation
4. Orthotolidine test

Select the correct answer using the code given below:

(a) 1 only
(b) 1 and 3 only
(c) 1, 2 and 3 only
(d) 1, 2, 3 and 4

EXPLANATION:

Orthotolidine Test

In this test, 10 ml of chlorinated sample of water is taken after the required contact period, in a glass tube. To this 0.1ml of orthotolidine solution is added. The color formed is observed after 5 minutes. The formation of yellow color normally indicates the presence of chlorine (either combined or free) in the water. The more yellow the color, the greater, is the chlorine residual.

Assessment of nutritional status
Methodology in clinical practice

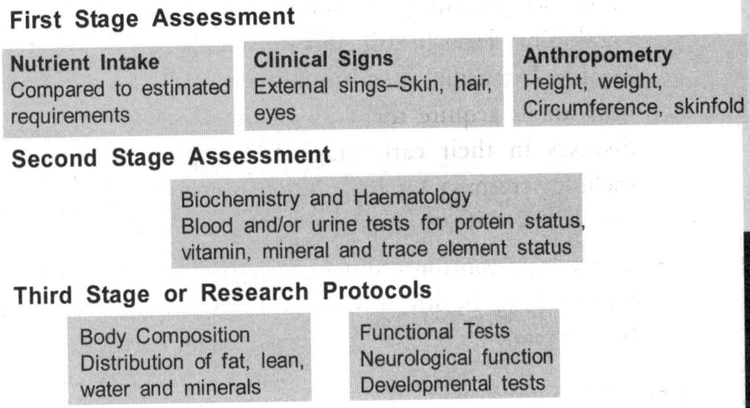

Ans. (C) i.e., 1, 2 and 3 only

103. Retrospective cohort studies have the following features except:

(a) Outcomes have occurred before the start of the study
(b) Generally more expensive than prospective studies
(c) Results are obtained more quickly
(d) Investigator goes back in time to select study groups

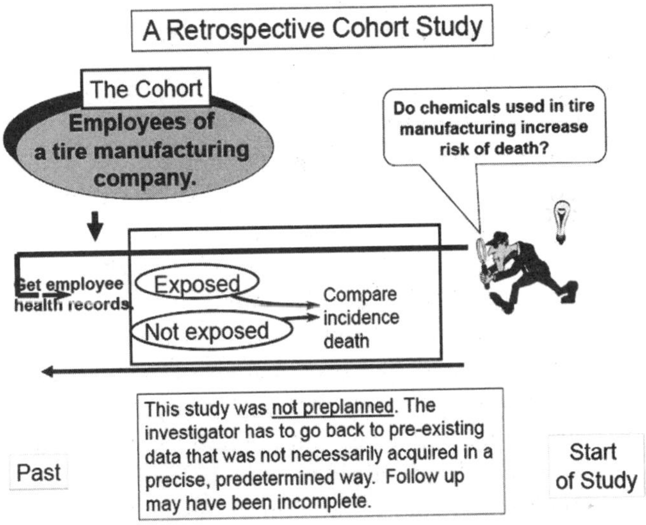

EXPLANATION:

A **retrospective cohort study**, also called a **historic cohort study**, is a longitudinal cohort study used in medical and psychological research. A cohort of individuals that share a common exposure factor is compared to another group of equivalent individuals not exposed to that factor, to determine the factor's influence on the incidence of a condition such as disease or death.

Ans. (B) i.e., Generally more expensive than prospective studies

104. What is the correct sequence of the following levels of prevention?

1. Specific protection
2. Early diagnosis and prompt treatment
3. Disability limitation and rehabilitation
4. Health promotion

Select the correct sequence from the code given below:

(a) 1, 2, 3, 4 (b) 4, 1, 2, 3 (c) 2, 3, 4, 1 (d) 3, 4, 1, 2

EXPLANATION:

Levels of Prevention

- **Primary prevention**—those preventive measures that prevent the onset of illness or injury before the disease process begins. Examples include immunization and taking regular exercise.
- **Secondary prevention**—those preventive measures that lead to early diagnosis and prompt treatment of a disease, illness or injury to prevent more severe problems developing. Here health educators such as Health Extension Practitioners can help individuals acquire the skills of detecting diseases in their early stages. Examples include screening for high blood pressure and breast self examination

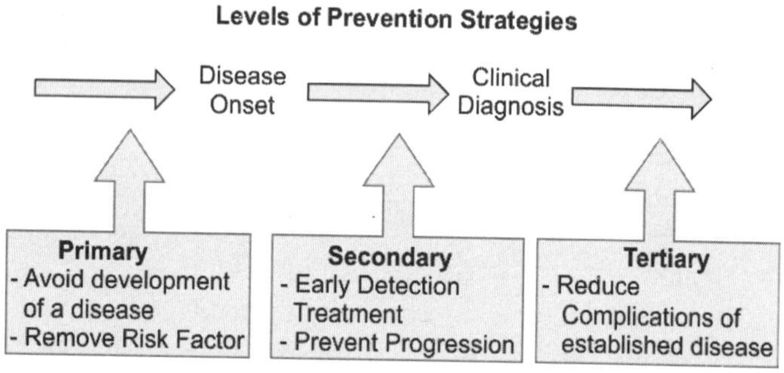

- **Tertiary prevention**—those preventive measures aimed at rehabilitation following significant illness. At this level health services workers can work to retrain, re-educate and rehabilitate people who have already developed an impairment or disability.

Ans. (B) i.e., 4, 1, 2, 3

105. Which of the following items are among the uses of epidemiology?

(a) To study historically the rise and fall of the diseases
(b) To arrive at community diagnosis
(c) To identify syndromes
(d) All of these

EXPLANATION:

Epidemiology is the study and analysis of the distribution (who, when, and where) and determinants of health and disease conditions in defined populations. It is the cornerstone of public health, and shapes policy decisions and evidence based practice by identifying risk factors for disease and targets for preventive healthcare. Epidemiologists help with study design, collection, and statistical analysis of data, amend interpretation and dissemination of results (including peer review and occasional systematic review). Epidemiology has helped develop methodology used in clinical research, public health studies, and, to a lesser extent, basic research in the biological sciences

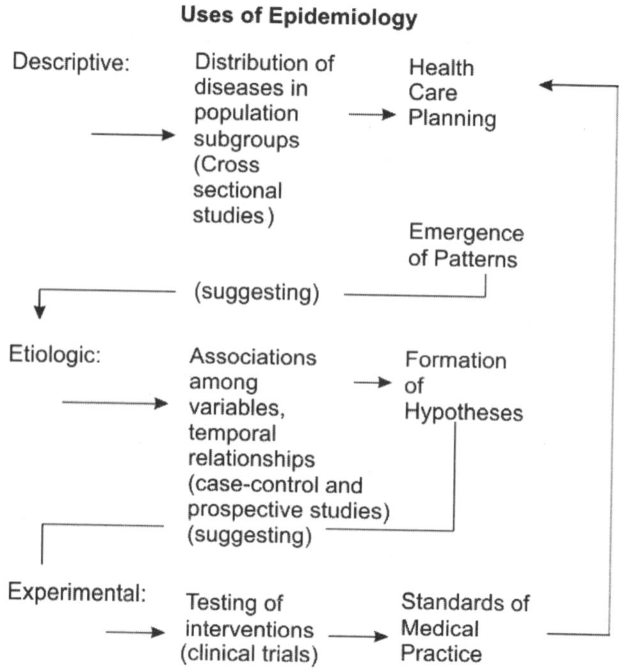

Ans. (D) i.e., All of these

106. Consider the following statements regarding folic acid:

1. It is needed for normal development of blood cells in the marrow
2. It has a role in synthesis of nucleic acids
3. It is resistant to boiling

Which of the above statements is/are correct?

(a) 1 only (b) 1 and 2 (c) 1 and 3 (d) 2 and 3

EXPLANATION:

Folic acid

- Folic acid and vitamin B_{12} are hemopoietic vitamins required for RBC formation.
- **Folic acid** is known as vitamin B_9 needed for the **synthesis**, repair, and methylation of **DNA.**

Ans. (B) i.e., 1 and 2

107. **The maternal and child health care indicator that gives a good indicator of the extent of pregnancy wastage as well as the quantity and quality of health care available to the mother and new born is:**

(a) Maternal Mortality Rate (b) Still Birth Rate

(c) Infant Mortality Rate (d) Perinatal Mortality Rate

EXPLANATION:

Perinatal mortality (PNM), also **perinatal death,** refers to the death of a fetus or neonate and is the basis to calculate the **perinatal mortality rate.** Variations in the precise definition of the perinatal mortality exist, specifically concerning the issue of inclusion or exclusion of early fetal and late neonatal fatalities. The World Health Organization defines perinatal mortality as the "number of stillbirths and deaths in the first week of life per 1,000 total births, the perinatal period commences at 22 completed weeks (154 days) of gestation, and ends seven completed days after birth".

Mortality in and around infancy

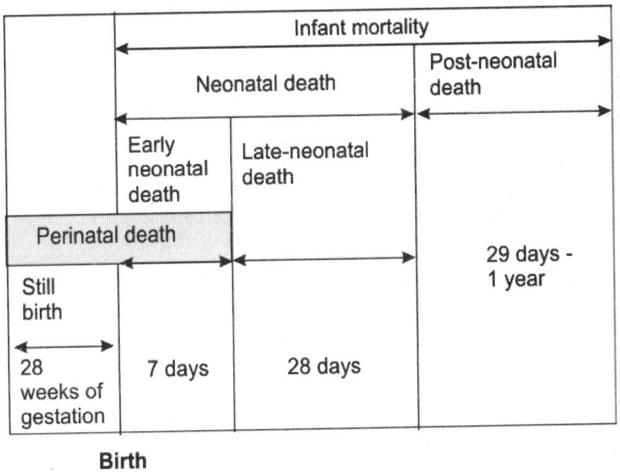

Ans. (D) i.e., Perinatal Mortality Rate

108. **To control Mansonoides mosquitoes, the most effective method is:**

(a) Oiling of water (b) Larvicidal insecticides

(c) Avoidance of water collections (d) Removal of water plants

EXPLANATION:

Mansonia mosquitoes are big, black or brown mosquitoes with sparkling on their wings and legs. They breed in ponds and lakes containing certain aquatic plants, especially the floating type like *Pistia stratiotes* and water hyacinth. The eggs are laid in star shaped clusters on the undersurface of leaves of these plants. The larvae and pupae are found attached to the rootlets of these plants by their siphon tubes. They obtain their air supply from these rootlets. When about to become adult, these pupae come to the surface of water and the fully formed adults emerge and escape. The control of *Mansonoia* mosquitoes is easy by removal or destruction of the aquatic host plants by herbicides.

Mosquito	Diseases
• Anopheles	• Malaria
• Culex	• Filaria, Japanese encephalitis
• Aedes	• Dengue, chickungunya, yellow fever
• Mansonoides	• Brugian filariasis

Ans. (D) i.e., Removal of water plants

109. What is the fertility indicator that gives the approximate magnitude of completed family size?

(a) General Fertility Rate
(b) Age Specific Fertility Rate
(c) Total Fertility Rate
(d) Gross Reproduction Rate

EXPLANATION:

The **total fertility rate** (TFR), sometimes also called the **fertility rate, absolute/potential natality, period total fertility rate** (PTFR), or **total period fertility rate** (TPFR) of a population is the average number of children that would be born to a woman over her lifetime if:

1. She were to experience the exact current age specific fertility rates (ASFRs) through her lifetime, and
2. She were to survive from birth through the end of her reproductive life.

Definition of Terms

- **Fertility** = Production a live birth (natality)
- **Infertility** = Inability to produce a live birth
- **Parity** = Number of children born alive to a woman
- **Gravidity** = Number of pregnancies a woman has had whether or not they produce a live birth
- **Fecundity** = Physiological capacity to conceive (reproductive potential)
- **Infecundity** (sterility) = Inability of a woman to conceive a pregnancy
  - o ***Primary sterility*** = Never able to conceive a pregnancy
  - o ***Secondary sterility*** = Inability to conceive afer one or more children have been born
- **Fecundability** = Probability that a woman will conceive during a menstrual cycle

Ans. (C) i.e., Total Fertility Rate

110. For a child aged four years, an Anganwadi Worker detects that the weight is lower than expected. What should the Anganwadi Worker do first regarding the malnutrition detected in the child?

(a) Refer the child to the nearby Health Centre
(b) Refer the child a nearby nutritional rehabilitation centre
(c) Give nutritional counselling to the mother
(d) Start fortnightly deworming

EXPLANATION:

The Ministry of Women and Child Development has laid down guidelines for the responsibilities of Anganwadi workers (AWW). These include showing community support and active participation in executing this programme, to conduct regular quick surveys of all families, organize preschool activities, provide health and nutrition education to families especially pregnant women on how to breastfeed, etc., motivating families to adopt family planning, educating parents about child growth and development, assist in the implementation and execution of Kishori Shakti Yojana (KSY) to educate teenage girls and parents by organizing social awareness programmes etc., identify disabilities in children, and so on.

Ans. (C) i.e., Give nutritional counselling to the mother

111. Which of the following anthropometrical measurements is/are carried out to assess the growth of children under five years of age?

1. Weight measurement
2. Height measurement
3. Mid upper arm circumference

Select the correct answer using the code given below:

(a) 1 only (b) 1 and 2 only
(c) 2 and 3 only (d) 1, 2 and 3

EXPLANATION:

Assessment of growth of children

- In children, parameters used to measure growth are weight in kilograms, height in meters and head and chest circumferences. Assessment can be longitudinal where serial measurement of the same child is recorded over different periods of time or cross sectional where recorded measurement is compared to that of his peers.
- Mid upper arm circumference and calf circumference indicate the status of muscle development. Mid calf and mid upper arm are heavily muscled and is approximately circular.

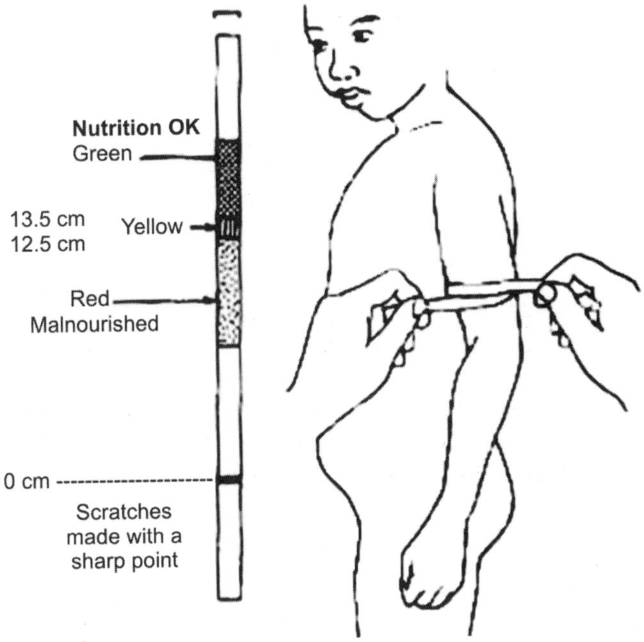

Ans. (D) i.e., 1, 2 and 3

112. Which of the following is included in detecting a child with severe acute malnutrition?

1. Weight for age Z score less than minus three SD
2. Bilateral pitting oedema
3. Weight for height Z score less than minus three SD
4. Mid upper arm circumference of less than 12 cm.

Select the correct answer using the code given below:

(a) 1 and 3 only (b) 2 and 3 only (c) 3 and 4 only (d) 1, 2, 3 and 4

EXPLANATION:

Severe acute malnutrition is defined by a very low weight for height (below -3z scores of the median WHO growth standards), by visible severe wasting, or by the presence of nutritional oedema. Decreasing child mortality and improving maternal health depend heavily on reducing malnutrition, which is responsible, directly or indirectly, for 35% of deaths among children under five.

	Moderate Malnutrition	Severe Malnutrition
Symmetrical oedema	No	Yes (oedematous malnutrition)
Weight-for-height	SD score between –2 and –3	SD score < –3 Severe wasting
Height-for-age	SD score between –2 and –3	SD score < –3 Severe wasting

Ans. (B) i.e., 2 and 3 only

113. Which of the following statements is/are correct regarding Essential Obstetric Care under the Reproductive, Maternal, Newborn and Child Health care Programme?

1. Early registration of pregnancy
2. Provision of first referral units
3. Provision of safe delivery practices
4. Provision of at least four postnatal checkups

Select the correct answer using the code given below:

(a) 1 and 2 only (b) 1 and 3 only (c) 2 and 3 only (d) 1, 2, 3 and 4

EXPLANATION:

Reproductive, Maternal, Newborn, and Child Health (RMNCH) covers the health concerns and interventions across the life course involving women before and during pregnancy; newborns, that is, the first 28 days of life; and children to their fifth birthday.

Ans. (B) i.e., 1 and 3 only

114. **A pregnant woman visits a medical officer for an antenatal check up. The woman mentions that she had received two doses of Tetanus Toxoid vaccine three years ago. Which of the following steps should the medical officer take with regard to administration of Tetanus Toxoid vaccine as per the Government of India recommended schedule?**

(a) Tetanus Immunoglobulin should be administered in the third trimester of pregnancy

(b) Two doses of Tetanus Toxoid vaccine should be administered with an interval of four weeks between the two doses

(c) Only one dose of Tetanus Toxoid vaccine is required

(d) No Tetanus Toxoid vaccine is required

2017

EXPLANATION:

To maximize the maternal antibody response and passive antibody transfer to the infant, the national immunization schedule in India recommends the 2 doses of tetanus toxoid (TT) for unknown immunization status of pregnant women i.e. the first dose of tetanus toxoid should be administered as soon as pregnancy is detected, second dose of tetanus toxoid is administered after 4 weeks and if a mother received 2 TT doses in the last pregnancy and mother gets again pregnant within 3 year than only one dose of TT is recommended and that dose is called booster dose.

Tetanus vaccine (Tetanus Toxoid)	
• Formalin-inactivated tetanus toxin, protein antigen	
• Schedule	Initially three or four doses + booster
	Booster every 10 years
• Efficacy	Approximately 100%
• Duration	Approximately 10 years
• Vaccine content	Same for children and adults
• Preferable administered with diphtheria toxoid as DTP, DTaP, DT, Td or Tdap	

Ans. (C) i.e., Only one dose of Tetanus Toxoid vaccine is required

115. With reference to quarantine measures to prevent the spread of a disease, which of the following statements is/are correct?

1. In addition to human beings, quarantine measures are at times also applied to an aircraft or a train or a container etc.
2. The duration of the quarantine period is equivalent to the minimum incubation period for the disease

Select the correct answer using the code given below:

(a) 1 only (b) 2 only (c) Both 1 and 2 (d) Neither 1 nor 2

EXPLANATION:

A **quarantine** is used to separate and restrict the movement of people; it is a 'a restraint upon the activities or communication of persons or the transport of goods designed to prevent the spread of disease or pests', for a certain period of time. This is often used in connection to disease and illness, such as those who may possibly have been exposed to a communicable disease. The term is often erroneously used to mean medical isolation, which is "to separate ill persons who have a communicable disease from those who are healthy".

Ans. (A) i.e., 1 only

116. Which is the first step in carrying out an Adverse Event Following Immunization (AEFI)?

(a) Formulate a working hypothesis
(b) Observe the immunization service in action
(c) Confirm information in report
(d) Collect data about the suspected vaccine

EXPLANATION:

Adverse event following immunization is any untoward medical occurrence which follows immunization and which does not necessarily have a causal relationship with the usage of the vaccine. If not rapidly and effectively dealt with, can undermine confidence in a vaccine and ultimately have dramatic consequences for immunization coverage and disease incidence.

- **At the end AEFI = Adverse event following immunization**
  - o A medical incident
  - o Takes place after an immunization
  - o Causes concern
  - o Is believed to be caused by immunization
- **AEFI can be categorized into:**
  - o Vaccine reaction
  - o Programme error
  - o Coincidental
  - o Injection reaction
  - o Unknown

Ans. (C) i.e., Confirm information in report

2017

117. At the end of an immunization session, you found that a reconstituted BCG vaccine vial has around two doses left in it. What should be done in such a situation?

(a) Can reuse the remaining two doses during the next immunization session
(b) Discard the vial in a black coloured bin
(c) Discard the vial in a red coloured bin
(d) Take decision depending upon the Vaccine Vial Monitor (VVM) status

EXPLANATION:

Colour	Waste Description
Yellow*	Human tissues, organs, body parts, items contaminated by blood/body fluids, soiled cotton and dressing, soiled plaster casts, etc.
Red*	Catheters, tubes, cannulae, syringes, plastic IV bottles and sets, used gloves, infected plastics, specimen containers, lab waste, microbiology cultures, used or discarded bags of blood/ blood products, vaccines, etc.
Blue*	Glass items, needles, syringes, scalpels, blades, used and unused sharps, etc.
Black*	Discarded medicines, discarded cytotoxic drugs, etc.

Ans. (C) i.e., Discard the vial in a red coloured bin

118. With reference to Vaccine Vial Monitors (VVM) being used on vaccine vials, which of the following statements is/are correct?

1. It gives information about heat exposure over a period of time
2. It directly indicates vaccine potency

Select the correct answer using the code given below:

(a) 1 only (b) 2 only (c) Both 1 and 2 (d) Neither 1 nor 2

EXPLANATION:

A **vaccine vial monitor** (VVM) is a thermochromic label put on vials containing vaccines which gives a visual indication of whether the vaccine has been kept at a temperature which preserves its potency. The labels were designed in response to the problem of delivering vaccines to developing countries where the cold chain is difficult to preserve, and where formerly vaccines were being rendered inactive and administered ineffectively due to their having been denatured by exposure to ambient temperature.

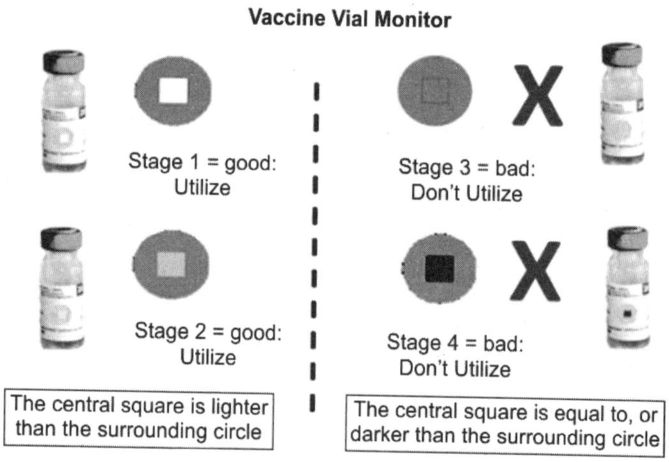

Ans. (A) i.e., 1 only

119. Why is matching done in a case control study?

1. To remove the effect of known confounders
2. To remove the effect of unknown confounders
3. To eliminate selection bias
4. To eliminate interviewer's bias

Select the correct answer using the code given below:

(a) 1 only (b) 2 and 3
(c) 1, 3 and 4 (d) 4 only

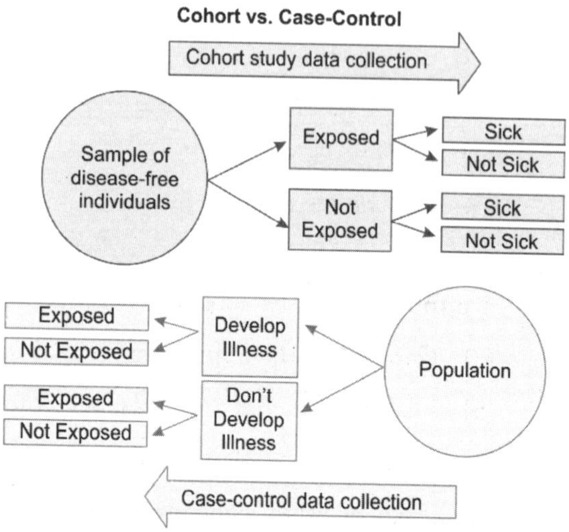

EXPLANATION:

Case control studies assign confounders to both groups, cases and controls, equally. For example, if somebody wanted to study the cause of myocardial infarct and thinks that the age is a probable confounding variable, each 67-year old infarct patient will be matched with a healthy 67-year old "control" person. In case control studies, matched variables most often are the age and sex.

Ans. (A) i.e., 1 only

120. Which of the following vaccines has NOT been introduced in the Universal Immunization Programme in India?

(a) Pentavalent vaccine
(b) MMR vaccine
(c) Injectable polio vaccine
(d) Cervical cancer vaccine

EXPLANATION:

Universal Immunization Programme is a vaccination program launched by the Government of India in 1985. It became a part of Child Survival and Safe Motherhood Programme in 1992 and is currently one of the key areas under **National Rural Health Mission** (NRHM) since 2005.

National Immunization Schedule (Jan. 2011)

Age	Vaccines
Pregnant Women	TT (2 doses/Booster)
Birth	BCG, OPV-O, Hep B
6 weeks	DPT-1, OPV-1, Hep B
10 weeks	DPT-2, OPV-2, Hep B
14 weeks	DPT-3, OPV-3, Hep B
9 months	Measles
16–24 months	DPT Booster, OPV – Booster, MCV (Measles Containing Vaccine), JE*
5 years	DPT Booster 2
10 years	TT
16 years	TT

Ans. (D) i.e., Cervical cancer vaccine

CHAPTER

4 CMS EXAMINATION 2017

PAPER - 1

1. **Which of the following is NOT correct?**
   (a) Hepatitis A does not lead to massive hepatic necrosis
   (b) Hepatitis B vaccination is part of universal childhood vaccination
   (c) Hepatitis C is commonest cause of transfusion transmitted hepatitis
   (d) Hepatitis E carries very high mortality in pregnant women

EXPLANATION

Hepatitis A is an infectious disease of the *liver* caused by the (HAV). Many cases have few or no symptoms, especially in the young. The time between infection and symptoms, in those who develop them, is between two and six weeks. When symptoms occur, they typically last eight weeks and may include nausea, vomiting, diarrhea, jaundice, fever, and abdominal pain. Around 10–15% of people experience a recurrence of symptoms during the six months after the initial infection. Acute liver failure may rarely occur, with this being more common in the elderly.

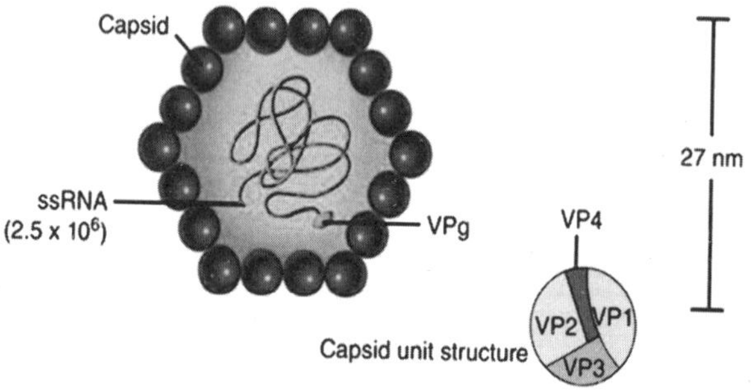

Ans. (A) i.e., Hepatitis A does not lead to massive hepatic necrosis

2. **Which of the following antihypertensive drugs is CONTRAINDICATED in pregnancy?**
   (a) Hydralazine
   (b) Amlodipine
   (c) Labetalol
   (d) Ramipril

EXPLANATION

Use of ACEI/Angiontensin Converting Enzyme inhibitors in the first trimester is associated with a risk of major congenital malformations, particularly affecting the cardiovascular and central nervous systems.

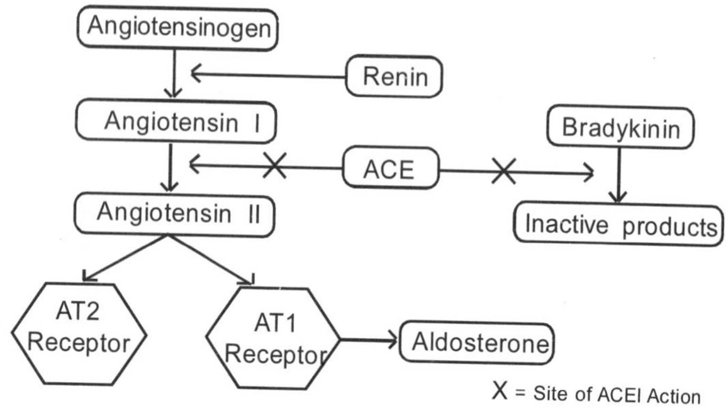

Ans. (B) i.e., Amlodipine

3. Which of the following LEAST predisposes to infective endocarditis?

(a) Ventricular septal defect
(b) Atrial septal defect
(c) Patent ductus arteriosus
(d) Tetralogy of Fallot

EXPLANATION

Due to the communication between the atria that occurs in ASDs, disease entities or complications from the condition are possible. Patients with an uncorrected atrial septal defect may be at increased risk for developing a cardiac arrhythmia, as well as more frequent respiratory infections.

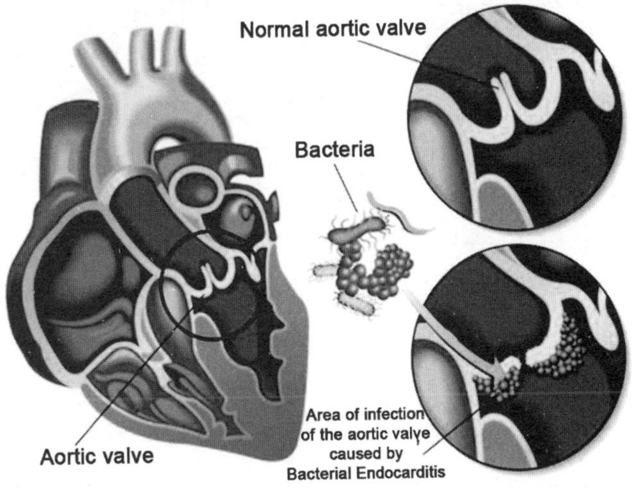

Ans. (B) i.e., Atrial septal defect

4. A 60-year old male with Marfan's syndrome comes to emergency department with severe generalised tearing pain localised to chest anteriorly and inter scapular region, sweating and weakness. On examination, his BP is 200/140mmHg. X-ray chest shows widening of superior mediastinum. ECG shows sinus tachycardia. What is the most likely diagnosis?

(a) Acute pulmonary embolism
(b) Dissection of aorta
(c) Acute myocardial infraction
(d) Acute pericarditis

2017

EXPLANATION

Aortic dissection is more common in those with a history of high blood pressure, a number of connective tissues disorder that affect blood vessel wall strength such as Marfans syndrome, a bicuspid aortic valve, and previous heart surgery.

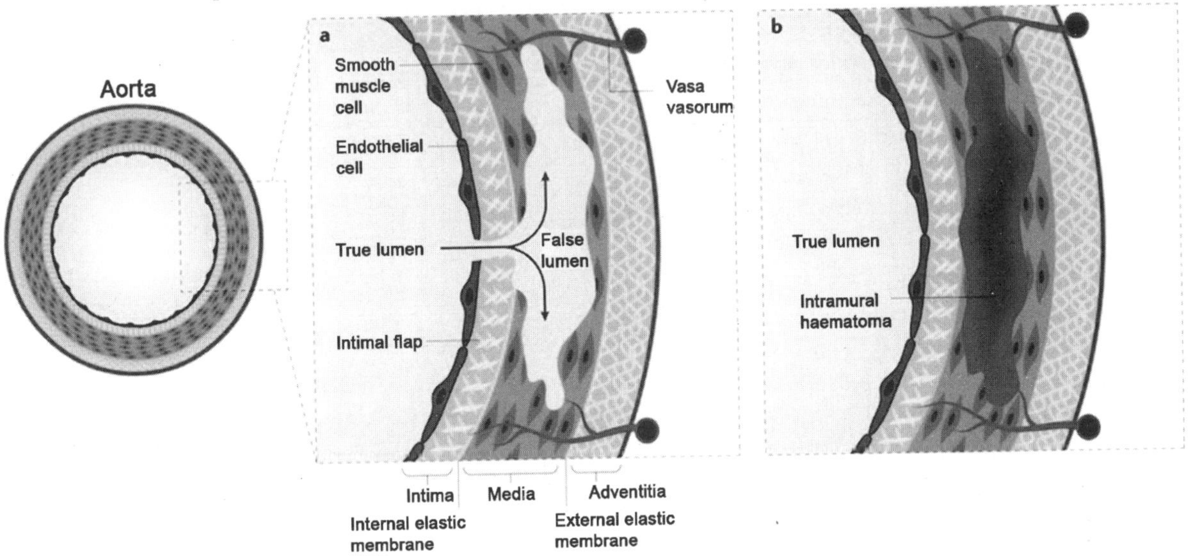

Ans. (B) i.e., Dissection of aorta

5. A patient who is allergic to penicillin can be prescribed which of the following drugs for prophylaxis of acute rheumatic fever?

(a) Ciprofloxacin
(b) Erythromycin
(c) Cotrimoxazole
(d) Tetracycline

EXPLANATION

Penicillin is given in cases of ARF to ensure eradication of streptococci that may persist in the upper respiratory tract. It may be advisable to use im benzathine penicillin G. Patients with a reliably documented penicillin allergy may be treated with oral erythromycin.

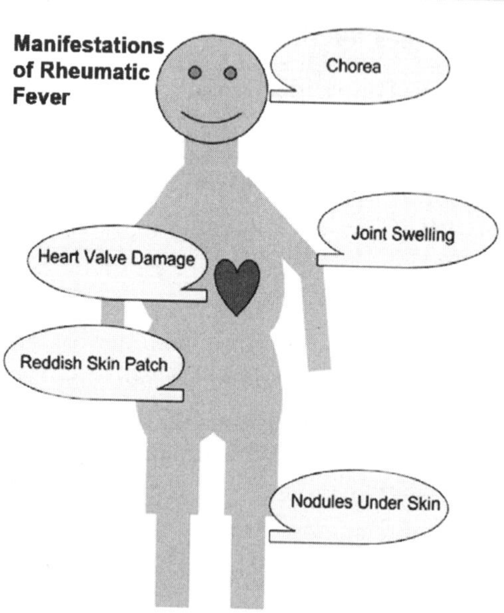

Ans. (B) i.e., Erythromycin

6. **QT interval is prolonged in:**

(a) Hypocalcaemia
(b) Hyperkalaemia
(c) Hypermagnesaemia
(d) Digoxin therapy

EXPLANATION

In hypocalcemia, intermittent QT prolongation, or intermittent prolongation of the QTc (corrected QT interval) on the EKG (electrocardiogram) is noted. The implications of intermittent QTc prolongation predisposes to life threatening cardiac electrical instability (and this is therefore a more critical condition than constant QTc prolongation). This type of electrical instability puts the patient at high risk of torsades de pointes, a specific type of ventricular tachycardia which appears on an EKG (or ECG) as something which looks a bit like a sine wave with a regularly increasing and decreasing amplitude. (Torsades de pointes can cause death, unless the patient can be medically or electrically cardioverted and returned to a normal cardiac rhythm.)

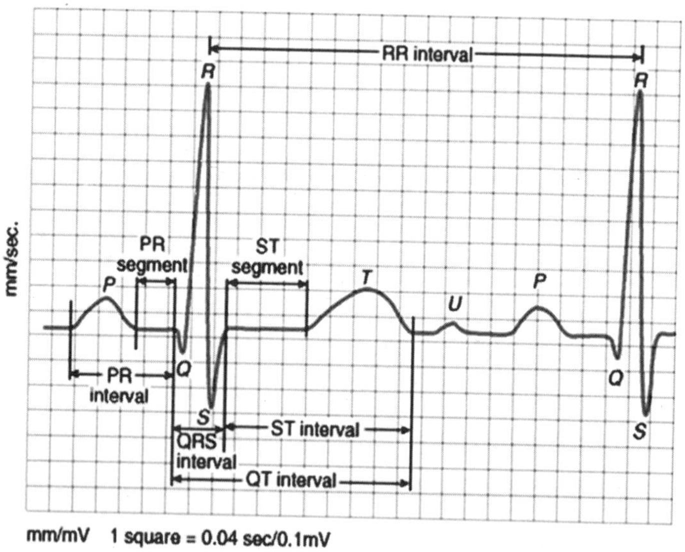

Ans. (A) i.e., Hypocalcaemia

7. **Differential cyanosis is seen in:**

(a) Atrial septal defect with pulmonary arterial hypertension
(b) Ventricular septal defect with pulmonary arterial hypertension
(c) Patent ductus arteriosus with pulmonary arterial hypertension
(d) Fallot tetralogy

2017

EXPLANATION

Differential cyanosis is the bluish coloration of the lower but not the upper extremity and the head. This is seen in patients with a patent dutcus arteriosus. Patients with a large ductus develop progressive pulmonary vascular disease, and pressure overload of the right ventricle occurs. As soon as pulmonary pressure exceeds aortic pressure, shunt reversal (right to left shunt) occurs. The upper extremity remains pink because the brachiocephalic trunk, left common carotid trunk and the left subclavian trunk is given off proximal to the PDA.

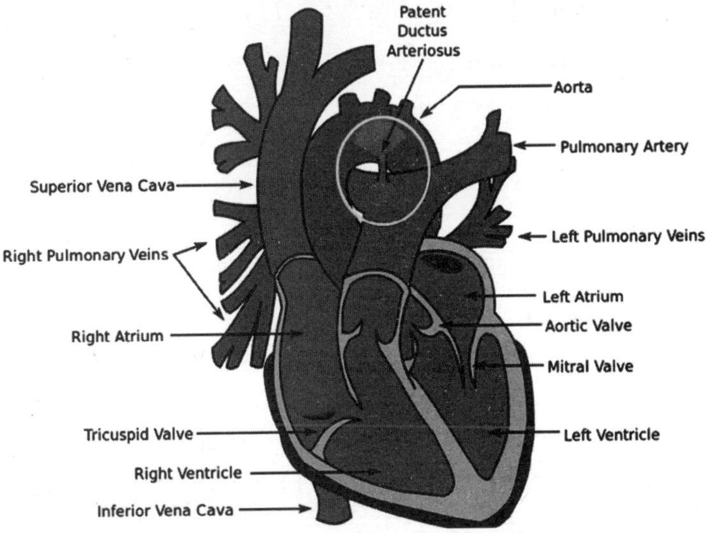

Ans. (C) i.e., Patent ductus arteriosus with pulmonary arterial hypertension

8. **Wilson's disease is characterised by all except:**

(a) Increased urinary copper
(b) Increased hepatic copper
(c) Deposition of copper in Descemet's membrane
(d) Increased serum ceruloplasmin

EXPLANATION

Levels of ceruloplasmin are abnormally low (<0.2g/L) in 80–95% of cases of Wilsons disease. The combination of neurological symptoms, Kayser–Fleischer rings and a low ceruloplasmin level is considered sufficient for the diagnosis of Wilson's disease.

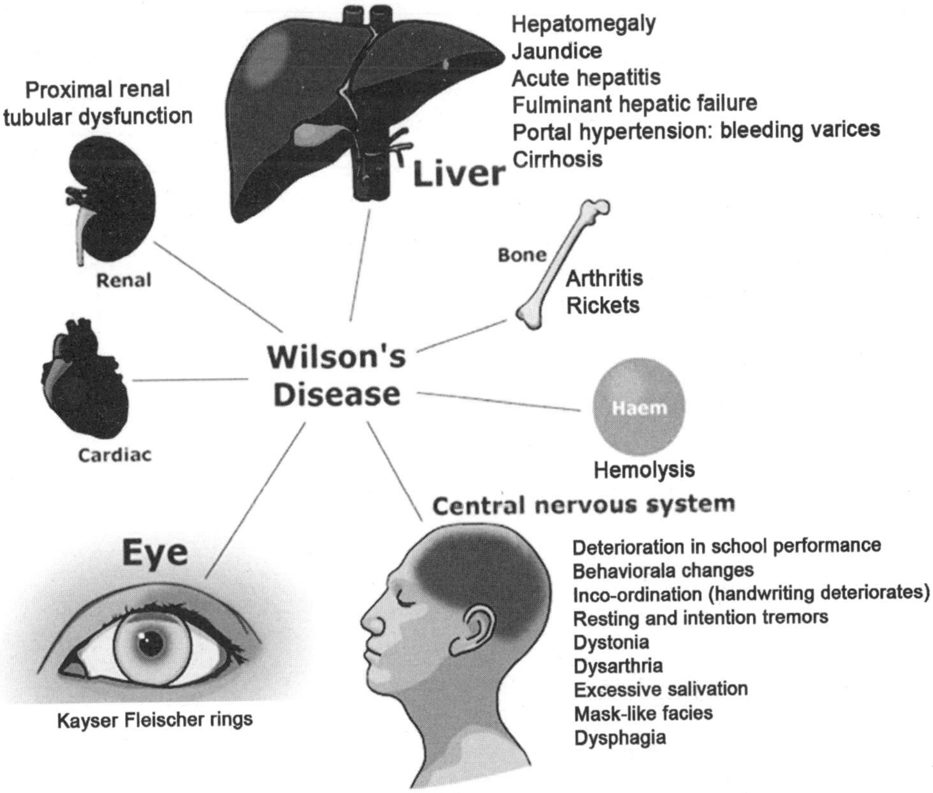

Ans. (D) i.e., Increased serum ceruloplasmin

9. Following drugs are used for *H.Pylori* eradication except:

(a) Amoxycillin
(b) Bismuth subsalicylate
(c) Tetracycline
(d) Cephalexin

EXPLANATION

Cefalexin can treat certain bacterial infections, including those of the middle ear, bone and joint, skin, and urinary tract. It may also be used for certain types of pneumonia, strep throat, and to prevent bacterial endocarditis. Cefalexin is not effective against infections caused by methicillin resistant staphylococcus aureus (MRSA), *Enterococcus*, or *Pseudomonas*.

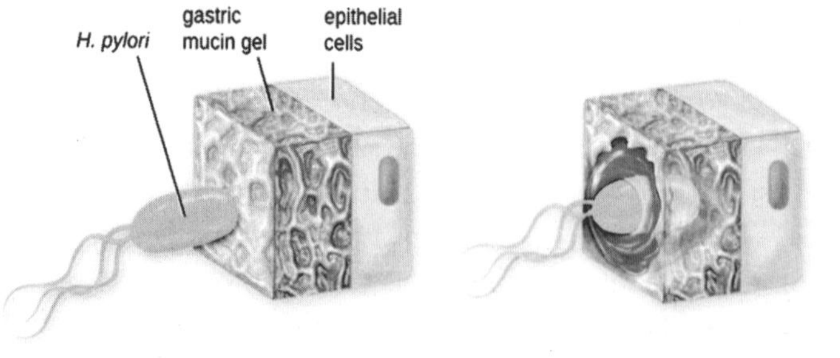

Contact with stomach acid keeps the mucin lining the epithelial cell layer in a spongy gel-like state. This consistency is impermeable to the bacterium *H. pylori*.

The bacterium releases urease, which neutralizes the stomach acid. This causes the mucin to liquefy, and the bacterium can swim right through it.

Ans. (D) i.e., Cephalexin

10. A 45-year old female comes to you with dysphagia. She is found to have anaemia and koilonychia. Most likely diagnosis is:

(a) Plummer Vinson syndrome
(b) Boerhaave syndrome
(c) Carcinoma oesophagus
(d) Reflux oesophagitis

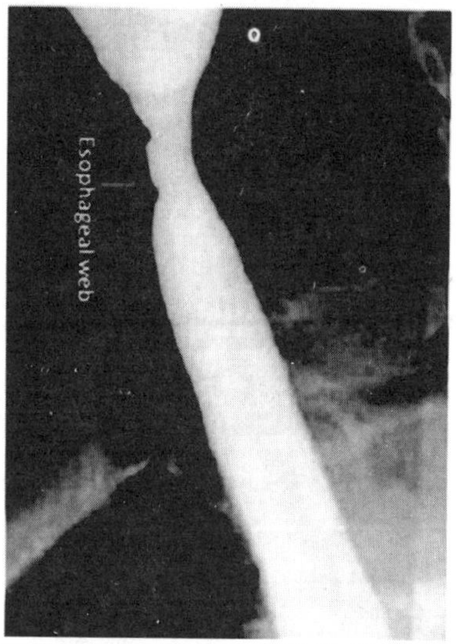

EXPLANATION

Plummer Vinson Syndrome (PVS), also called Paterson–Brown–Kelly syndrome or sideropenic dysphagia, is a rare disease characterized by difficulty in swallowing, iron deficieincy anemia, glossitis, cheilosis and esophageal webs. Treatment with iron supplementation and mechanical widening of the esophagus generally provides an excellent outcome.

Ans. (A) i.e., Plummer Vinson syndrome

11. Chest tube insertion should be considered in a patient with parapneumonic effusion include the following except:

(a) Loculated pleural effusion
(b) Positive Gram stain/culture of pleural fluid
(c) Pleural effusion is less than 10 mm thickness on decubitus
(d) Pleural fluid pH less than 7.20

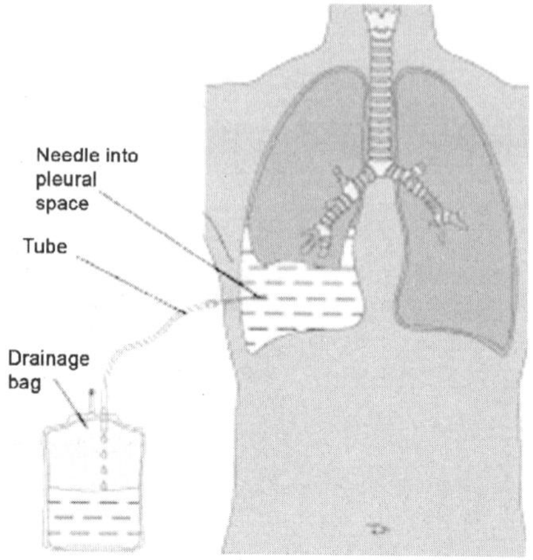

EXPLANATION

A parapneumonic effusion is a type of pleural effusion that arises as a result of a pneumonia, lung abscess, or bronchiectasis. There are three types of parapneumonic effusions: uncomplicated effusions, complicated effusions, and empyema. Small effusions (ie, <10mm thickness) will usually resolve with antibiotics alone.

Ans. (C) i.e., Pleural effusion is less than 10mm thickness on decubitus

12. A patient underwent hip replacement surgery. On fourth post operative day, he had dyspnoea, pleuritic pain and haemoptysis. Most likely diagnosis is:

(a) Pulmonary embolism (b) Pneumonia
(c) Pulmonary oedema (d) Pericarditis

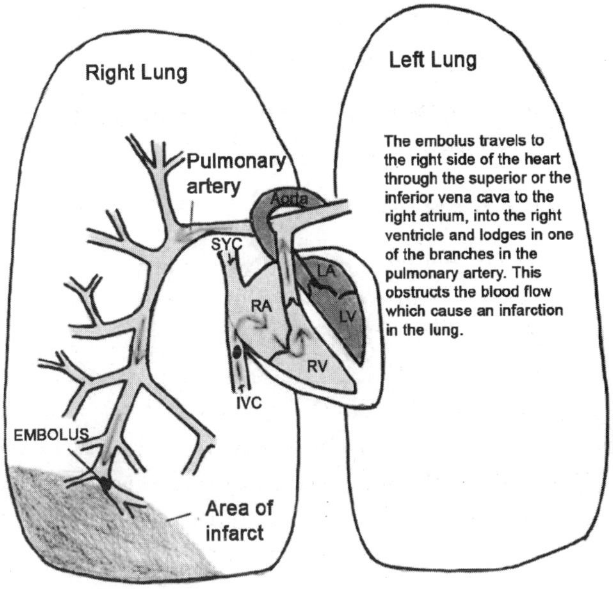

EXPLANATION

Symptoms of pulmonary embolism are typically sudden in onset and may include one or many of the following: dyspnea (shortness of breath), tachypnea (rapid breathing), chest pain of a "pleuritic" nature (worsened by breathing), cough and hemoptysis (coughing up blood). More severe cases can include signs such as cyanosis (blue discoloration, usually of the lips and fingers), collapse, and circulatory instability because of decreased blood flow through the lungs and into the left side of the heart. About 15% of all cases of sudden death are attributable to PE.

Ans. (A) i.e., Pulmonary embolism

13. A 55-year old male with a history of chronic obstructive pulmonary disease was rushed to emergency department with increasing shortness of breath, fever and a productive cough with yellow green sputum. He has difficulty in communicating because of his inability to complete a sentence. Measurement of arterial blood gas shows pH 7.3, $PaCO_2$ 68mmHg, HCO_3 28mmol/L, and PaO_2 60mmHg. How would you interpret this?

(a) Respiratory acidosis, uncompensated (b) Respiratory alkalosis, uncompensated
(c) Respiratory acidosis, partially compensated (d) Respiratory alkalosis, partially compensated

EXPLANATION

Normal pH: 7.35–7.45; Normal $PaCO_2$: 4.7–6 & Normal HCO_3: 22–24

Abnormality		pH	CO_2	HCO_3	Examples
Respiratory acidosis	Uncompensated	↓	↑	→	Severe Asthma
	Partially compensated	↓	↑	↑	Pneumonia
	Fully compensated	→	↑	↑	Hypoventilation
Respiratory alkalosis	Uncompensated	↑	↓	→	Hyperventilation
	Partially compensated	↑	↓	↓	Panic attack
	Fully compensated	→	↓	↓	Aspirin poisoning
Metabolic acidosis	Uncompensated	↓	→	↓	Diabetic ketoacidosis
	Partially compensated	↓	↓	↓	Lactic acidosis
	Fully compensated	→	↓	↓	Alcohol, salicylate
Metabolic alkalosis	Uncompensated	↑	→	↑	Loss of acid: severe
	Partially compensated	↑	↑	↑	Vomiting
	Fully compensated	→	↑	↑	Loss of potassium

Ans. (C) i.e., Respiratory acidosis, partially compensated

14. A 40-years old woman presents with hematuria, ecchymoses and menorrhagia of six months duration. What is the most likely diagnosis?

(a) Haemophilia A
(b) Haemophilia B
(c) Idiopathic thrombocytopaenic purpura
(d) Henoch Schonlein purpura

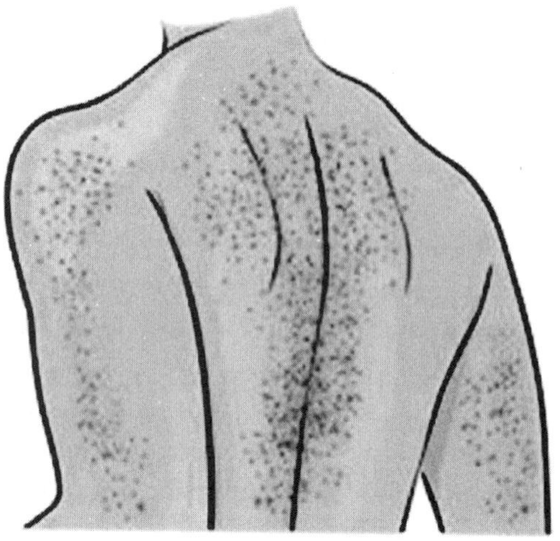

EXPLANATION

Signs of ITP include the spontaneous formation of bruises (purpura) and petechiae (tiny bruises), especially on the extremities, bleeding from the nostrils and/or gums, and menorrhagia (excessive menstrual bleeding), any of which may occur if the platelet count is below 20,000 per µl. A very low count (<10,000 per µl) may result in the spontaneous formation of hematomas (blood masses) in the mouth or on other mucous membranes.

Ans. (C) i.e., Idiopathic thrombocytopaenic purpura

15. Which of the following heavy metal poisoning strictly affects motor nerve?

(a) Cadmium (b) Mercury (c) Lead (d) Thallium

EXPLANATION

Peripheral Neuropathy

Demyelinating pathology	Axonal pathology
• Guillain-Barré syndrome	• Alcohol
• Chronic inflammatory demyelinating polyneuropathy (CIDP)	• Diabetes mellitus (± demyelinating picture)
• Amiodarone	• Vasculitis
• Hereditary sensorimotor neuropathies (HSMN) type I	• Vit. B_{12} deficiency (± demyelinating picture)
• Paraprotein neuropathy	• Hereditary sensorimotor neuropathies (HSMN) type II

Predominately motor loss	Predominately sensory loss
• Guillain-Barré syndrome	• Diabetes
• Porphyria	• Uremia
• Lead poisoning	• Leprosy
• HSMN – Charcot-Marie-Tooth	• Alcoholism
• CIDP	• Vitamin B_{12} deficiency
• Diphtheria	• Amyloidosis

Ans. (C) i.e., Lead

16. A patient develops skin necrosis 3 days after being started on warfarin for deep vein thrombosis. What is the most likely cause?

(a) Antiphospholipid antibody syndrome
(b) Protein C deficiency
(c) Disseminated intravascular coagulation
(d) Thrombotic thrombocytopaenic purpura

EXPLANATION

Protein C is vitamin K dependent. Patients with Protein C deficiency are at an increased risk of developing skin necrosis while on warfarin. Protein C has a short half life (8 hour) compared with other vitamin K dependent factors and therefore is rapidly depleted with warfarin initiation, resulting in a transient hypercoagulable state.

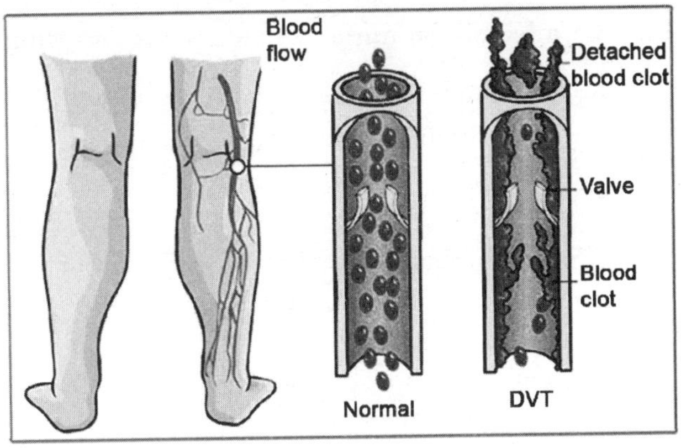

Ans. (B) i.e., Protein C deficiency

17. A 15-year old boy is brought to emergency with two days history of headache, vomiting and altered sensorium. His BP is 70mmHg systolic and he has ecchymoses on his skin. Most likely organism causing his condition is:

(a) Haemophilus influenzae
(b) Listeria monocytogenes
(c) *Neisseria meningitidis*
(d) Streptococcus pneumoniae

EXPLANATION

Waterhouse Friderichsen Syndrome can be caused by a number of different organisms. When caused by Neisseria meningitidis, WFS is considered the most severe form of meningococcal sepsis. The onset of the illness is nonspecific with fever, rigors, vomiting, and headache. Soon a rash appears; first macular, not much different from the rose spots of typhoid, and rapidly becoming petechial and purpuric with a dusky gray color. Low blood pressure (hypotension) develops and rapidly leads to septic shock. The cyanosis of extremities can be extreme and the patient is very prostrated or comatose. In this form of meningococcal disease, meningitis generally does not occur.

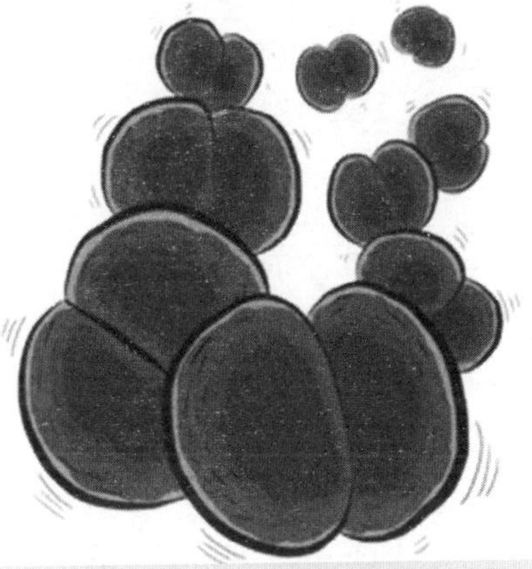

Ans. (C) i.e., *Neisseria meningitidis*

18. A child presents with episode of hematuria soon after respiratory tract infection. What is the most likely diagnosis?

(a) IgA nephropathy
(b) Wegener granulomatosis
(c) Post streptococcal glomerulonephritis
(d) Churg Strauss syndrome

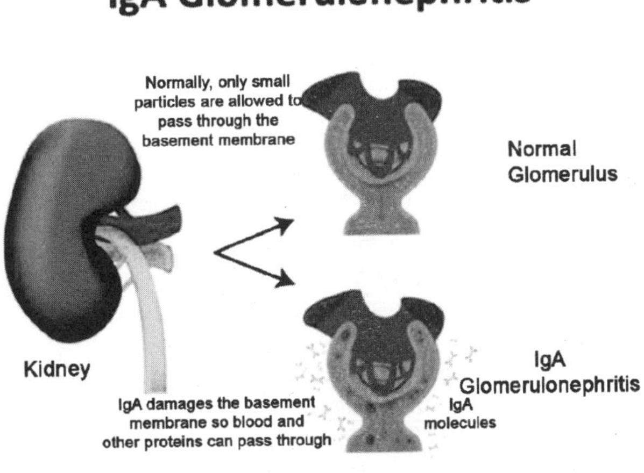

EXPLANATION

The classic presentation (in 40–50% of the cases) of IgA nephropathy is episodic hematuria, which usually starts within a day or two of a non specific upper respiratory tract infection (hence *synpharyngitic*), as opposed to post streptococcal glomerulonephritis, which occurs some time (weeks) after initial infection. Less commonly gastrointestinal or urinary infection can be the inciting agent.

Ans. (A) i.e., IgA nephropathy

19. **In microalbuminuria, 24 hours urinary albumin is:**

(a) 8–10mg (b) 30–300mg
(c) 300–3000mg (d) > 3000mg

EXPLANATION

Microalbuminuria can be diagnosed from a 24-hour urine collection (between 30–300 mg/24 hours) or, more commonly, from elevated concentration in a spot sample (20 to 200 mg/L). Both must be measured on at least two of three measurements over a two- to three-month period. An albumin level above the upper limit values is called "macroalbuminuria", or sometimes just albuminuria.

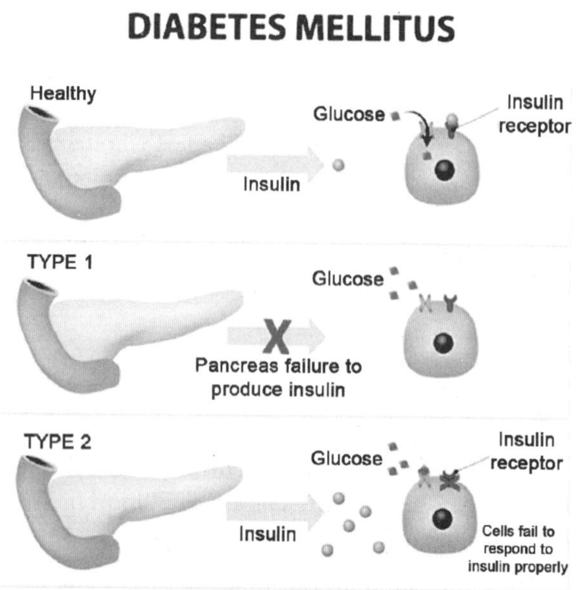

Ans. (B) i.e., 30–300mg

20. **Following are complications of acute renal failure except:**

(a) Intravascular volume overload (b) Hyponatraemia
(c) Hyperkalaemia (d) Metabolic alkalosis

EXPLANATION

Metabolic acidosis is a condition that occurs when the body produces excessive quantities of acid or when the kidneys are not removing enough acid from the body. If unchecked, metabolic acidosis leads to acidemia, i.e., blood pH is low (less than 7.35) due to increased production of hydrogen ions by the body or the inability of the body to form bicarbonate (HCO_3^-) in the kidney. Causes include

- M-Methanol
- U-Uremia (Kidney failure)
- D-Diabetic ketoacidosis
- P-Paraldehyde
- I-Infection, Iron, Isoniazid, Inborn errors of metabolism
- L-Lactic acidosis
- E-Ethylene glycol (Note: Ethanol is sometimes included in this mnemonic, as well, although the acidosis caused by ethanol is actually primarily due to the increased production of lactic acid found in such intoxication).
- S-Salicylates

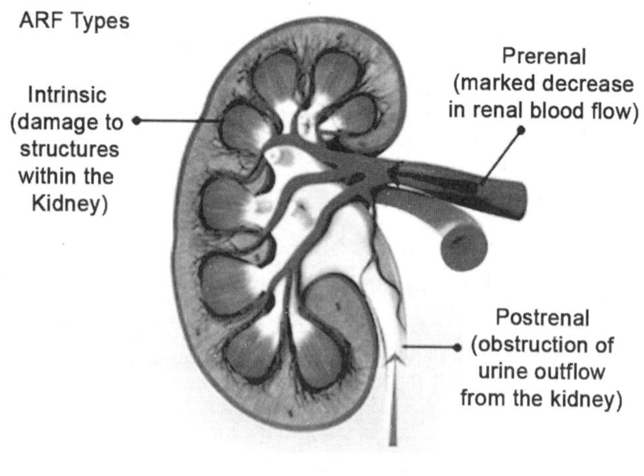

Ans. (D) i.e., Metabolic alkalosis

21. **Deficiency of which vitamin causes subacute combined degeneration of spinal cord?**

(a) Vitamin B_1 (b) Vitamin B_6 (c) Vitamin B_2 (d) Vitamin B_{12}

2017

EXPLANATION

Subacute combined degeneration of spinal cord, also known as Lichtheim's disease, refers to degeneration of the posterior and lateral columns of the spinal cord as a result of vitamin B_{12} deficiency (most common), vitamin E deficiency, and copper deficiency. It is usually associated with pernicious anemia.

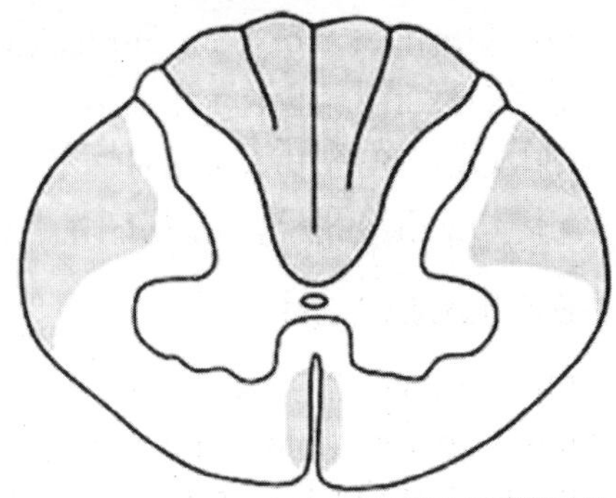

Ans. (D) i.e., Vitamin B_{12}

22. Obstructive lung function tests are seen in which of the following conditions?

(a) Obesity
(b) Kyphoscoliosis
(c) Pleural effusion
(d) Asthma

EXPLANATION

Pulmonary function testing is a diagnostic and management tool used for a variety of reasons, such as:

- Chronic shortness of breath
- Asthma
- Chronic obstructive pulmonary disease
- Restrictive lung disease
- Preoperative testing
- Impairment or disability

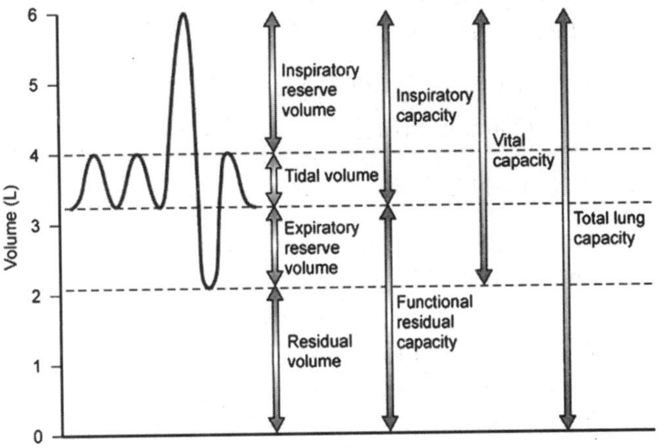

Ans. (D) i.e., Asthma

23. In which of the following conditions is there an increase in lung diffusion capacity?

(a) Emphysema
(b) Idiopathic pulmonary fibrosis
(c) Alveolar haemorrhage
(d) Pulmonary oedema

EXPLANATION

Lung conditions that increase lung diffusion capacity

1. Alveolar hemorrhage Goodpasture's syndrome, polycythemia, left to right intracardiac shunts, due increase in volume of blood exposed to inspired gas.
2. Asthma due to better perfusion of apices of lung. This is caused by increase in pulmonary arterial pressure and/or due to more negative pleural pressure generated during inspiration due to bronchial narrowing.

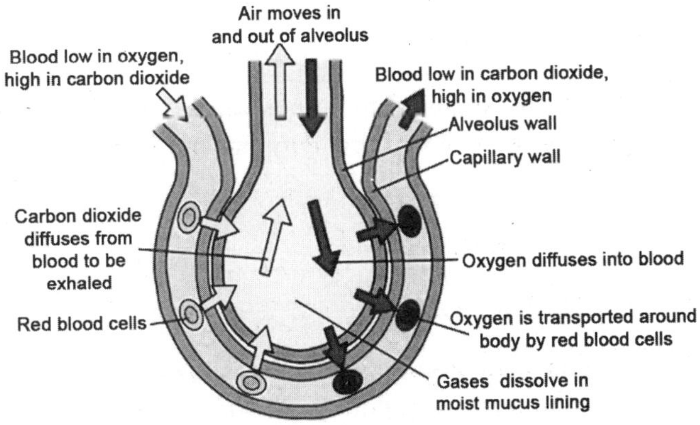

Ans. (C) i.e., Alveolar haemorrhage

24. Which one of the following statements is correct?

(a) Omalizumab is an antileukotriene

(b) Omalizumab is a blocking antibody that neutralises circulating IgE

(c) Omalizumab is a newer long acting anticholinergic agent

(d) Omalizumab is once a day long acting beta 2 agonistic

EXPLANATION

Omalizumab is a recombinant DNA derived humanized IgG1k monoclonal antibody that specifically binds to free human immunoglobulin E (IgE) in the blood and interstitial fluid and to membrane bound form of IgE (mIgE) on the surface of mIgE expressing B lymphocytes. Unlike an ordinary anti IgE antibody, it does not bind to IgE that is already bound by the high affinity IgE receptor (FcεRI) on the surface of mast cells, basophils, and antigen presenting dendritic cells.

Ans. (B) i.e., Omalizumab is a blocking antibody that neutralises circulating IgE

25. Widespread concave ST segment elevation and PR depression in most leads except aVR lead favours the diagnosis of:

(a) Acute myocardial infarction

(b) Pericarditis

(c) Digoxin toxicity

(d) Hypertrophic obstructive cardiomyopathy

EXPLANATION

The preferred initial diagnostic testing in a suspected case of pericarditis is the ECG, which may demonstrate a 12 lead electrocardiogram with diffuse, non specific, concave ("saddle shaped"), ST segment elevations in all leads except aVR and V1 and PR segment depression possible in any lead *except aVR*; sinus tachycardia, and low voltage QRS complexes can also be seen if there is subsymptomatic levels of pericardial effusion. The PR depression is often seen early in the process as the thin atria are affected more easily than the ventricles by the inflammatory process of the pericardium.

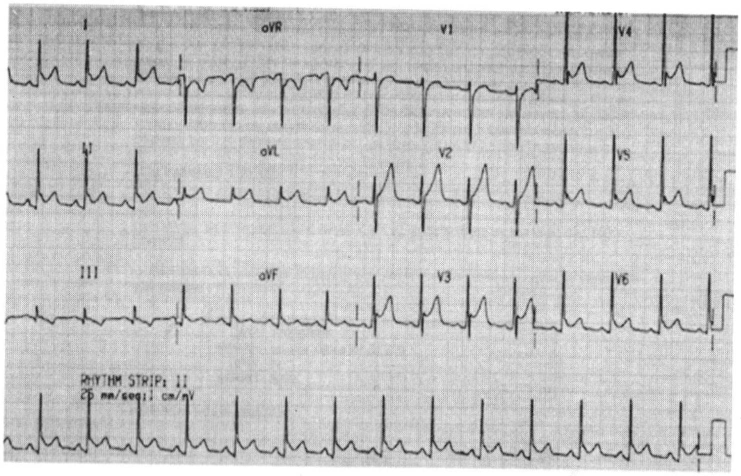

Ans. (B) i.e., Pericarditis

26. A known case of lepromatous leprosy was initiated on treatment. She developed painful erythmatous papules with fever and lymphadenopathy. What is the likely reactional state?

(a) Type 1 lepra reaction

(b) Type 2 lepra reaction

(c) Lucio's phenomenon

(d) Lupus pernio

EXPLANATION

Erythema nodosum (EN), also known as subacute migratory panniculitis of Vilanova and Piñol, is an inflammatory condition characterized by inflammation of the fat cells under the skin, resulting in tender red nodules or lumps that are usually seen on both shins. EN may also be due to excessive antibody production in lepromatous leprosy leading to deposition of immune complexes.

2017

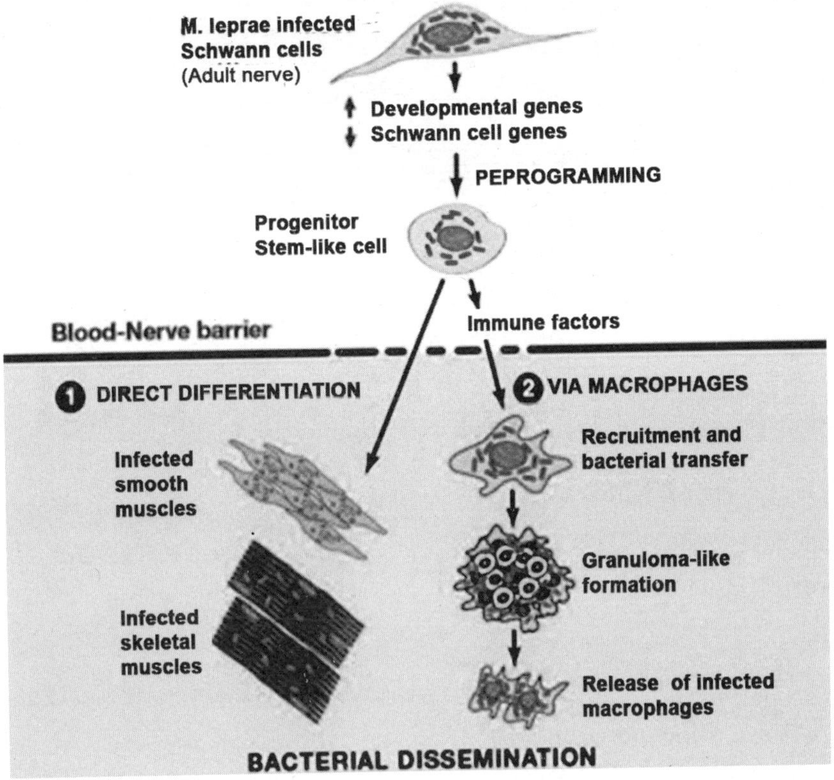

Ans. (B) i.e., Type 2 lepra reaction

27. **Which of the following is NOT true regarding congestive cardiac failure in the elderly?**
    (a) Incidence rises with age
    (b) Common causes include coronary artery disease and hypertension
    (c) Diastolic dysfunction is often present
    (d) Loop diuretics are usually well tolerated

EXPLANATION

Diuretics have been a mainstay of treatment for treatment of fluid accumulation, and include diuretics classes such as loop diuretics, thiazide like diuretic, and potassium sparing diuretic. Although widely used, evidence on their efficacy and safety is limited, with the exception of mineralocorticoid antagonist such as spironolactone. Mineralocorticoid antagonists in those under 75 years old appear to decrease the risk of death.

Mechanism of Action of Loop Diuretic

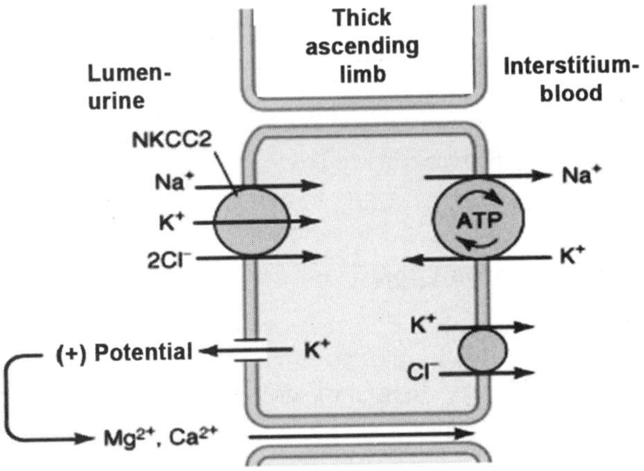

Ans. (D) i.e., Loop diuretics are usually well tolerated

28. **Multidrug resistant tuberculosis is defined as:**
    (a) At least resistance to three or more antitubercular drugs
    (b) At least resistance to Isoniazid, Streptomycin and Ethambutol
    (c) At least resistance to Isoniazid and Rifampicin
    (d) At least resistance to Streptomycin and Rifampicin

EXPLANATION

Multidrug resistant tuberculosis (MDR-TB) is a form of tuberculosis (TB) infection caused by bacteria that are resistant to treatment with at least two of the most powerful first line anti TB drugs, isoniazid and rifampin. Some forms of TB are also resistant to second line medications, and are called extensively drug resistant TB (XDR-TB).

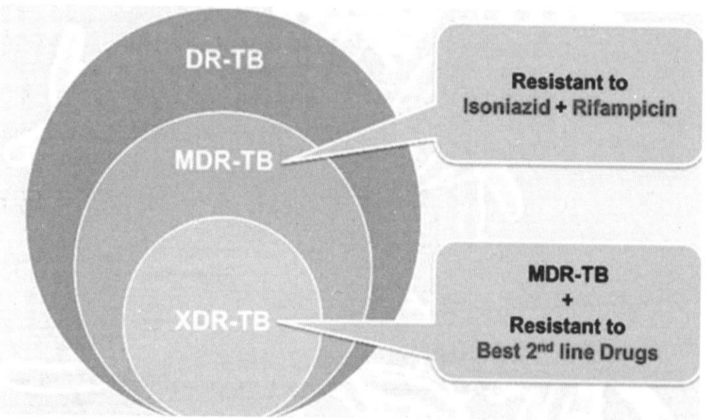

Ans. (C) i.e., At least resistance to Isoniazid and Rifampicin

29. Aortic stenosis is associated with:

(a) Pulsus paradoxus

(b) Pulsus parvus et tardus

(c) Pulsus alternates bisferens

(d) Pulsus bigeminus

EXPLANATION

Pulsus tardus et parvus, also pulsus parvus et tardus, slow rising pulse and anacrotic pulse, is a pulse with a weak/small (parvus), and late (tardus) relative to its expected characteristics. It is caused by a stiffened aortic valve that makes it progressively harder to open, thus requiring increased generation of blood pressure in the left ventricle. It is seen in aortic valve stenosis.

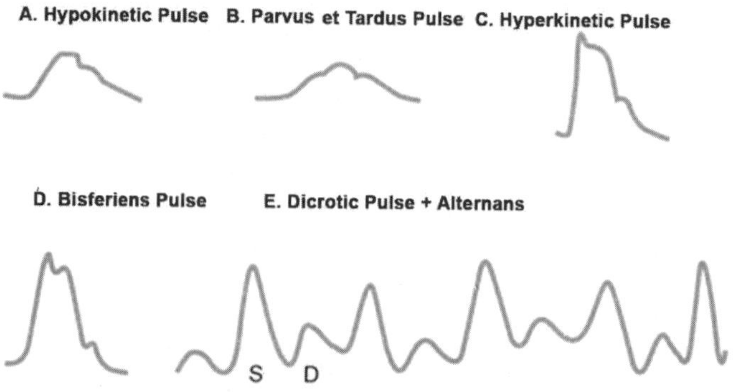

Ans. (B) i.e., Pulsus parvus et tardus

30. Which of the following is associated with hypercoagulable state?

1. Protein C deficiency 2. Antiphospholipid syndrome 3. Homocysteinemia

Select the correct answer using the code given below:

(a) 1 only (b) 2 and 3 only (c) 1 and 3 only (d) 1, 2 and 3

EXPLANATION

Hypercoagulable states

- The rare forms of congenital thrombophilia are typically caused by a deficiency of natural anticoagulants. They are classified as "type I" and are more severe in their propensity to cause thrombosis. The main ones are antithrombin III deficiency, protein C deficiency and protein S deficiency.
- A number of acquired conditions augment the risk of thrombosis. A prominent example is Antiphospholipid syndrome, which is caused by antibodies against constituents of the cell membrane, particularly lupus anticoagulant (first found in people with the disease systemic lupus erythematosus but often detected in people without the disease), anticardiolipin antibodies, and anti-beta2-glycoprotein 1 antibodies; it is therefore regarded as an autoimmune disease.
- There is an association between the blood levels of homocysteine and thrombosis, although this has not been reported consistently in all studies.

Congenital & Acquired hypercoagulable states

Congenital	Acquired
1. Protein C deficiency	1. Antiphospholipid antibody syndrome
2. Protein S deficiency	2. Malignancy
3. Antithrombin deficiency	3. Surgery/Trauma
4. Factor V leiden	4. Pregnancy/Oral contraceptives
5. Prothrombin gene G20210A mutation	5. Prolonged immobilization
6. Hyper-homocysteinemia	6. Older age
7. Dysfibrinolysis	

Ans. (D) i.e., 1, 2 and 3

31. A 20-year old male walked into outpatient department with high grade fever, cough and chest pain for one day. Chest X-ray showed consolidation of left upper zone. His respiratory rate is 22/minute, pulse rate 96/minute, BP systolic 120mmHg and blood urea 18 mg/dl. What is his CURB score?

(a) 0 (b) 1 (c) 2 (d) 3

EXPLANATION

CURB-65

Symptom	Points
Confusion	1
BUN > 7 mmol/l	1
Respiratory rate $\geq$ 30	1
SBP < 90 mmHg, DBP $\leq$ 60 mmHg	1
Age $\geq$ 65	1

Ans. (A) i.e., 0

32. Which of the following conditions is an autosomal dominant disorder?
(a) G-6PD deficiency
(b) Sickle cell disease
(c) Fanconi anaemia
(d) Marfan syndrome

EXPLANATION

Marfan syndrome/MFS is an autosomal dominant disorder. About 75% of the time, the condition is inherited from a parent, while 25% of the time it is a new mutation. It involves a mutation to the gene that makes fibrillin, which results in abnormal connective tissue. Diagnosis is often based on the Ghent criteria.

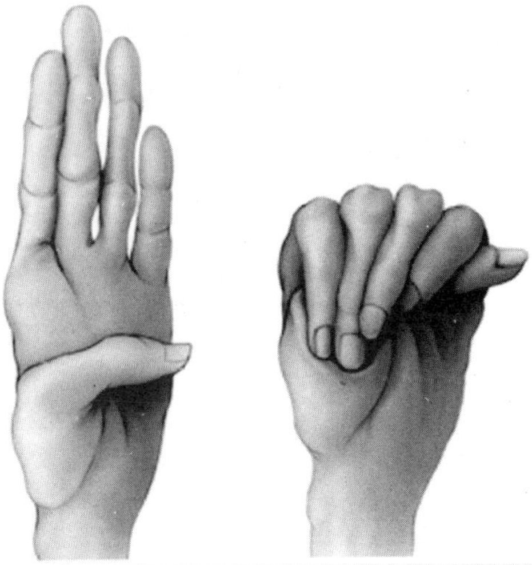

Ans. (D) i.e., Marfan syndrome

33. Consider the following statements regarding the treatment of bronchial asthma:

1. Tablets of β2 adrenoceptor agonist are better than aerosol therapy
2. Inhaled corticosteroids are contraindicated in acute severe asthma

3. **Oral steroids may be necessary for severe acute asthma**
4. **Anticholinergic bronchodilators are muscarinic antagonists**
5. **Salmeterol and formoterol are highly selective and potent long acting β2 adrenoceptor agonists**

Which of the statements given above are true?

(a) 1, 4 and 5 only (b) 3, 4 and 5 only (c) 1, 2 and 5 only (d) 1, 2 and 3 only

EXPLANATION

Treatment of bronchial asthma

- Corticosteroids are generally considered the most effective treatment available for long term control. Inhaled forms such as beclomethasone are usually used except in the case of severe persistent disease, in which oral corticosteroids may be needed.
- Ipratropium exhibits broncholytic action by reducing cholinergic influence on the bronchial musculature. It blocks muscarinic acetylcholine receptors, without specificity for subtypes, and therefore promotes the degradation of cyclic guanosine monophosphate (cGMP), resulting in a decreased intracellular concentration of cGMP.

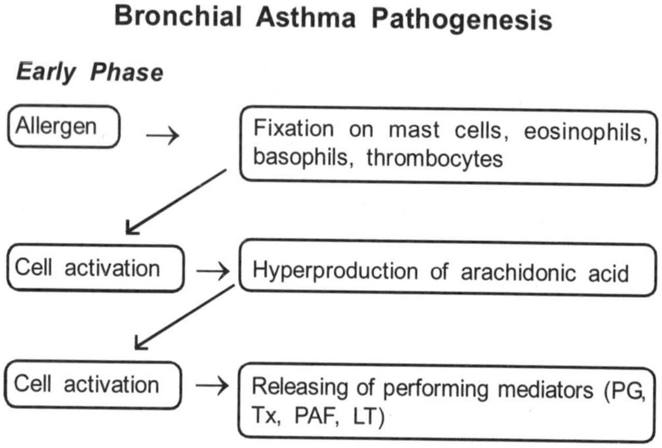

- Long acting beta-adrenoceptor agonists (LABA) such as Salmeterol and formoterol can improve asthma control, at least in adults, when given in combination with inhaled corticosteroids.

Ans. (B) i.e., 3, 4 and 5 only

2017

34. **Acute massive pulmonary embolism is manifested by the following except:**

(a) Reduced PaO_2 and reduced $PaCO_2$
(b) Pulmonary opacities in chest X-ray
(c) SIQIIITIII with RBBB in ECG
(d) Reduced cardiac output and acute right heart failure

EXPLANATION

Chest X-rays in PE are rarely normal, but usually lack signs that suggest the diagnosis of PE (for example, Westermark sign, Hampton's hump).

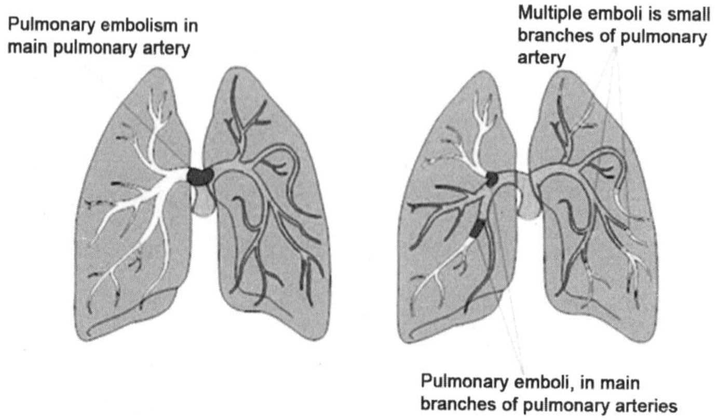

Ans. (B) i.e., Pulmonary opacities in chest X-ray

35. **The side effects of isoniazid include the following except:**

(a) Hepatitis
(b) Rash
(c) Peripheral neuropathy
(d) Hyperuricaemia

EXPLANATION

The principal drugs that contribute to hyperuricemia by decreased excretion are the primary antiuricosurics. Other drugs and agents include diuretics, salicylates, pyrazinamide, ethambutol, nicotinic acid, cyclosporin, 2-ethylamino-1, 3, 4-thiadiazole, and cytotoxic agents.

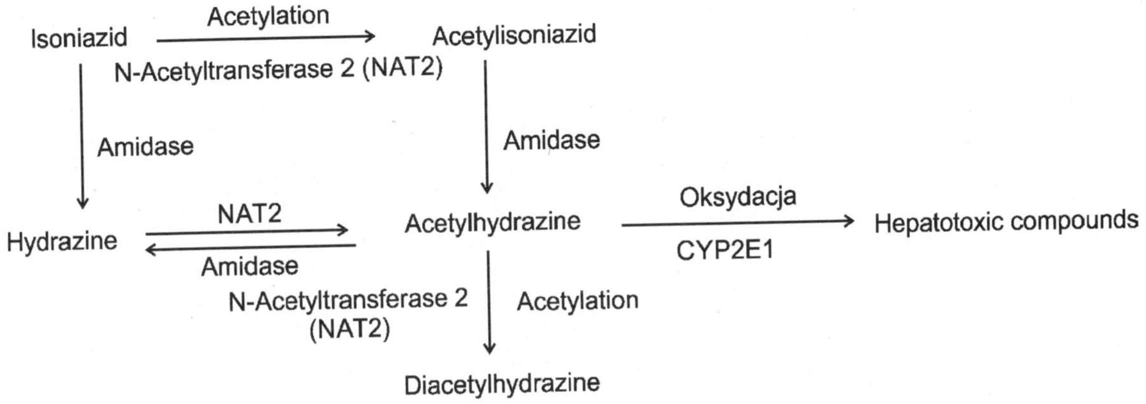

Ans. (D) i.e., Hyperuricaemia

36. **A patient of COPD develops a large pneumothorax during a violent bout of coughing. The most appropriate management would be:**

1. Simple aspiration 2. Tube thoracostomy 3. Pleurodesis

Which of the above is/are correct?

(a) 1 and 2
(b) 2 and 3
(c) 1 and 3
(d) 2 only

EXPLANATION

Management of pneumothorax

- In a larger pneumothorax, or if there is shortness of breath, the air may be removed with a syringe or a chest tube connected to a one way valve system.
- Occasionally, surgery may be required if tube drainage is unsuccessful, or as a preventive measure, if there have been repeated episodes. The surgical treatments usually involve pleurodesis (in which the layers of pleura are induced to stick together) or pleurectomy (the surgical removal of pleural membranes).

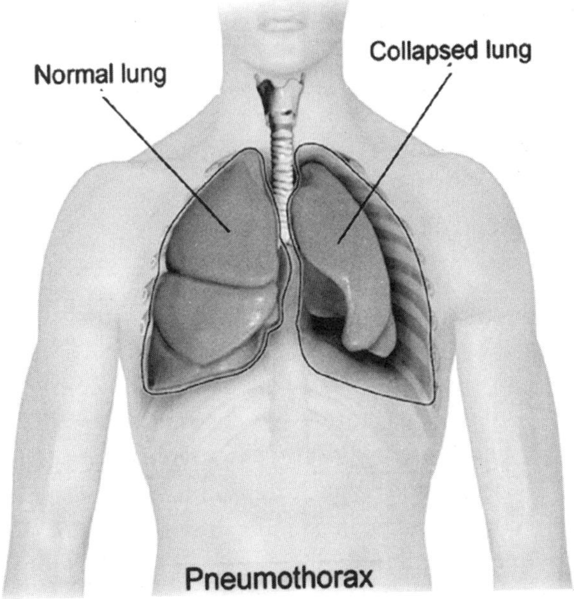

Ans. (B) i.e., 2 and 3

37. **Carbon dioxide tension ($PaCO_2$) in arterial blood at sea level is:**

(a) Less than 25mm of Hg
(b) 25–35mm of Hg
(c) 35–45mm of Hg
(d) 45–55mm of Hg

EXPLANATION

As carbon dioxide concentrations continue to increase ($PaCO_2$ > 45mmHg), a condition known as respiratory acidosis occurs. Respiratory alkalosis ($PaCO_2$ < 35mmHg) occurs when there is too little carbon dioxide in the blood.

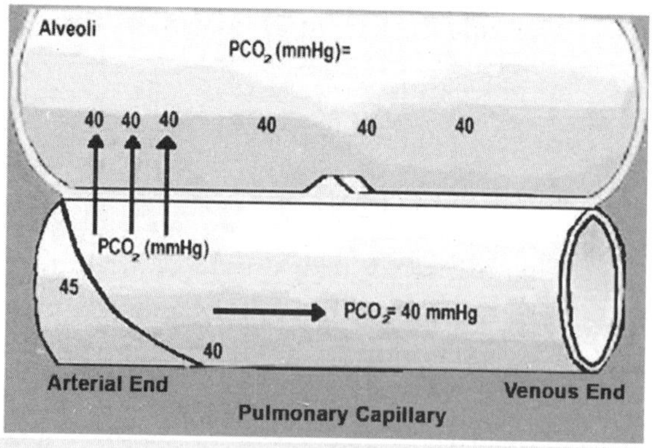

Ans. (C) i.e., 35–45 mm of Hg

38. The volume of fresh air entering the alveoli each minute is called as:

(a) Dead space
(b) Diffusing capacity
(c) Alveolar ventilation
(d) Ventilation perfusion

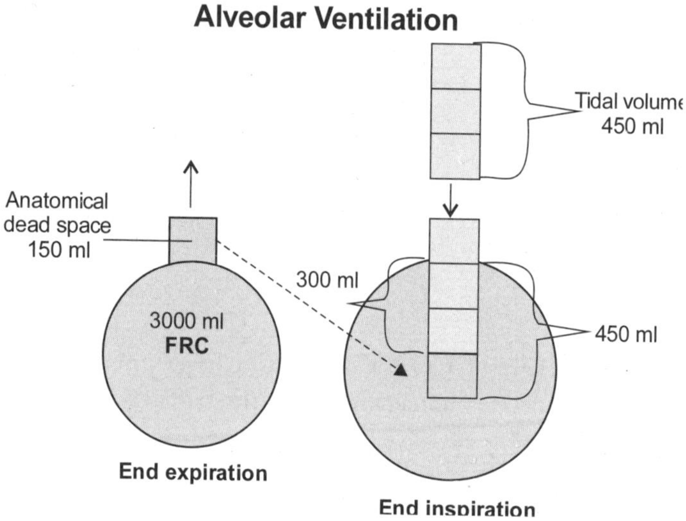

EXPLANATION

Alveolar ventilation refers to the amount of gas that reaches the **alveoli** during a breath. Deadspace **ventilation** refers to the rest of the gas taken in during a breath that stays in spaces not capable of gas exchange, like the trachea and conducting airways.

Ans. (C) i.e., Alveolar ventilation

39. Exacerbations of bronchial asthma that occur with little or no warning are called:

(a) Brittle asthma
(b) Acute severe asthma
(c) Poorly controlled asthma
(d) Nocturnal asthma

EXPLANATION

Brittle asthma is a type of **asthma** distinguishable from other forms by recurrent, severe attacks. There are two subtypes divided by symptoms: Type 1 and Type 2, depending on the stability of the patient's maximum speed of expiration, or peak expiratory flow rate (PEFR).

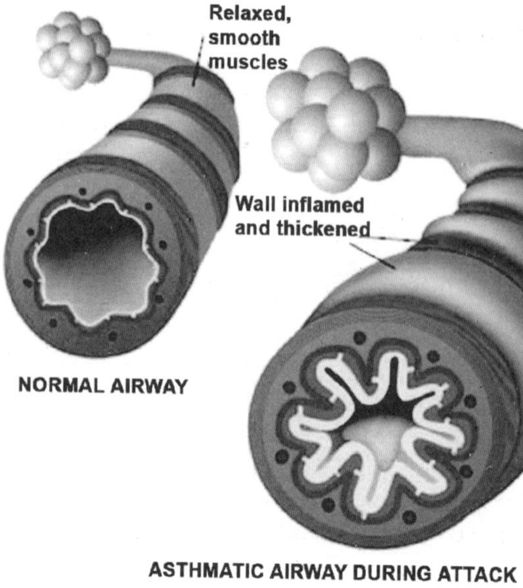

Ans. (A) i.e., Brittle asthma

2017

40. **Which of the following constituents of antacid can cause constipation?**

(a) Magnesium hydroxide (b) Aluminium hydroxide
(c) Calcium carbonate (d) Sodium bicarbonate

EXPLANATION

Aluminium hydroxide antacids can cause constipation, because the aluminium ions inhibit the contractions of smooth muscle cells in the gastrointestinal tract, slowing peristalsis and lengthening the time needed for stool to pass through the colon.

Ans. (B) i.e., Aluminium hydroxide

41. **"TIPS" procedure in the treatment of cirrhosis liver stands for:**

(a) Transvenous intrahepatic portal shunt (b) Transvenous intraabdominal portal shunt
(c) Transjugular intrahepatic portosystemic shunt (d) Transjugular intrahepatic peritoneal shunt

EXPLANATION

Transjugular intrahepatic portosystemic shunt (TIPS or TIPSS) is an artificial channel within the liver that establishes communication between the inflow portal vein and the outflow hepatic vein. It is used to treat portal hypetension (which is often due to liver cirrhosis) which frequently leads to intestinal bleeding, life threatening esophageal bleeding (esophageal varices) and the buildup of fluid within the abdomen (ascites).

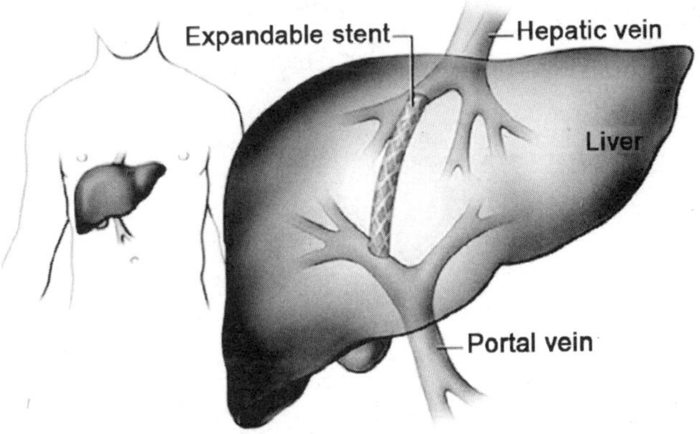

Ans. (C) i.e., Transjugular intrahepatic portosystemic shunt

42. **The drug of choice in the treatment of oesophageal candidiasis is:**

(a) Fluconazole (b) Nystatin oral suspension
(c) IV amphotericin (d) Griseofulvin

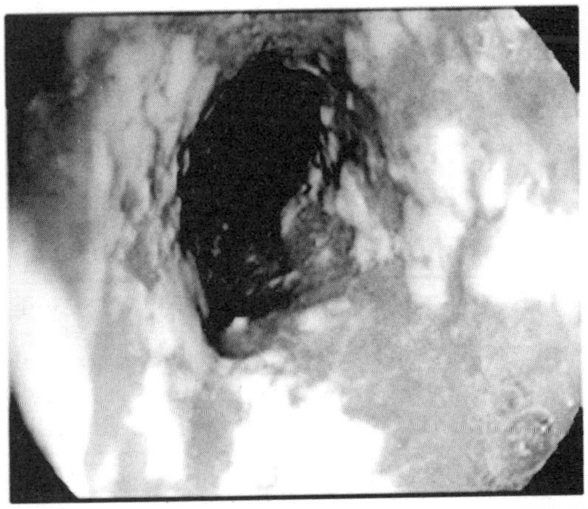

EXPLANATION

Fluconazole is an antifungal medication used for a number of fungal infections. This includes candidiasis, blastomycosis, coccidiodomycosis, cryptococcoisis, histoplasmosis, dermatophytosis, and pityriasis versicolor. It is also used to prevent candidiasis in those who are at high risk such as following organ transplantation, low birth weight babies, and those with low blood neutrophil count.

Ans. (A) i.e., Fluconazole

43. **Which of the following statements is NOT true regarding neuroleptic malignant syndrome?**

(a) Caused by haloperidol
(b) Characterized by muscle rigidity and hyperthermia
(c) There is stimulation of central dopamine receptors in hypothalamus
(d) Treated by IV dantrolene

2017

2017

EXPLANATION

In NMS, the mechanism is thought to depend on decreased levels of dopamine activity due to:

- Dopamine receptor blockade
- Genetically reduced function of dopamine receptor D_2

Clinical Features of Neuroleptic Malignant Syndrome

Hyperthermia	**Autonomic Disturbances**
(38° to 42°C)	Labile blood pressure
Neurologic Signs	Tachycardia
Rigidity	Tachypnea
Akinesia	Pallor
Dyskinesias	Incontinence
Tremors	Profuse diaphoresis
Masklike facies	Sialorrhea
Chorea	**Altered Consciousness**
Trismus	Mutism
Dystonic reactions	Stupor
Dysarthria	Obtundation
Dysphagia	Coma
Abnormal reflexes	
Opisthotonus	
Tiptoe walking	
Seizures	
Babinski responses	

Ans. (C) i.e., There is stimulation of central dopamine receptors in hypothalamus

44. Type IV renal tubular acidosis may be caused by all of the following except:

(a) Low molecular weight heparin
(b) NSAIDS
(c) Penicillin
(d) Trimethoprim

EXPLANATION

Drugs causing type IV RTA (aldosterone resistance): NSAIDs, ACE inhibitors and ARBs, Eplerenone, Spironolactone, Trimethoprim, Pentamidine.

	RTA Type I	RTA Type II	RTA Type IV
Primary defect	**Impaired ability to excrete H^+ in distal tubule**	**Impaired HCO_3 reabsorption in proximal tubule**	**Decreased secretion of aldosterone or decreased effect**
Minimum urine pH	pH > 5.5	pH < 5.5	pH < 5.5.
Stones	Yes	No	No
Hyperchloremic acidosis	Yes	Yes	Yes
Serum potassium	Low–normal	Low–normal	High
Plasma bicarbonate	< 10 meq/L	12–20 meq/L	> 17 meq/L

RTA: Renal tubular acidosis, HCO_3: Bicarbonate

Ans. (C) i.e., Penicillin

45. **Treatment options available for management of renal artery stenosis is/are:**

(a) Medical treatment for hypertension by antihypertensive drugs
(b) Angioplasty, with or without stenting
(c) Renal artery bypass surgery
(d) All of these

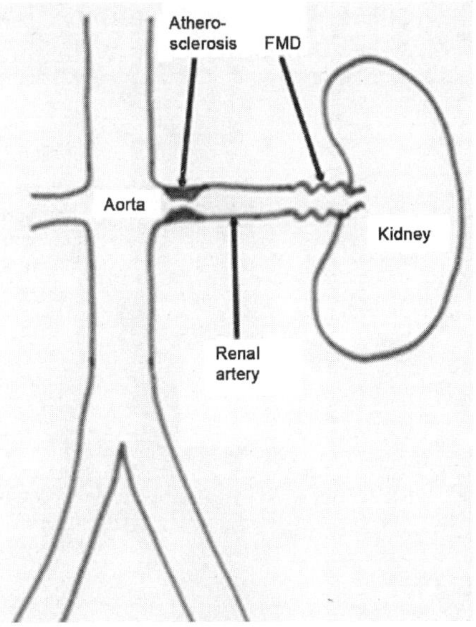

EXPLANATION

Atherosclerotic RAS is initially treated with medications, including diuretics, and medicine for control of blood pressure. When high grade renal artery stenosis is documented and blood pressure cannot be controlled with medication, or if renal function deteriorates, surgery may be resorted to. The most commonly used procedure is a minimally invasive angioplasty with or without stenting.

Ans. (D) i.e., All of these

46. **A reversible cause of dementia is:**

(a) Alzheimer disease
(b) Huntington chorea
(c) Parkinson disease
(d) Subdural haematoma

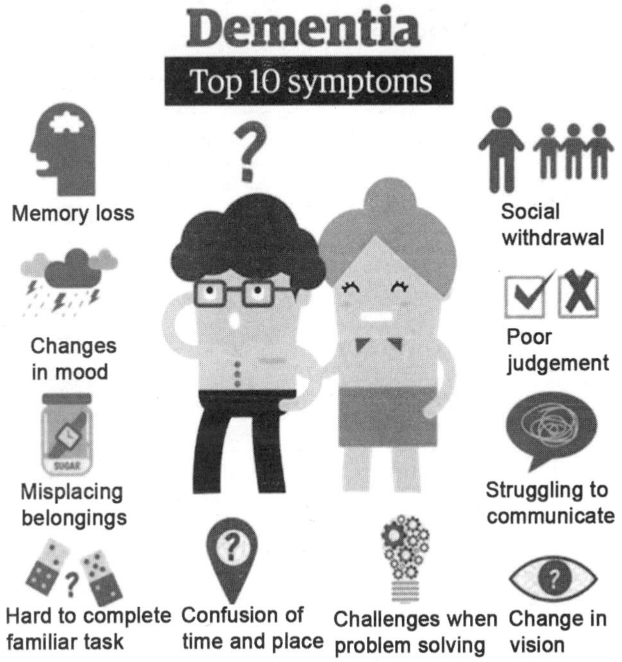

EXPLANATION

The most common type of dementia is Alzheimer's disease, which makes up 50% to 70% of cases. Other common types include vascular dementia (25%), Lewy body dementia (15%), and frontotemporal dementia. Less common causes include normal pressure hydrocephalus, Parkinson's disease, syphilis, and Creutzfeldt–Jakob disease among others. There are four main causes of easily reversible dementia: hypothyroidism, vitamin B_{12} deficiency, Lyme disease, and neurosyphillis.

Ans. (D) i.e., Subdural haematoma

47. **In Wallenberg syndrome, where is the site of lesion?**

(a) Lateral medulla
(b) Medial medulla
(c) Pontomedullary junction
(d) Dorsal midbrain

EXPLANATION

Lateral medullary syndrome is a neurological disorder causing a range of symptoms due to ischemia in the lateral part of the medulla oblongata in the brainstem. The ischemia is a result of a blockage in the posterior inferior cerebellar artery or one of its branches. Lateral medullary syndrome is also called Wallenberg syndrome, posterior inferior cerebellar artery syndrome, PICA syndrome, Vertebral artery syndrome, and Wallenberg's syndrome.

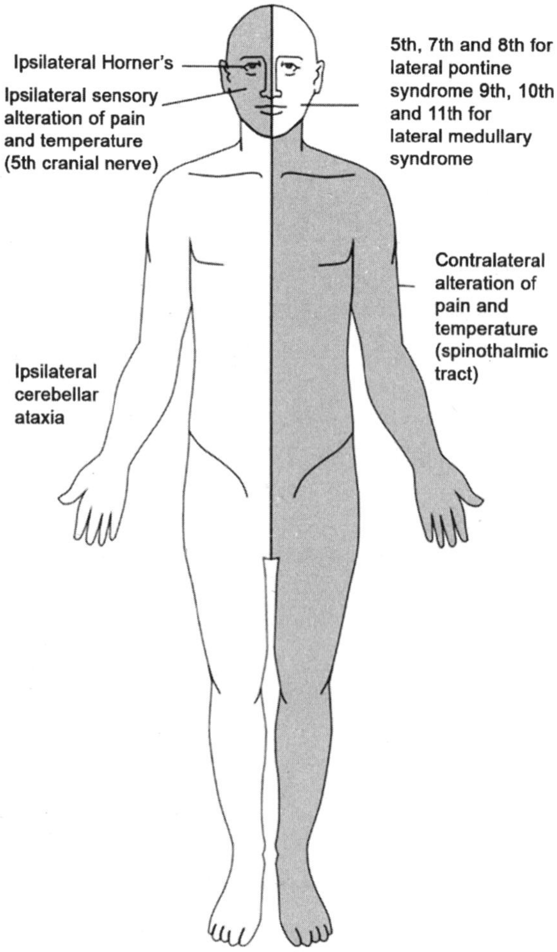

Ans. (A) i.e., Lateral medulla

48. The following are features of polycythaemia vera except:

(a) Elevated red cell mass
(b) Normal arterial oxygen saturation
(c) Splenomegaly
(d) Elevated plasma erythropoietin levels

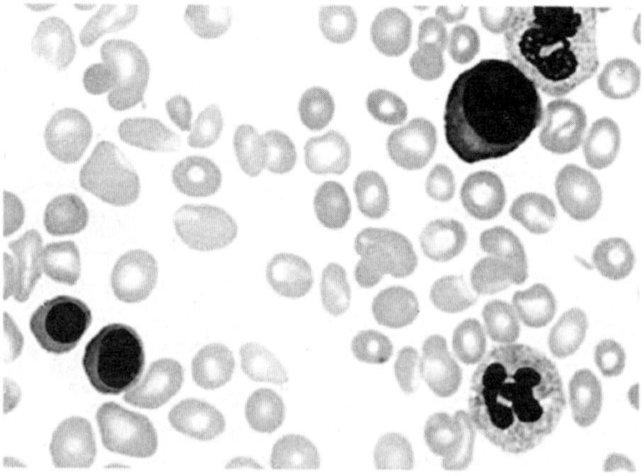

EXPLANATION

Because polycythemia vera results from an essential decrease in erythrocyte production, patients have a low erythropoietin (EPO) level.

Ans. (D) i.e., Elevated plasma erythropoietin levels

49. Which of the following conditions is associated with cigarette smoking?

(a) Non specific interstitial pneumonia
(b) Acute interstitial pneumonia
(c) Cryptogenic organizing pneumonia
(d) Desquamative interstitial pneumonia

EXPLANATION

Desquamative interstitial pneumonia is a form of idiopathic interstitial pneumonia featuring elevated levels of macrophages. Its name is derived from the former belief that these macrophages were pneumocytes that had desquamated. It is associated with patients with a history of smoking.

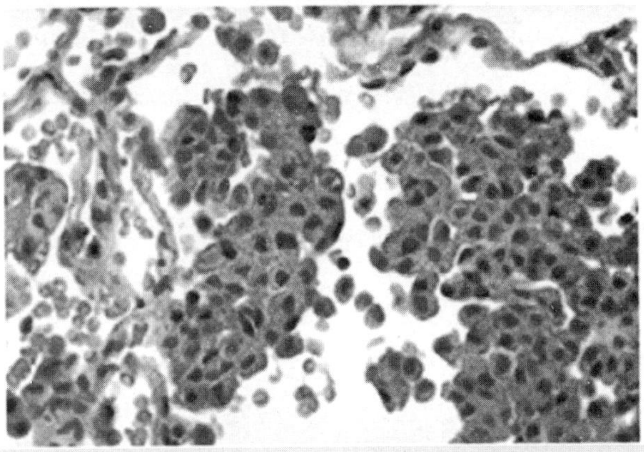

Ans. (D) i.e., Desquamative interstitial pneumonia

50. Which of the following is NOT true of Wilson disease?

(a) There is hepatolenticular degeneration
(b) Autosomal recessive transmission
(c) Serum ceruloplasmin is increased
(d) Urinary copper is increased

EXPLANATION

Levels of ceruloplasmin are abnormally low (<0.2 g/L) in 80–95% of cases of Wilson disease.

Ans. (C) i.e., Serum ceruloplasmin is increased

51. A 55-year old patient on treatment for pulmonary tuberculosis with Rifampicin, Isoniazid, Pyrazinamide and Ethambutol complain of pain in large and small joints. Which one of the following investigations will you order?

(a) Serum creatinine
(b) Serum amylase
(c) SGOT/SGPT
(d) Serum uric acid

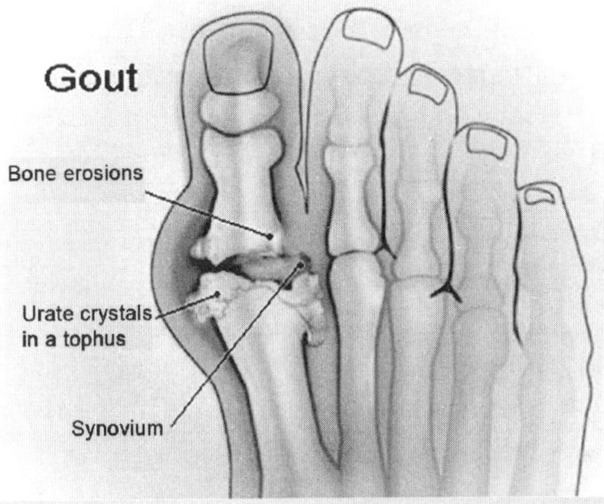

EXPLANATION

Gout is a form of inflammatory arthritis characterized by recurrent attacks of a red, tender, hot, and swollen joint. Pain typically comes on rapidly in less than twelve hours. The joint at the base of the big toe is affected in about half of cases. It may also result in tophi, kidney stones, or urate nephropathy.

Ans. (D) i.e., Serum uric acid

52. The following diseases can cause bullous lesions in the skin except:

(a) Pemphigus
(b) Impetigo
(c) Toxic epidermal necrolysis
(d) Pityriasis rosea

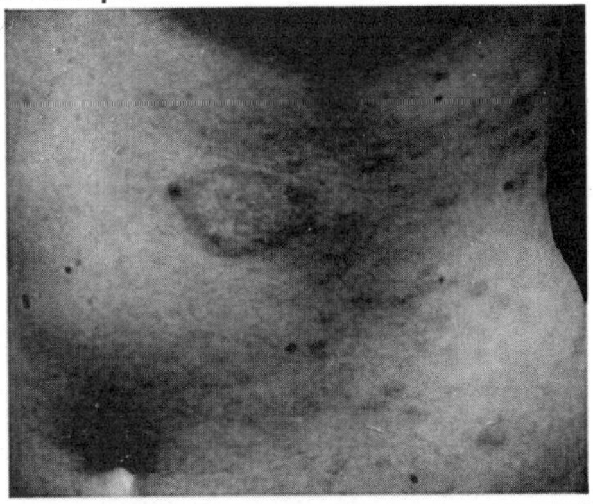

EXPLANATION

Pityriasis rosea is a type of skin rash. Classically, it begins with a single red and slightly scaly area known as a "herald patch". This is then followed, days to weeks later, by a pink whole body rash. It typically lasts less than three months and goes away without treatment.

Ans. (D) i.e., Pityriasis rosea

2017

53. **Which of the following disorder is autosomal recessive?**

(a) Cystic fibrosis
(b) Nail patella syndrome
(c) Myotonic dystrophy
(d) Huntington disease

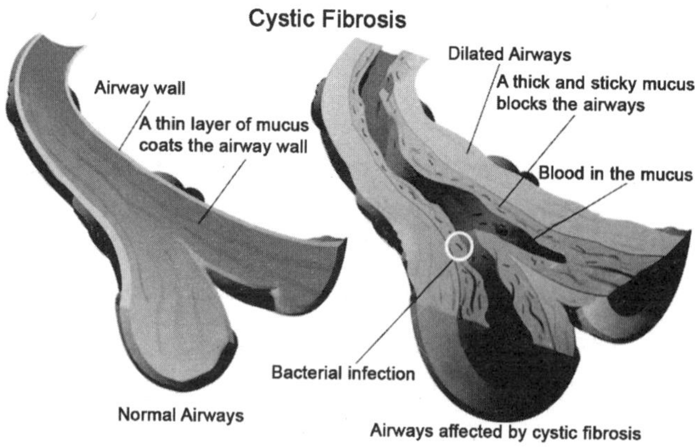

EXPLANATION

CF is inherited in an autosomal recessive manner. It is caused by the presence of mutations in both copies of the gene for the cystic fibrosis transmembrane conductance regulator (CFTR) protein.

Ans. (A) i.e., Cystic fibrosis

54. **Which one of the following is the most appropriate treatment for overdose aspirin ingestion?**

(a) Acetazolamide
(b) Sodium bicarbonate
(c) Allopurinol
(d) N-acetyl-cysteine

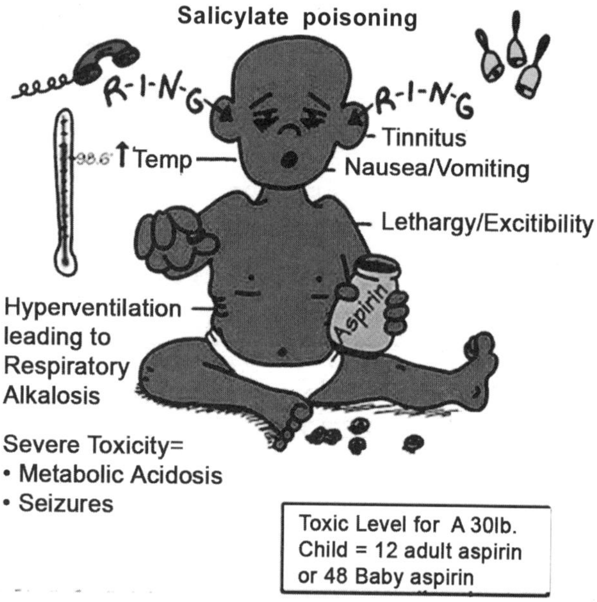

EXPLANATION

Toxicity of aspirin is managed with a number of potential treatments, including activated charcoal, intravenous dextrose and normal saline, sodium bicarbonate, and dialysis. The diagnosis of poisoning usually involves measurement of plasma salicylate, the active metabolite of aspirin, by automated spectrophotometric methods. Plasma salicylate levels in general range from 30–100 mg/l after usual therapeutic doses, 50–300 mg/l in people taking high doses and 700–1400 mg/l following acute overdose.

Ans. (B) i.e., Sodium bicarbonate

55. **Killer T cells which are responsible for defence against intracellular pathogen are expressed by which of the following CD phenotypes?**

(a) CD 2 (b) CD 5
(c) CD 8 (d) CD 10

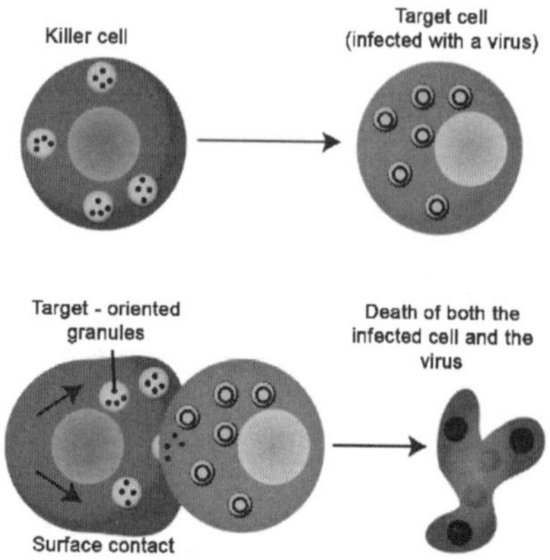

EXPLANATION

Natural killer T-cells/NKT cells include both NK 1.1$^+$ and NK1.1$^-$, as well as CD4$^+$, CD4$^-$, CD8$^+$ and CD8$^-$ cells.

Ans. (C) i.e., CD 8

56. **Intravenous immunoglobulin therapy is approved in the following conditions except:**

(a) Kawasaki disease
(b) Severe rheumatoid arthritis
(c) Guillain Barre syndrome
(d) Dermatomyositis

EXPLANATION

The goals of treatment of rheumatoid arthritis/RA are to reduce pain, decrease inflammation, and improve a person's overall functioning. This may be helped by balancing rest and exercise, the use of splints and braces, or the use of assistive devices. Pain medications, steroids, and NSAIDs are frequently used to help with symptoms. Disease modifying antirheumatic drugs (DMARDs), such as hydroxychloroquine and methotrexate, may be used to try to slow the progression of disease.

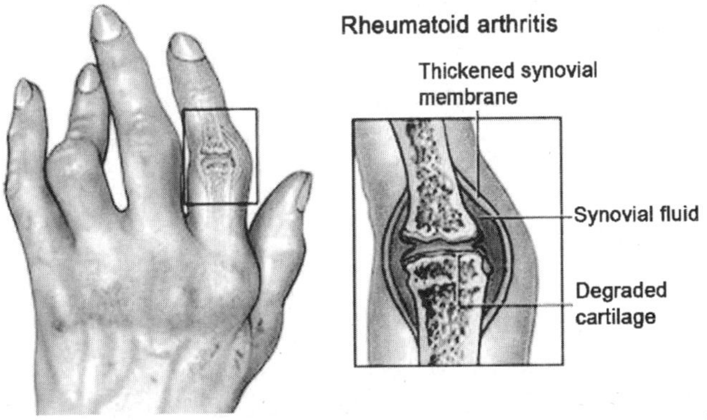

Ans. (B) i.e., Severe rheumatoid arthritis

57. **Which of the following does NOT cause small vessel vasculitis?**

(a) Churg Strauss Syndrome
(b) Henoch Schonlein purpura
(c) Kawasaki disease
(d) Granulomatosis with polyangiitis

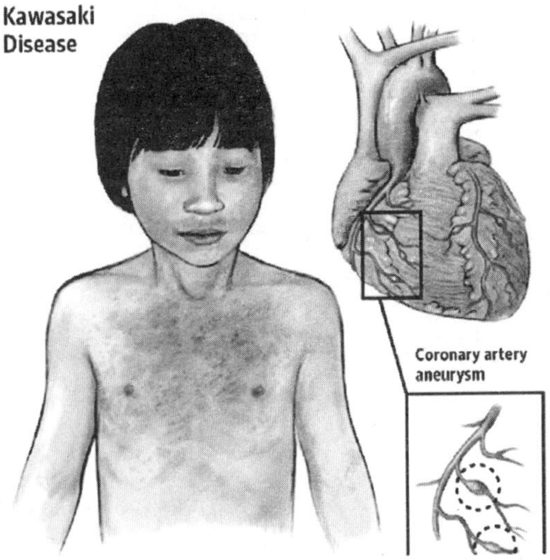

EXPLANATION

Kawasaki disease complications have been described, such as aneurysm of other arteries: aortic aneurysm, with a higher number of reported cases involving the abdominal aorta, axillary artery aneurysm, brachiocephalic artery aneurysm, aneurysm of iliac and femoral arteries, and renal artery aneurysm. Other vascular complications can occur such as increased wall thickness and decreased distensibility of carotid arteries, aorta, and brachioradial artery.

Ans. (C) i.e., Kawasaki disease

58. **Most common cells in peripheral blood smear of chronic myeloid leukemia are:**

(a) Myeloblasts
(b) Promyelocytes
(c) Metamyelocytes
(d) Neutrophils

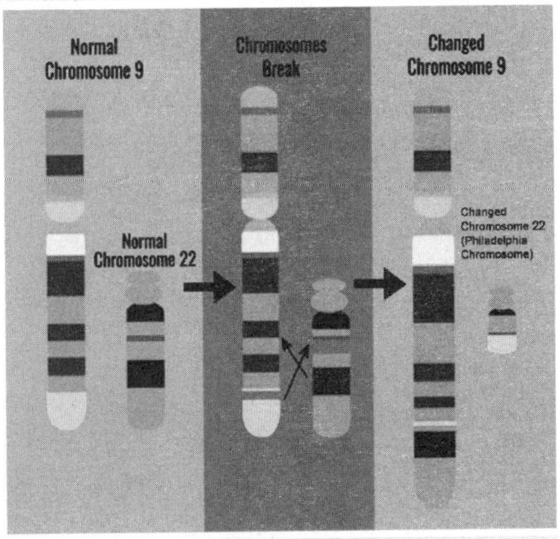

EXPLANATION

CML is often suspected on the basis of a complete blood count, which shows increased granulocytes of all types, typically including mature myeloid cells. Basophils and eosinophils are almost universally increased; this feature may help differentiate CML from a leukemoid reaction.

Ans. (D) i.e., Neutrophils

59. Consider the following statements about infective endocarditis:

1. Modified Duke criteria are used for clinical diagnosis
2. Echocardiographic findings form one of the major Duke criteria
3. Presence of one major and two minor criteria is considered as diagnostic of endocarditis
4. Presence of glomerulonephritis is a minor Duke criterion

Which of the statements given above are correct?

(a) 1, 2 and 3 only (b) 1, 2 and 4 only (c) 3 and 4 only (d) 1, 2, 3 and 4

EXPLANATION

Infective endocarditis

- Established in 1994 by the Duke Endocarditis Service and revised in 2000, the Duke criteria are a collection of major and minor criteria used to establish a diagnosis of infective endocarditis. According to the Duke criteria, diagnosis of infective endocarditis can be definite, possible, or rejected.
- Evidence of endocardial involvement with positive echocardiogram is a major criteria
- Immunological problems is a minor criteria: glomerulonephritis, Osler's nodes, Roth's spots, Rheumatoid factor

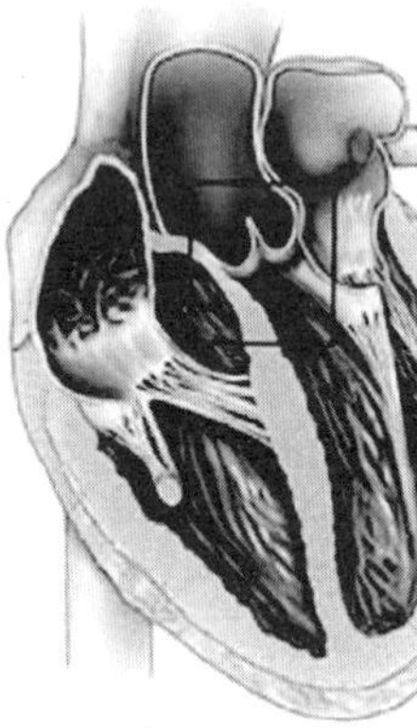
Cross section of the heart

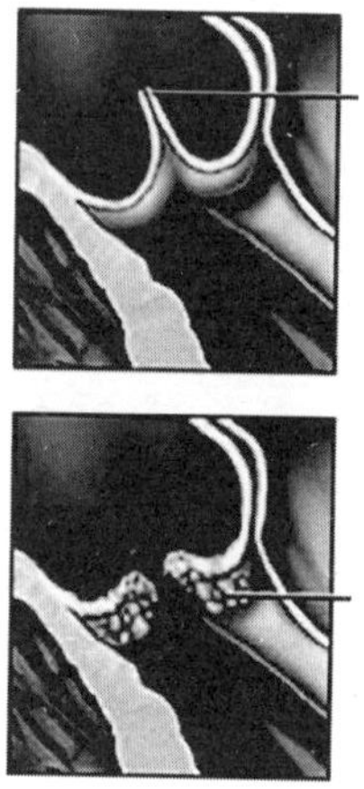

Ans. (B) i.e., 1, 2 and 4 only

60. A 16-year old had an acute episode of dyspnoea, wheezing and coughing during early morning hours. The episode resolved spontaneously. What is the likely diagnosis?

(a) Pulmonary oedema (b) Asthma (c) Panic attack (d) Pneumonia

EXPLANATION

Asthma is characterized by recurrent episodes of wheezing, shortness of breath, chest tightness, and coughing. Sputum may be produced from the lung by coughing but is often hard to bring up. During recovery from an attack, it may appear pus like due to high levels of white blood cells called eosinophils. Symptoms are usually worse at night and in the early morning or in response to exercise or cold air.

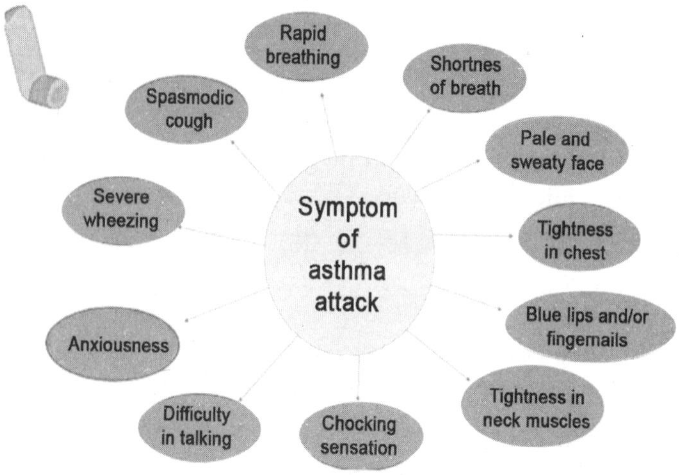

Ans. (B) i.e., Asthma

61. An elderly patient had cerebrovascular accident which was diagnosed as ischaemic in nature. Which of the following is a contraindication for thrombolysis?

1. Onset of symptoms to time of drug administration is ≤ 4.5 hours
2. Gastrointestinal bleeding in preceding 21 days

Select the correct answer using the code given below:

(a) 1 only (b) 2 only (c) Both 1 and 2 (d) Neither 1 nor 2

EXPLANATION

Absolute contraindications to thrombolytic therapy include dissecting aortic aneurysm, pericarditis, stroke, or neurosurgical procedures within 6 months or known **intracranial neoplasm.** Relative contraindications include major surgery or **bleeding** within 6 weeks, known **bleeding** diathesis, and severe uncontrolled hypertension.

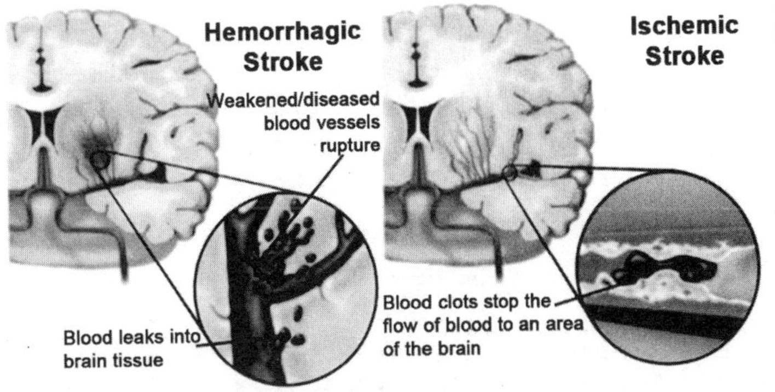

Ans. (B) i.e., 2 only

62. Consider the following insulin preparations:

1. Aspart 2. Glulisine 3. Detemir 4. Regular

Which of the above are considered short acting insulin?

(a) 1 and 2 only
(b) 3 and 4 only
(c) 1, 2 and 4 only
(d) 1, 2, 3 and 4

EXPLANATION

Fast acting insulin

- *Rapid Acting Insulin Analogs* (Insulin Aspart, insulin Lyspro, Insulin Glulisine) which have an onset of action of 5 to 15 minutes, peak effect in 1 to 2 hours and duration of action that lasts 4–6 hours.
- *Regular Human Insulin* which has an onset of action of 1/2 hour to 1 hour, peak effect in 2 to 4 hours, and duration of action of 6 to 8 hours.

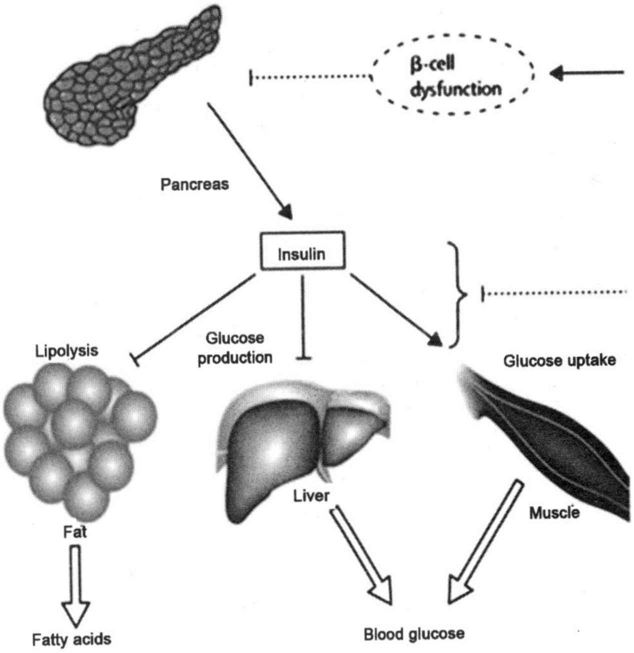

Ans. (C) i.e., 1, 2 and 4 only

63. A middle aged male known smoker presented with recurrent sinusitis, haemoptysis, haematuria, arthralgia and palpable purpura. What is the most likely diagnosis?

(a) Wegener granulomatosis
(b) Goodpasture syndrome
(c) Polyarteritis nodosa
(d) Systemic lupus erythematosus

EXPLANATION

Wegener granulomatosis/Granulomatosis with polyangiitis (GPA)

- Initial signs are extremely variable, and diagnosis can be severely delayed due to the nonspecific nature of the symptoms. In general, rhinitis is the first sign in most people
- Lungs: pulmonary nodules (referred to as "coin lesions"), infiltrates (often interpreted as pneumonia), cavitary lesions, pulmonary haemorrhage causing haemoptysis, and rarely bronchial stenosis.
- Kidney: rapidly progressive glomerulonephritis (75%), leading to chronic kidney failure
- Arthritis: Pain or swelling (60%), often initially diagnosed as rheumatoid arthritis
- Skin: subcutaneous nodules (granulomas) on the elbow, purpura, various others

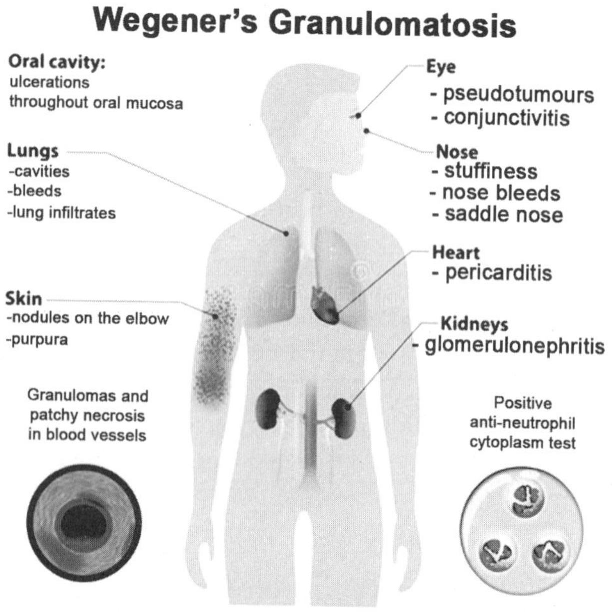

Ans. (A) i.e., Wegener granulomatosis

2017

64. **A patient presents with diarrhoea, steatorrhea and weight loss. Which of the following diseases is LEAST possible?**

(a) Whipple disease (b) Tropical sprue
(c) Celiac disease (d) Menetrier disease

EXPLANATION

Individuals with the Menetrier disease present with upper abdominal pain (epigastric), at times accompanied by nausea, vomiting, loss of appetite, edema, and weight loss. A small amount of gastrointestinal bleeding may occur, which is typically due to superficial mucosal erosions; large volume bleeding is rare. 20% to 100% of patients, depending on time of presentation, develop a protein losing gastropathy accompanied by low blood albumin and edema

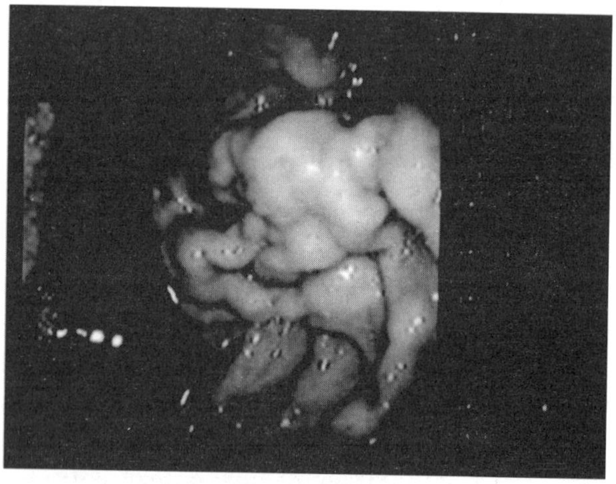

Menetrier's disease

Ans. (D) i.e., Menetrier disease

65. **Consider the following statements regarding post streptococcal glomerulonephritis (PSGN) :**

1. Immunosupressive therapy is effective
2. PSGN develops one to three weeks after streptococcal pharyngitis
3. PSGN develops two to six weeks after impetigo
4. The classic presentation is acute nephritis

Which of the statements given above are correct?

(a) 1, 2 and 3 only (b) 2, 3 and 4 only
(c) 1 and 4 only (d) 1, 2, 3 and 4

EXPLANATION

Post streptococcal glomerulonephritis

- Acute proliferative glomerulonephritis (post streptococcal glomerulonephritisis) is caused by an infection with streptococcus bacteria, usually three weeks after infection, usually of the pharynx or the skin, given the time required to raise antibodies and complement proteins.
- Among the signs and symptoms of acute proliferative glomerulonephritis are the following:
- Hematuria
- Oliguria
- Edema
- Hypertension
- Fever (headache, malaise, anorexia, nausea).

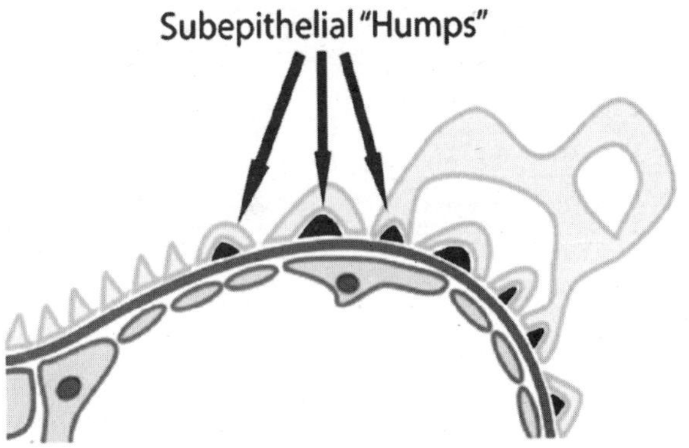

Acute Post-Strep GN

Ans. (B) i.e., 2, 3 and 4 only

66. A patient with long term implantable cardioverter defibrillator device developed neck and facial swelling, hoarseness of voice, nasal congestion, dysphagia and haemoptysis.

The facial swelling increased on supine position. This patient most likely developed:

(a) Cardiac tamponade
(b) Intracardiac thrombosis
(c) Superior vena cava obstruction
(d) Pulmonary thromboembolism

2017

EXPLANATION

Superior vena cava syndrome

- Shortness of breath is the most common symptom, followed by face or arm swelling.
- Difficulty breathing
- Headache
- Facial swelling
- Venous distention in the neck and distended veins in the upper chest and arms
- Upper limb edema
- Lightheadedness
- Cough
- Edema (swelling) of the neck, called the *collar of Stokes*

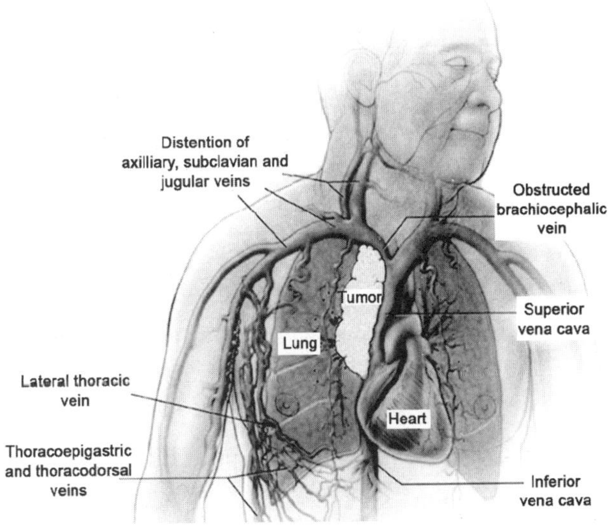

Ans. (C) i.e., Superior vena cava obstruction

67. A patient of AIDS developed ophthalmoplegia, ataxia and global confusion. He is likely to have the deficiency of:

(a) Biotin (b) Niacin
(c) Pyridoxine (d) Thiamine

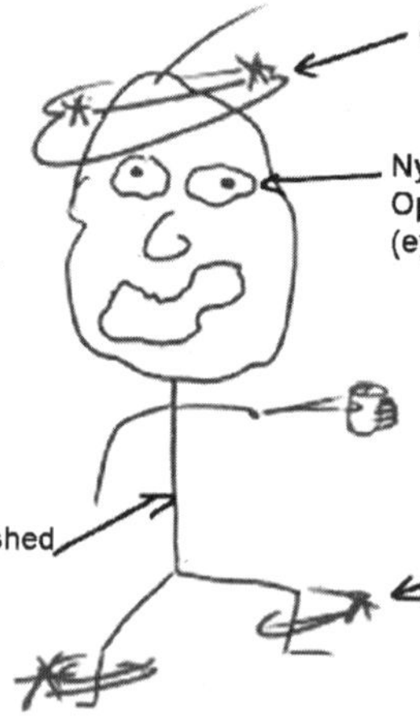

EXPLANATION

Wernicke encephalopathy (WE) also **Wernicke's encephalopathy** is the presence of neurological symptoms caused by biochemical lesions of the central nervous system after exhaustion of B-vitamin reserves, in particular thiamine (vitamin B_1). Classically, Wernicke encephalopathy is characterised by the triad – ophthalmoplegia, ataxia, and confusion. However, only 10% of patients exhibit all three features, and other symptoms may also be present.

Ans. (D) i.e., Thiamine

68. **An elderly male presents with persistent productive cough with large volume purulent sputum production. He has had several episodes in the past. He also had digital clubbing. He is a case of:**

(a) Empyema (b) Bronchiectasis
(c) Bronchopneumonia (d) Necrotising pneumonia

EXPLANATION

Some people with bronchiectasis may have a cough productive of frequent green/yellow mucus (sputum), up to 240ml (8 oz) daily. Bronchiectasis may also present with coughing up blood (hemoptysis) in the absence of sputum, called "dry bronchiectasis". Sputum production may also occur without coloration. People with bronchiectasis may have bad breath indicative of active infection. Frequent bronchial infections and breathlessness are two possible indicators of bronchiectasis. Crepitations and expiratory rhonchi may be heard on auscultation. Nail clubbing is rare.

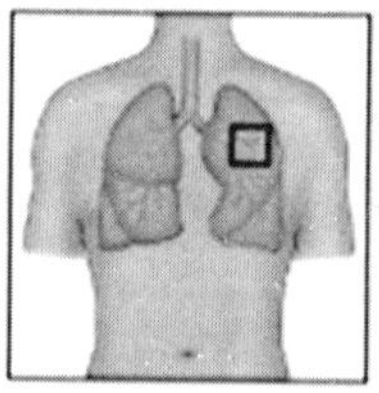

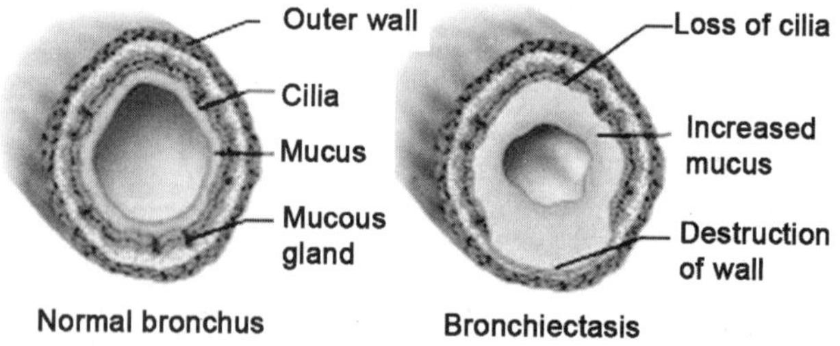

Ans. (B) i.e., Bronchiectasis

69. **A chemical factory worker has acute onset dyspnoea with fever, chills, and malaise, following a few hours of exposure to a new chemical. These symptoms resolve in four to five days after removal from exposure. He is likely to have:**

(a) Hypersensitivity pneumonitis
(b) Atypical pneumonia
(c) Cryptogenic organising pneumonia
(d) Non specific interstitial pneumonia

EXPLANATION

Hypersensitivity pneumonitis (HP; also called **allergic alveolitis**, **bagpipe lung**, or **extrinsic allergic alveolitis**, EAA) is an inflammation of the alveoli within the lung caused by hypersensitivity to inhaled organic dusts. Sufferers are commonly exposed to the dust by their occupation or hobbies. In the acute form of HP, symptoms may develop 4–6 hours following heavy exposure to the provoking antigen. Symptoms include fever, chills, malaise, cough, chest tightness, dyspnea, rash, swelling and headache. Symptoms resolve within 12 hours to several days upon cessation of exposure.

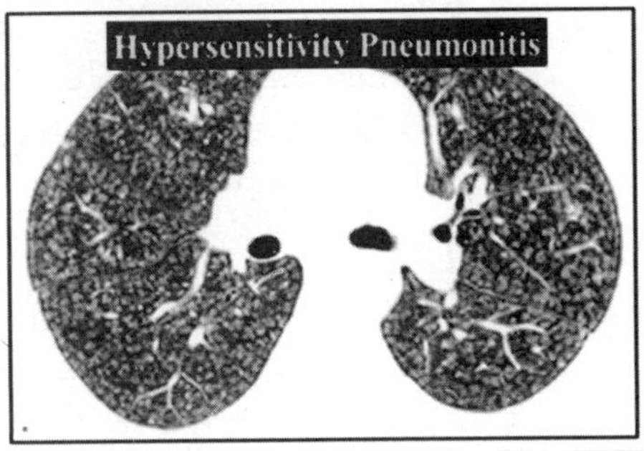

Ans. (A) i.e., Hypersensitivity pneumonitis

70. A 25-year old man presents with nausea, vomiting and diarrhoea with crampy abdominal pain. He gives history of consumption of rice preparation in his last meal. What is the likely organism causing the above complaints?

(a) Clostridium perfringens
(b) Bacillus cereus
(c) Staphylococcus aureus
(d) Campylobacter jejuni

EXPLANATION

The 'emetic' form of Bacillus foodborne illness is commonly caused by rice cooked for a time and temperature insufficient to kill any spores present, then improperly refrigerated. It can produce a toxin, cereulide, which is not inactivated by later reheating. This form leads to nausea and vomiting one to five hours after consumption. It can be difficult to distinguish from other short term bacterial foodborne intoxications such as by *Staphylococcus aureus.*

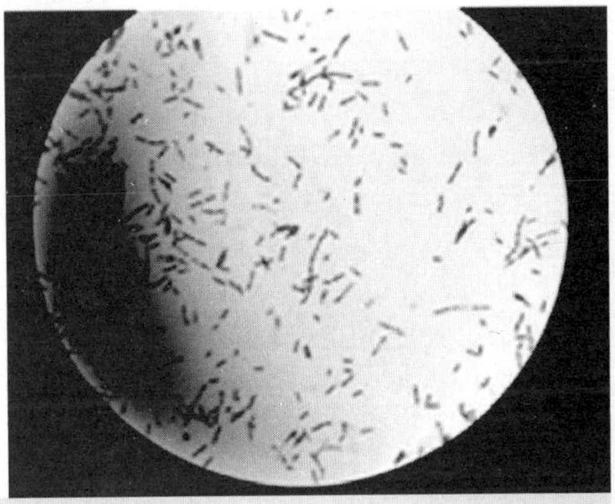

Ans. (B) i.e., *Bacillus cereus*

2017

71. A five year old child was diagnosed with nephrotic syndrome, 18 months back. He was treated and successfully went into remission at that time. Following, the initial episode, the child has had 3 relapses, each of which was successfully treated with oral prednisolone (60mg/m 2/24h) until remission, followed by 40mg/m 2 single dose, alternate days for four weeks. What is the diagnosis?

(a) Nephrotic syndrome, infrequent relapses
(b) Nephrotic syndrome, frequent relapses
(c) Nephrotic syndrome, steroid dependent
(d) Nephrotic syndrome, steroid resistant

EXPLANATION

Infrequent relapser **nephrotic syndrome**: Patients having less than two **relapses** within 6 months or less than four **relapses** within 12 months of response.

Definitions, derived from international study of kidney disease in children (ISKDC)

Relapse	: Urinary proteins ++ or more with albustix on 3 consecutive days.
Frequent relapses	: Two or more relapses within six months of initial response or four or more relapses within any 12 months period.
Steroid dependence	: Two consecutive relapses occurring during corticosteroid treatment or within 14 days after its cessation.
Steroid resistance	: Failure to achieve response in spite of 4 weeks of treatment with prednisolone (60 mg/M sq/day).
Remission	: Urinary protein = 0/trace on albustix on three consecutive days.

Ans. (A) i.e., Nephrotic syndrome, infrequent relapses

72. A 7-year old girl presents to you with non specific abdominal pain, mild abdominal distension, and not growing well. The child weighs 14kg and height is 95cm. Systemic examination is normal. The haemoglobin was 7.5g/dL (microcytic hypochromic RBCs) and has not responded to iron therapy. Which of the following will be the first investigation you will like to do for diagnosing the condition?

(a) Bone marrow aspiration
(b) Tissue transglutaminase antibodies
(c) Lower GI contrast examination
(d) Colonoscopy/sigmoidoscopy

EXPLANATION

Coeliac disease, also spelled **celiac disease**, is a long term autoimmune disorder that primarily affects the small intestine. Classic symptoms include gastrointestinal problems such as chronic diarrhoea, abdominal distention, malabsorption, loss of appetite and among children failure to grow normally. This often begins between six months and two years of age. Non classic symptoms are more common, especially in people older than two years. For most children and adults, the best way to screen for celiac disease is with the Tissue Transglutaminase IgA antibody, plus an IgA antibody in order to ensure that the patient generates enough of this antibody to render the celiac disease test accurate.

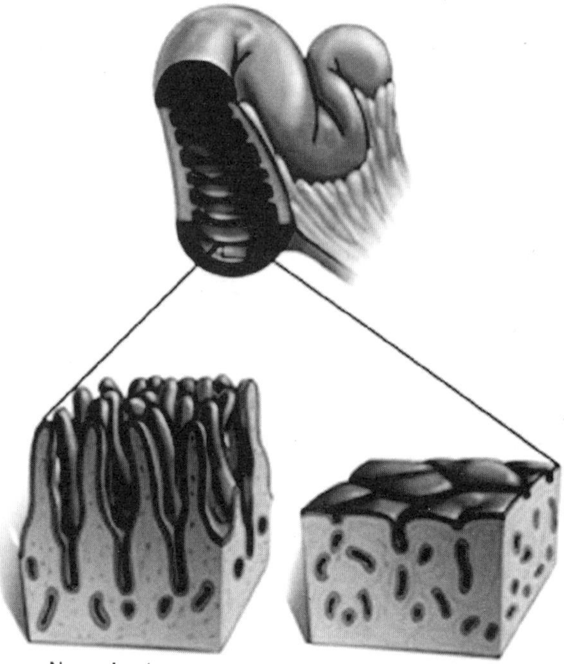

Ans. (B) i.e., Tissue transglutaminase antibodies

73. **A seven year old boy weighing 20 kg presented with bleeding from upper GI tract (haemetemasis) for last 18 hours. On examination, PR-86/m, RR-16/m and BP-100/70mmHg; and spleen is palpable 5 cm below costal margin. There is no other abnormality. Liver function tests are normal. What is the next best step in management?**

(a) Fluid resuscitation with crystalloids
(b) Intravenous vasopressin
(c) Intravenous propranolol
(d) Transdermal nitroglycerine

EXPLANATION

Esophageal varices result can from portal hypertension, regardless of the age group. The increased resistance to blood flow through the portal system is due to prehepatic, intrahepatic, and suprahepatic obstruction, but the most common causes of portal hypertension in children include portal vein thrombosis (prehepatic) and biliary atresia (intrahepatic).

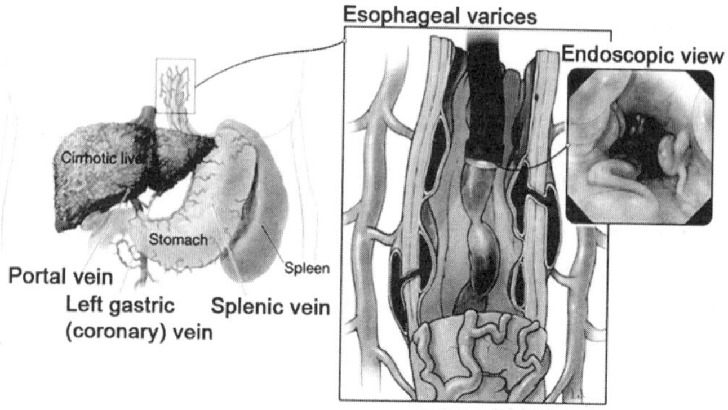

Ans. (B) i.e., Intravenous vasopressin

74. A seven years old girl presents in emergency room with hypertension, lethargy, headache, seizures, and visual disturbances. Fundus examination reveals haemorrhages and exudates. Which of the following treatment regimen will be the most appropriate for this child?

(a) Sublingual nifedipine
(b) Intravenous labetalol infusion
(c) Intravenous minoxidi
(d) Furosemide

EXPLANATION

Labetalol is effective in the management of hypertensive emergencies, postoperative hypertension, pheochromocytoma associated hypertension, and rebound hypertension from beta blocker withdrawal.

Classification of β-blockers

	Non-selective	β_1-selective
No Intrinsic Sympathomimetic Activity (ISA)	• Tertalol • **Propranolol** • Timolo • Sotalol • Nadolol	• **Atenolol** • Bisoprolol • Betaxolol • Esmolol • **Metoprolol** • **(Nebivolol)** • Bevantolol
Intrinsic Sympathomimetic Activity (ISA)	• Alprenolol • Pindolol • Oxprenolol • Carteolol • Penbutalol	• Acebutolol • Celiprolol
Hydrophilic	• Nadolol • Sotalol	• **Atenolol** • Celiprolol
With Alpha blocking activity	• Labetalol • **Carvedilol** • Bucindolol	

Ans. (B) i.e., Intravenous labetalol infusion

2017

75. On routine newborn screening at day 3 of life, the baby was found to have TSH level 40mU/L. What should be the next step?

(a) Repeat thyroid profile within one week
(b) Start child on thyroxine immediately
(c) Repeat thyroid profile after four weeks
(d) Repeat thyroid profile/start thyroxine, if the child has clinical features of congenital hypothyroidism, otherwise wait and watch

EXPLANATION

TSH concentrations in children are normally higher than in adults. In 2002, the NACB recommended age related reference limits starting from about 1.3 to 19μIU/mL for normal term infants at birth, dropping to 0.6–10μIU/mL at 10 weeks old, 0.4–7.0μIU/mL at 14 months and gradually dropping during childhood and puberty to adult levels, 0.3–3.0μIU/mL

Classification of Congenital Hypothyroidism

- **Permanent Congenital Hyperthyroidism**

  Thyroid Dysgenesis
  - — Athyrosis
  - — Dystopic or ectopic thyroid
  - — Thyroid hypoplasia

  Thyroid dyshormonogenesis
  - — Iodide transport defects
  - — Iodide organification defects
  - — Thyroglobulin synthesis defects
  - — Iodotyrosine deiodinase defects

  Thyrotropin resistance syndromes

  Thyroid hormone resistance syndromes

  Thyrotropin or thyroid releasing hormone deficiency
- **Transient Congenital Hypothyroidism**

  Prenatal use of iodine-containing drugs and compounds
  - — Potassium iodide (asthma)
  - — Povidone-iodine (disinfection)
  - — Amidarone (arrhythmia)
  - — Contrast agents (amniofetography)

  Postnatal use of iodine-containing compounds
  - — Povidone-iodine
  - —Radiographic contrast agents

  Maternal antithyroid drugs

  Maternal antithyroid antibodies

Ans. (A) i.e., Repeat thyroid profile within one week

2017

76. A five year old girl is brought to you with history of fever for seven days associated with rash, anorexia, myalgia and petechial haemorrhages. Which of the following investigations will be most appropriate for making a diagnosis of dengue fever?

(a) Detection of NS1 antigen
(b) Platelet count
(c) IgG capture ELISA
(d) Detection of IgM antibodies for dengue

EXPLANATION

Detection of NS1 during the febrile phase of a primary infection may be greater than 90% sensitive however is only 60–80% in subsequent infections. Tests for dengue virus-specific antibodies, types IgG and IgM, can be useful in confirming a diagnosis in the later stages of the infection. Both IgG and IgM are produced after 5–7 days. The highest levels (titres) of IgM are detected following a primary infection, but IgM is also produced in reinfection. IgM becomes undetectable 30–90 days after a primary infection, but earlier following re-infections.

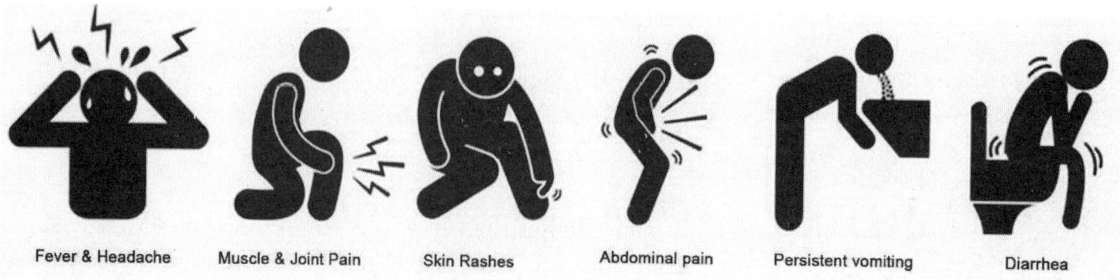

Ans. (D) i.e., Detection of IgM antibodies for dengue

77. An eight year old boy was diagnosed to have *P.vivax* malaria and was treated with appropriate dosages of chloroquine. The fever subsided but recurred after 3 weeks. Peripheral smear was again positive for P.vivax. This child should now be treated as a case with

(a) Relapse
(b) Recrudescence
(c) Either relapse/recrudescence
(d) Fresh infection

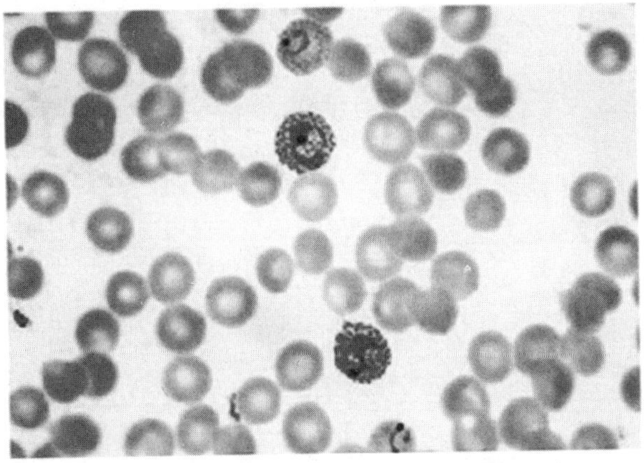

EXPLANATION

The *Plasmodium* parasites, which are responsible for malaria, can persist in the blood without causing apparent symptoms for a few months (recrudescence). Relapse in this context occurs due to activation of hypnozoites in the liver.

Ans. (C) i.e., Either relapse/recrudescence

78. **A two day old neonate is brought with cyanosis, single second heart sound, and pansystolic murmur on the left sternal border. ECG reveals left axis deviation, right atrial overload and left ventricular hypertrophy. What is the most likely diagnosis?**

(a) Tetrology of Fallot
(b) Tricuspid atresia
(c) Transposition of great arteries
(d) Total anomalous pulmonary venous connection

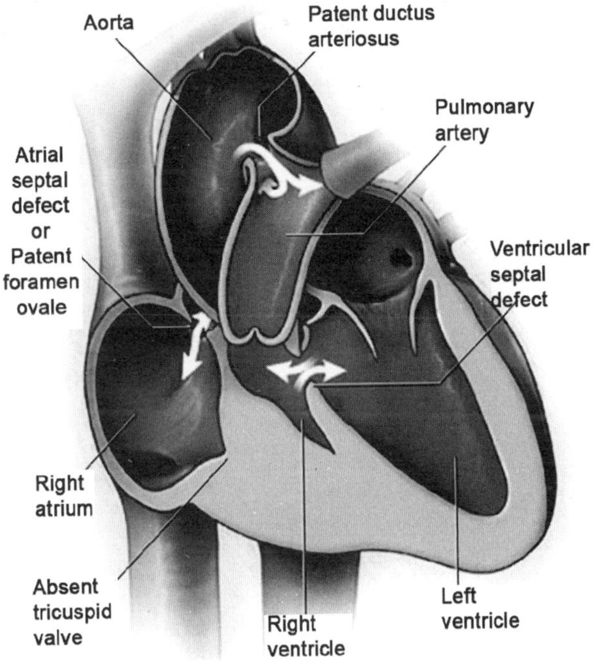

EXPLANATION

Tricuspid atresia

- Progressive cyanosis
- Poor feeding
- Tachypnea over the first 2 weeks of life
- Holosystolic murmur due to the VSD
- Left axis deviation on electrocardiography and left ventricular hypertrophy (since it must pump blood to both the pulmonary and systemic systems)
- *Normal* heart size

Ans. (B) i.e., Tricuspid atresia

79. **A three year old girl is brought with complaint of not being able to ever stand or walk. She achieved head control at one year of age. Examination reveals generalised hypotonia, brisk knee jerk, and ankle clonus. What is the likely diagnosis?**

(a) Cerebral palsy
(b) Spinal muscular atrophy
(c) Congenital hypothyroidism
(d) Congenital myotonic dystrophy

EXPLANATION

Abnormal muscle tone, delayed motor development and persistence of primitive reflexes are the main early symptoms of CP. Symptoms and diagnosis typically occur by the age of 2, although persons with milder forms of cerebral palsy may be over the age of 5, if not in adulthood, when finally diagnosed. It is a developmental disability.

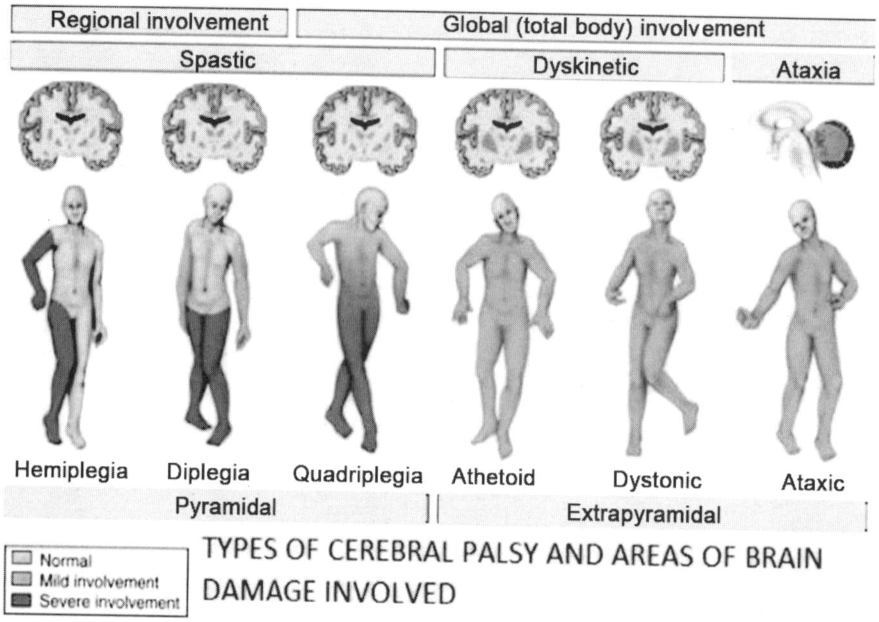

TYPES OF CEREBRAL PALSY AND AREAS OF BRAIN DAMAGE INVOLVED

Ans. (A) i.e., Cerebral palsy

80. A child presents with sensations of itching, burning and a probable foreign body beneath the eyelids. Examination reveals photophobia, large oval follicles within the conjunctiva and preauricular adenopathy. The most likely diagnosis is:

(a) Epidemic keratoconjunctivitis
(b) Vernal conjunctivitis
(c) Trachomatous conjunctivitis
(d) Phlyctenular conjunctivitis

EXPLANATION

Ocular signs/symptoms of Epidemic keratoconjunctivtis

- Conjunctival hyperemia/erythema (redness) of bulbar conjunctiva
- Conjunctival hyperemia/erythema (redness) of palpebral conjunctiva
- Ocular itchiness and irritation
- Chemosis (conjunctival edema)
- Photophobia
- Epiphora (excessive tearing)
- Foreign body sensation
- Blurred vision/loss of visual acuity
- Eyelid swelling
- Follicular reaction
- Clear or yellow discharge from the eye(s)
- Epithelial keratitis

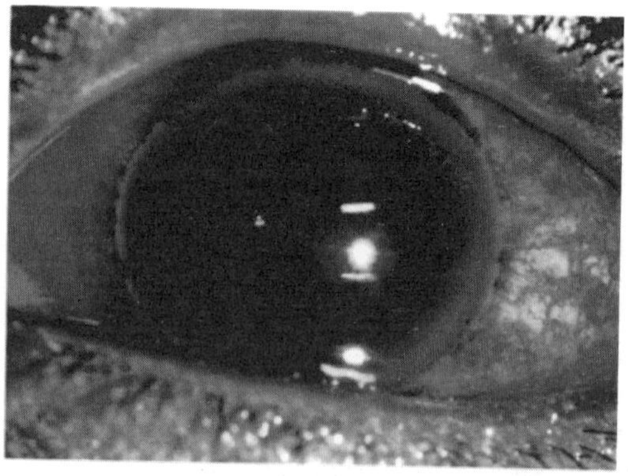

Epidemic keratoconjunctivitis can be transmitted through close contact and non-sterile eye examinations.

Systemic signs/symptoms of Epidemic keratoconjunctivtis

- Lymphadenopathy (swollen nymph nodes, specifically the preauricular lymph nodes)
- Fever
- Headache
- Fatigue

Ans. (A) i.e., Epidemic keratoconjunctivitis

81. A seven year old boy presents with acute onset of mild intermittent pain in the right groin and a limp. Abduction and internal rotation of the hip were restricted on the affected side. There was no fever. Radiographs of the pelvis were normal. The most likely diagnosis is :

(a) Transient monoarticular synovitis
(b) Legg Calve Perthes disease
(c) Slipped capital femoral epiphyses
(d) Osteochondritis dissecans

EXPLANATION

Transient synovitis causes pain in the hip, thigh, groin or knee on the affected side. There may be a limp (or abnormal crawling in infants) with or without pain. On clinical examination, the child typically holds the hip slightly bent, turned outwards and away from the middle line (flexion, external rotation and abduction). Active and passive movements may be limited because of pain, especially abduction and internal rotation. The hip can be tender to palpation.

Differential Diagnosis

Age	Painful limp	Painless limp
1–3 yr	1. Infection Septic arthritis/osteomyelitis/cellulitis/transient synovitis 2. Trauma 3. Primary or metastatic neoplasm	1. Developmental dyplasia of the hip 2. Neuromuscular disease — Cerebral palsy — Muscular dystrophy 3. Lower limb length discrepancy

Ans. (A) i.e., Transient monoarticular synovitis

82. A child is brought with history of ingestion of an unknown substance. On examination child has excess salivation, lacrimation, miosis, gastrointestinal cramps and emesis. What was the most likely substance ingested?

(a) Carbamates
(b) Phenothiazines
(c) Opioids
(d) Tricyclic antidepressants

Difference between OP & Carbamates

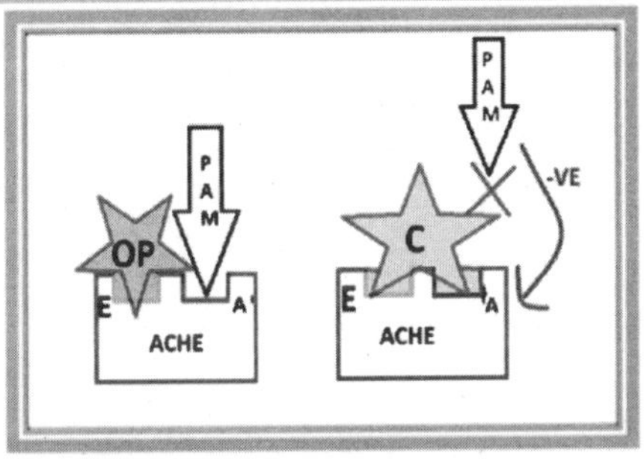

EXPLANATION

Carbamate insecticides target human melatonin receptors, along with inhibiting Acetylcholinesterase.

Ans. (A) i.e., Carbamates

2017

83. A term newborn presents with respiratory failure which is refractory to mechanical ventilation, surfactant replacement therapy, glucocorticoid administration and extra corporeal membrane oxygenation. The most likely diagnosis is:

(a) Surfactant Protein B deficiency
(b) Primary ciliary dyskinesia
(c) Persistent tachypnea of infancy
(d) Lymphocytic interstitial pneumonitis

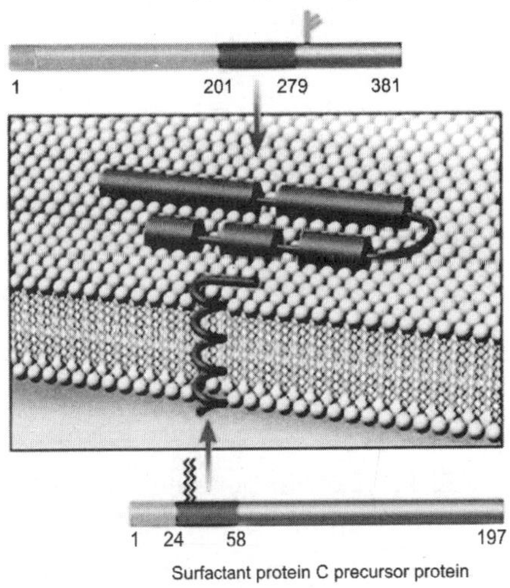

EXPLANATION

Surfactant protein B is an essential lipid associated protein found in pulmonary surfactant. Without it, the lung would not be able to inflate after a deep breath out. It rearranges lipid molecules in the fluid lining the lung so that tiny air sacs in the lung, called alveoli, can more easily inflate.

Ans. (A) i.e., Surfactant Protein B deficiency

84. A child after snake bite develops petechiae and ecchymosis on the skin. In addition, child develops bleeding from venipuncture site and oliguria. The most likely snake species is:

(a) Pit viper (b) Cobra
(c) Mamba (d) Python

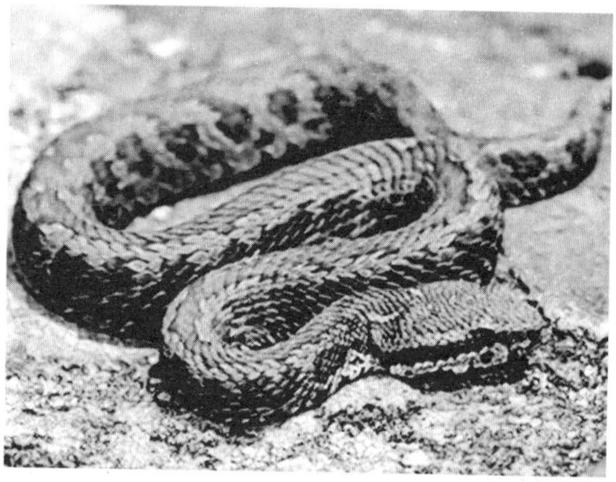

EXPLANATION

Trimeresurus venom varies in toxicity between species, but all are primarily hemotoxic and considered to be medically significant to humans.

Ans. (A) i.e., Pit viper

85. **A six year old boy presents with short neck, low hairline and restriction of neck movements. The child also has Sprengel anomaly, scoliosis, and fused cervical vertebrae. The most likely diagnosis is:**

(a) Atlantoaxial instability (b) Klippel Feil syndrome
(c) Noonan syndrome (d) Sandifer syndrome

EXPLANATION

The most common sign of the disorder is restricted mobility of the neck and upper spine. A short neck and low hairline at the back of the head may occur in some patients.

Associated abnormalities may include:

- Scoliosis (side to side curvature of the spine), which is abnormal curving of the spine. The spine sometimes appears as a "C" or an "S"
- Spina bifida, when the spinal canal and the back bone do not close completely during birth
- Anomalies of the kidneys and the ribs
- Cleft palate (hole in the roof of the mouth)
- Dental problems (late dentition, high risk of caries, oligo- and hypodontia)
- Respiratory problems
- Heart malformations
- Short stature
- Duane syndrome
- Srb's anomaly
- Approximately 35% of patients with Klippel–Feil syndrome will also have a congenital elevation of the scapula known as Sprengel's deformity

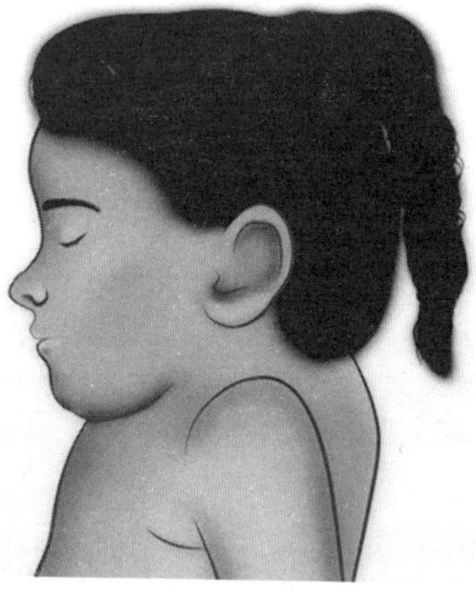

Ans. (D) i.e., Sandifer syndrome

86. **A 10-year old boy presents with recurrent bouts of nasal congestion, itching, sneezing, clear rhinorrhoea and conjunctival irritation. On examination he has conjunctival hyperaemia, allergic gape and a transverse nasal crease. Which of the following drugs is preferred for management of this child?**

(a) Diphenhydramine (b) Fluticasone
(c) Cetirizine (d) Ipratropium bromide

EXPLANATION

Fluticasone is a synthetic glucocorticoid which is used in some countries to treat nasal symptoms. Both the furoate and propanoate esters, fluticasone furoate and fluticasone propionate, are also used as topical anti inflammatories and inhaled corticosteroids, and are used much more commonly in comparison.

Ans. (B) i.e., Fluticasone

87. **A two year old child presents with partial albinism and susceptibility to infection. Peripheral smear examination reveals giant peroxidise positive lysosomal granules in granulocytes. Which of the following is most likely diagnosis?**
   (a) Angelman Syndrome
   (b) Hermansky Pudlak Syndrome
   (c) Waardenburg Syndrome
   (d) Chediak Higashi syndrome

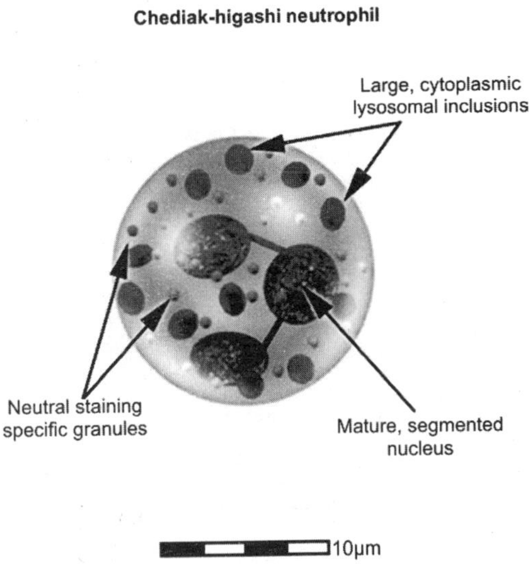

Chédiak–Higashi syndrome is a rare autosomal recessive disorder that arises from a mutation of a lysosomal trafficking regulator protein, which leads to a decrease in phagocytosis. The decrease in phagocytosis results in recurrent pyogenic infections, albinism and peripheral neuropathy.

Ans. (D) i.e., Chediak-Higashi syndrome

88. **A one year old child on exclusive milk feeds presents with constipation. On examination there is no fecal impaction. What is the next step in management?**
   (a) Oral lactulose
   (b) Increasing intake of vegetables and cereals
   (c) Colonic enemas using polyethylene glycol
   (d) Milk of Magnesia

EXPLANATION

Measures that may help include drinking enough fluids, eating more fiber

Ans. (B) i.e., Increasing intake of vegetables and cereals

89. **A six year old boy presents with generalized seizure disorder and hypo pigmented skin lesions. On examination he has tiny red nodules over the nose and cheeks. The most likely diagnosis is:**
   (a) Tuberous sclerosis
   (b) Sturge Weber disease
   (c) PHACE Syndrome
   (d) Neurofibromatosis

EXPLANATION

Tuberous sclerosis complex (TSC) is a rare multisystem genetic disease that causes benign tumors to grow in the brain and on other vital organs such as the kidneys, heart, liver, eyes, lungs, and skin. A combination of symptoms may include seizures, intellectual disability, developmental delay, behavioral problems, skin abnormalities, and lung and kidney disease. TSC is caused by a mutation of either of two genes, *TSC1* and *TSC2*, which code for the proteins hamartin and tuberin, respectively. These proteins act as tumor growth suppressors, agents that regulate cell proliferation and differentiation.

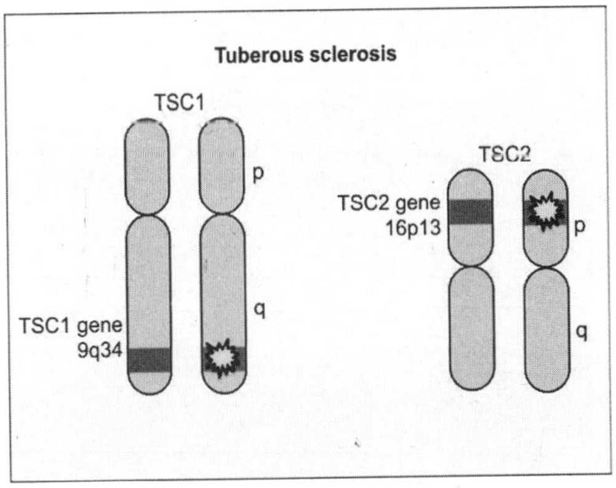

Ans. (A) i.e., Tuberous sclerosis

2017

90. **Which of the following can cause bilateral sensorineural hearing loss?**

(a) Histiocytosis (b) Cholesteatoma
(c) Loop diuretics (d) Glomus tumors

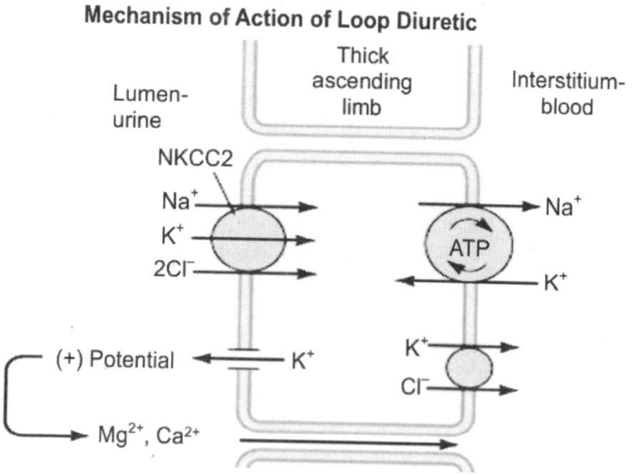

EXPLANATION

Ototoxic drugs include antibiotics such as gentamicin, loop diuretics such as furosemide and platinum based chemotherapy agents such as cisplatin. A number of nonsteroidal anti inflammatory drugs (NSAIDS) have also been shown to be ototoxic. This can result in sensorineural hearing loss, dysequilibrium, or both.

Ans. (C) i.e., Loop diuretics

91. **The joint sitting of Parliament for transacting a legislative business is presided over by:**

(a) The President of India
(b) The Vice President of India
(c) The Prime Minister of India
(d) The Speaker of Lok Sabha

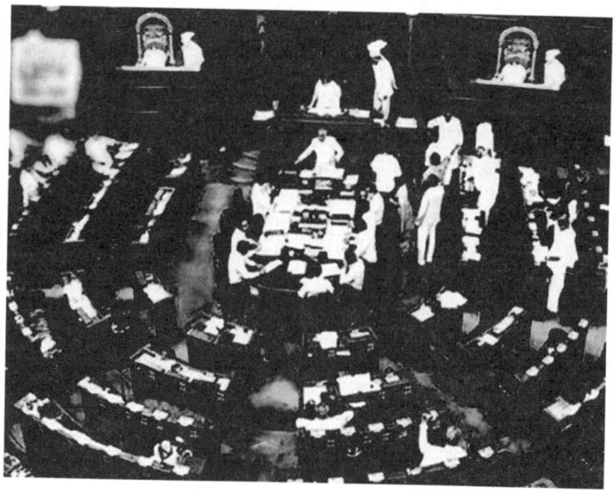

EXPLANATION

The **Speaker of the Lok Sabha** is the presiding officer of the Lok Sabha, the lower house of the Parliament of India. The speaker is elected in the very first meeting of the Lok Sabha following general elections. Serving for a term of five years, the Speaker chosen from amongst the members of the Lok Sabha, and is by convention a member of the ruling party or alliance.

Ans. (D) i.e., The Speaker of Lok Sabha

92. **Recently, a massive coral bleaching has been reported in the 'Great Barrier Reef'. It is located near the coast of:**

(a) Queensland (b) Maldives
(c) Hawaii (d) Andaman

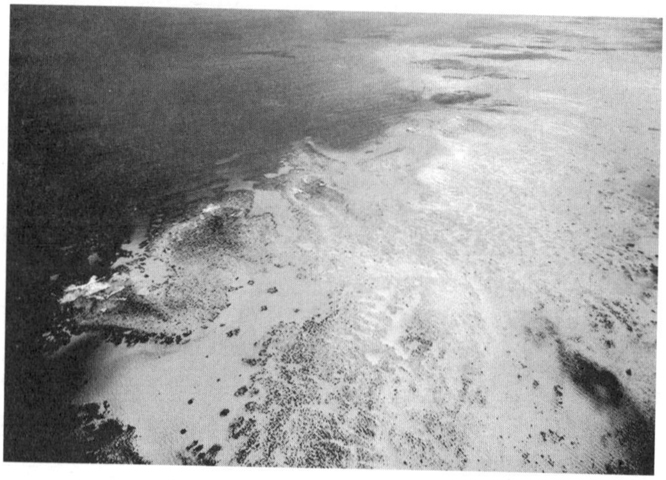

EXPLANATION

The **Great Barrier Reef** is the world's largest coral reef system composed of over 2,900 individual reefs and 900 islands stretching for over 2,300 kilometres (1,400 mi) over an area of approximately 344,400 square kilometres (133,000 sq mi). The reef is located in the Coral Sea, off the coast of Queensland, Australia.

Ans. (A) i.e., Queensland

93. **Who is the first Law Officer of the Government of India?**

(a) Chief Justice of India
(b) Attorney General of India
(c) Law Secretary
(d) Union Law Minister

EXPLANATION

The **Attorney General of India** is the Indian government's chief legal advisor, and its primary lawyer in the Supreme Court of India. He can be said as the lawyer from government's side. He is appointed by the President of India under Article 76(1) of the Constitution and holds office during the pleasure of the President. He must be a person qualified to be appointed as a Judge of the Supreme Court, also must have been a judge of some high court for five years or an advocate of some high court for ten years or an eminent jurist, in the opinion of the President and must be a citizen of India.

Attorney General

- The Attorney General for India is the Indian government's chief legal advisor, and Supreme Court of India.
- He is appointed by the President of India under Article 76(1) of the Constitution and holds office during the pleasure of the President.

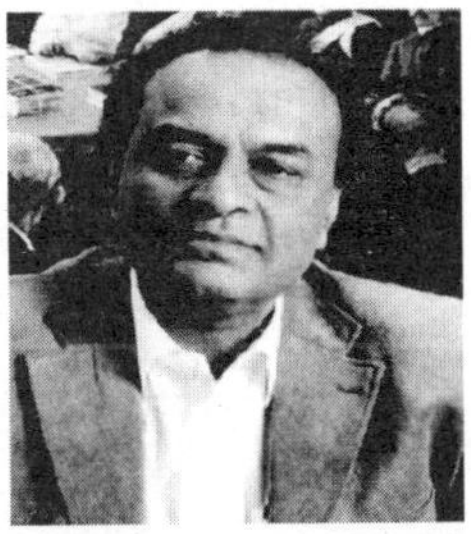

The 14th and Current Attorney general of India Mr. Mukul Rohatgi

Ans. (B) i.e., Attorney General of India

94. **In the context of Genetic Engineering, scientists have developed a new computational method called 'Target Finder' which can predict where non coding DNA interacts with genes. Which of the following is a likely advantage of this?**

(a) Artificial induction of beneficial mutations so as to develop high yielding varieties
(b) Finding new drug targets to treat some genetic diseases
(c) Rapid cloning of domesticated animals
(d) All of these

EXPLANATION

The computational method, called TargetFinder, can predict where non coding DNA—the DNA that does not code for proteins—interacts with genes. This technology helps researchers connect mutations in the so called genomic "dark matter" with the genes they affect, potentially revealing new therapeutic targets for genetic disorders.

Ans. (B) i.e., Finding new drug targets to treat some genetic diseases

2017

95. **Consider the following:**

1. Gold
2. Platinum
3. Silver

Which of the above is/are found in e-waste?

(a) 1 and 2 only
(b) 3 only
(c) 1, 2 and 3
(d) None

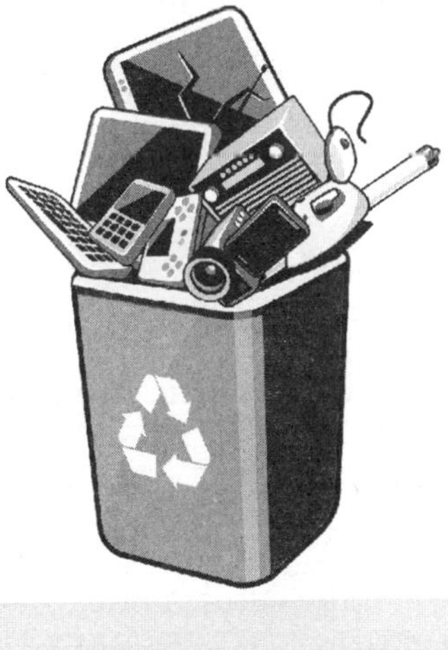

EXPLANATION

Raw materials in the e-waste scrap include metals such as gold, silver, copper, platinum and palladium

Ans. (C) i.e., 1, 2 and 3

96. "Boil a small quantity of khoya with some water, cool and add a few drops of iodine solution and see the formation of blue colour". This is the test to find the presence of which of the following?

(a) Fructose (b) Gram flour (c) Starch (d) Urea

EXPLANATION

Khoa is often adulterated with wheat or rice flour (starch). Hence iodine method is used to its direction; iodine solution gives intense blue colour with starch due to formation of unstable complex starch iodine compound.

Detection of starch in milk and milk products (khoya, chenna, paneer)

Testing method:

1. Boil 2–3 ml of sample with 5 ml of water.
2. Cool and add 2–3 drops of tincture of iodine.
3. Formation of blue colour indicates the presence of starch (in the case of milk, addition of water and boiling is not required).

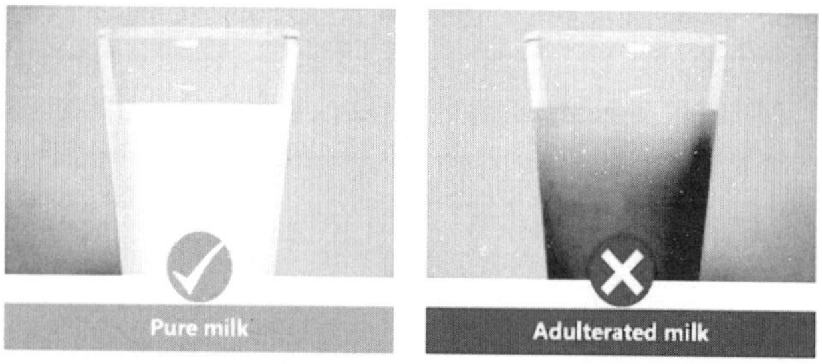

Ans. (C) i.e., Starch

97. Which of the following CANNOT be used as a biofertilizer in rice cultivation?

(a) Azolla (b) Azospirillum (c) Blue green algae (d) Rhizobium

EXPLANATION

Rhizobium is a genus of Gram negative soil bacteria that fix nitrogen. *Rhizobium* species form an endosymbiotic nitrogen fixing association with roots of legumes and *Parasponia.*

Ans. (D) i.e., Rhizobium

2017

98. Groundwater in many areas in West Bengal has been contaminated leading to a large number of cases of poisoning. What is the substance responsible for such cases?

(a) Arsenic (b) Cyanide (c) Polonium (d) Lead

EXPLANATION

Extensive arsenic contamination of groundwater has led to widespread arsenic poisoning in Bangladesh and neighboring countries. It is estimated that approximately 57 million people in the Bengal basin are drinking groundwater with arsenic concentrations elevated above the World Health Organization's standard of 10 parts per billion (ppb)

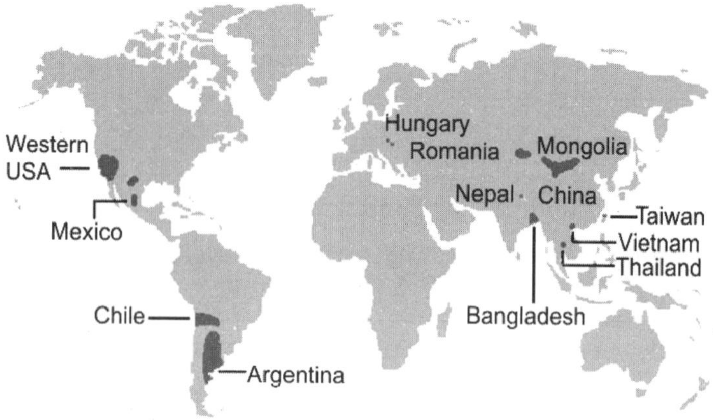

Ans. (A) i.e., Arsenic

99. For acquiring ethanol for blending with petrol, the oil companies in India depend on:

(a) Cosmetic industry (b) Food processing plants

(c) Fertilizer factories (d) Sugar mills

EXPLANATION

Ethyl alcohol or ethanol can either be produced by direct fermentation of cane juice or from molasses, which is a byproduct of the sugar manufacturing process. In India, ethanol can be produced only from molasses whereas, mills in Brazil produce ethanol directly from sugarcane juice. Ethanol can be used for potable alcohol industry, chemical industry and as a biofuel in vehicles (direct/blended with gasoline).

In India, ethanol is consumed primarily by portable alcohol industry, Oil marketing companies (for blending with petrol) and chemical industries.

What is ethanol?????....

The Fermentation of sugar crops (sugarcane, wheat, sorghum, maize, etc.), starch, cornstalks, vegetable leftover and fruits after distillation is known as **ETHANOL**.

Ethanol, or ethyl alcohol, has the chemical formula C_2H_3OH.

Ethanol has been used as a fuel for internal combustion engine.

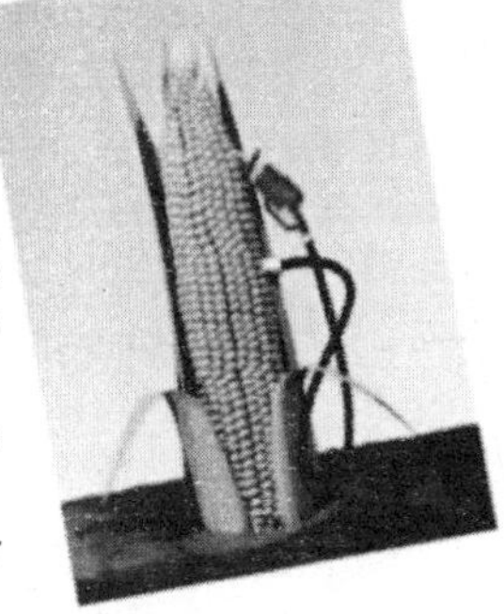

Ans. (D) i.e., Sugar mills

100. Consider the following statements:

Targeted Delivery of Financial and Other Subsidies, Benefits and Services Act, 2016 aims to

1. Strengthen the Pradhan Mantri Jan Dhan Yojana

2. Provide funds for the relief of farmers

Which of the statements given above is/are correct?

(a) 1 only (b) 2 only (c) Both 1 and 2 (d) Neither 1 nor 2

EXPLANATION

Targeted Delivery of Financial and Other Subsidies, Benefits and Services Act, 2016 is an Act to provide for, as a good governance, efficient, transparent, and targeted delivery of subsidies, benefits and services, the expenditure for which is incurred from the Consolidated Fund of India, to individuals residing in India through assigning of unique identity numbers to such individuals and for matters connected therewith or incidental thereto.

Aadhaar Act, 2016

- The passage of the Aadhaar Act, 2016 has received strong criticism.
- The government has introduced the Act as a 'money bill' under Article 110 of the Constitution of India.
- The Act lies well outside the confines of the Article.
- The Act warrants censure for its process.
- The Act takes away an individual's control of his/her own information.

Ans. (D) i.e., Neither 1 nor 2

101. The Pradhan Mantri Jan Dhan Yojna aims to promote:

(a) Financial inclusion

(b) Collateral security in housing for rural and urban poor

(c) Cashless financial transactions

(d) Financial literacy

EXPLANATION

Pradhan Mantri Jan Dhan Yojana (P.M.J.D.Y), Prime Minister's People Money Scheme is India's National Mission for Financial Inclusion to ensure access to financial services, namely Banking Savings & Deposit Accounts, Remittance, Credit, Insurance, Pension in an affordable manner. This financial inclusion campaign was launched by the Prime Minister of India Narendra Modi on 28 August 2014.

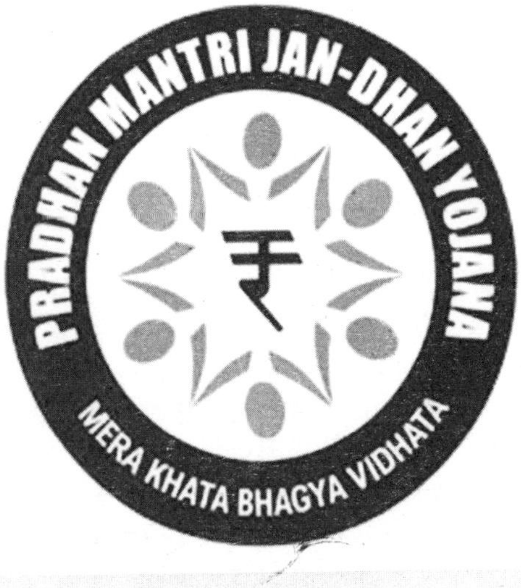

Ans. (A) i.e., Financial inclusion

102. The objective of the "Paramparagat Krishi Vikas Yojana" is to promote:

(a) Conservation of groundwater

(b) Cultivation of wild varieties of cereal crops

(c) Dryland farming

(d) Organic farming

EXPLANATION

Government is promoting organic farming through various schemes/programmes under National Mission for Sustainable Agriculture (NMSA)/Paramapragat Krishi Vikas Yojana (PKVY), Rashtriya Krishi Vikas Yojana (RKVY), Mission for Integrated Development of Horticulture (MIDH), National Mission on Oilseeds & Oil Palm (NMOOP), Network Project on Organic Farming of ICAR.

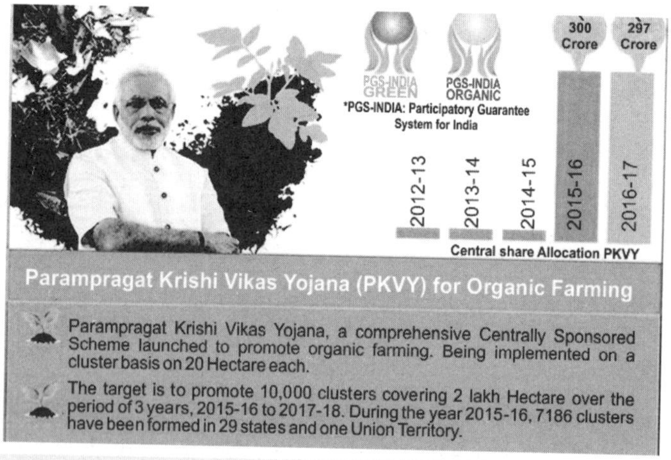

Ans. (D) i.e., Organic farming

103. Which among the following is a very water intensive crop?

(a) Grapes (b) Finger millet (c) Sugarcane (d) Wheat

EXPLANATION

Below is a table on thirsty/water intensive crops grown in India:

CROP	(Water requirement in litres/kg of crop)
Cotton	7,000–29,000
Rice	3,000–5,000
Sugarcane	1,500–3,000
Soya	2,000
Wheat	900
Potatoes	500

Ans.(C) i.e., Finger millet

104. Which of the following does nanoscience have applications?

1. Drug delivery
2. Electronics
3. Food processing
4. Water purification

Select the correct answer using the code given below:

(a) 1 and 2 only (b) 1 and 3 only (c) 2, 3 and 4 only (d) 1, 2, 3 and 4

EXPLANATION

Nanotechnology as defined by size is naturally very broad, including fields of science as diverse as surface science, organic chemistry, molecular biology, semiconductor physics, energy storage, microfabrication, molecular engineering, etc. The associated research and applications are equally diverse, ranging from extensions of conventional device physics to completely new approaches based upon molecular self assembly, from developing new materials with dimensions on the nanoscale to direct control of matter on the atomic scale. Nanotechnology may be able to create many new materials and devices with a vast range of applications, such as in nanomedicine, nanoelectronics, biomaterials energy production, and consumer products.

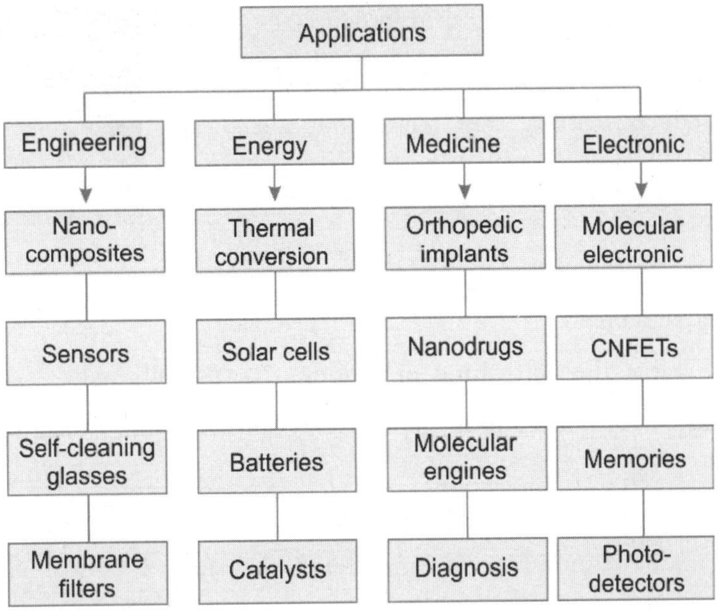

Ans. (D) i.e., 1, 2, 3 and 4

105. Which of the following is/are the exclusive powers of the Lok Sabha as compared to Rajya Sabha?

1. **Introducing money bills**
2. **Passing a motion of no confidence against the Council of Ministers**

Select the correct answer using the code given below:

(a) 1 only (b) 2 only (c) Both 1 and 2 (d) Neither 1 nor 2

EXPLANATION

The main business of the Lok Sabha may be consideration of a Bill or financial business or consideration of a resolution or a motion.

Ans. (C) i.e., Both 1 and 2

106. Who among the following do not participate in the election of the President of India?

(a) Elected members of Rajya Sabha
(b) Elected members of Vidhan Sabhas
(c) Elected members of Lok Sabha
(d) Elected members of Vidhan Parishads

EXPLANATION

The President is indirectly elected by an electoral college comprising the Parliament of India (both houses) and the Legislative Assemblies (Vidhan Sabha) of each of India's states and territories, who themselves are all directly elected. Vidhan parishad is also known as Legislative council.

Ans. (D) i.e., Elected members of Vidhan Parishads

107. There is a popular opposition to the use of "plastic microbeads". In the manufacture of which of the following are they used?

(a) Cosmetics
(b) Electronics
(c) Wooden furniture
(d) Synthetic textiles

EXPLANATION

Due to the increase in bans of microbeads in the USA, many cosmetic companies are also phasing out microbeads from their production lines. L'Oreal is planning to phase out polyethylene microbeads in the exfoliates, cleansers and shower gels from their products by 2017. Johnson and Johnson, who have already started to phase out microbeads at the end of 2015, will by 2017 not be producing any polyethylene microbeads in their products. Lastly, Crest phased out microbead plastics in its toothpastes by February 2016.

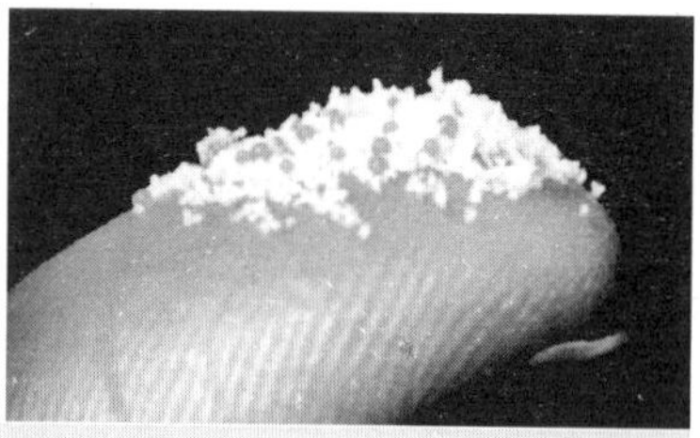

Ans. (A) i.e., Cosmetics

108. Consider the following statements:

1. **In certain parts of India, the cultivation of opium is legally allowed.**
2. **Opium gum is mixed with cluster bean gum in fracking technology that is used in the shale gas extraction.**

Which of the statements given above is/are correct?

(a) 1 only (b) 2 only (c) Both 1 and 2 (d) Neither 1 nor 2

EXPLANATION

Legal opium production in India is much more traditional. As of 2008, opium was collected by farmers who were licensed to grow 0.1 hectares (0.25 acres) of opium poppies, who to maintain their licences needed to sell 56 kilograms of unadulterated raw opium paste. The price of opium paste is fixed by the government according to the quality and quantity tendered. The average is around 1500 rupees (US$29) per kilogram.

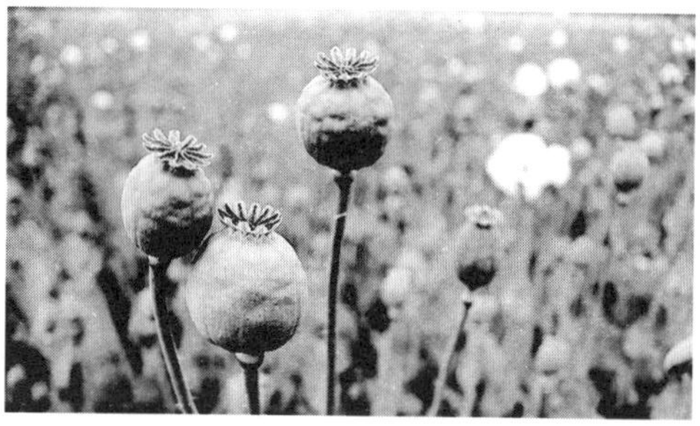

Ans. (A) i.e., 1 only

109. There is a worldwide protest against the use of hydrofluorocarbons. In which of the following household things are they used?

(a) Air conditioning machines (b) Cooking gas cylinders
(c) Gas geysers (d) Microwave ovens

EXPLANATION

Hydrofluorocarbons (HFCs), organic compounds that contain fluorine and hydrogen atoms, are the most common type of organofluorine compounds. They are commonly used in air conditioning and as refrigerants in place of the older chlorofluorocarbons such as R-12 and hydrochlorofluorocarbons such as R-21. They do not harm the ozone layer as much as the compounds they replace; however, they do contribute to global warming. Their atmospheric concentrations and contribution to anthropogenic greenhouse gase missions are rapidly increasing, causing international concern about their radiative forcing.

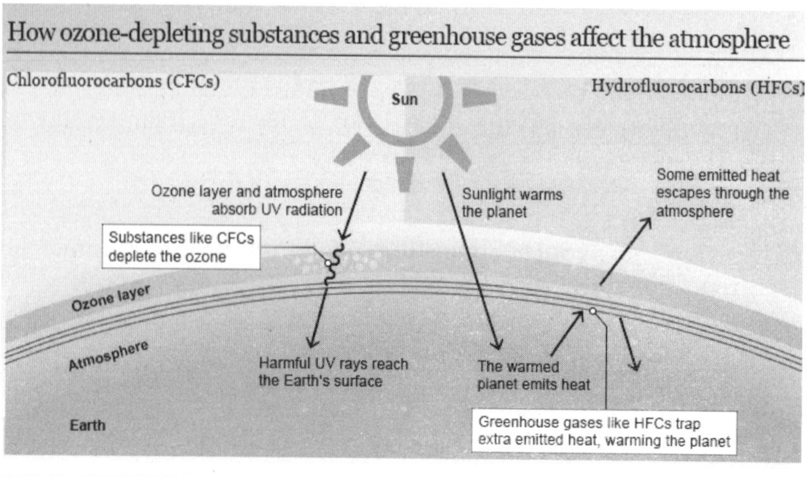

Ans. (A) i.e., Air conditioning machines

110. What is/are the objectives of Cartagena Protocol on Biosafety?

1. Establishing or promoting *in situ* conservation facilities for rare and endangered organisms
2. Maintaining the worldwide network of gene banks for all the known flora and fauna

Select the correct answer using the code given below:

(a) 1 only (b) 2 only (c) Both 1 and 2 (d) Neither 1 nor 2

EXPLANATION

The **Cartagena Protocol on Biosafety to the Convention on Biological Diversity** is an international agreement on biosafety as a supplement to the Convention on Biological Diversity effective since 2003. The Biosafety Protocol seeks to protect biological diversity from the potential risks posed by genetically modified organisms resulting from modern biotechnology.

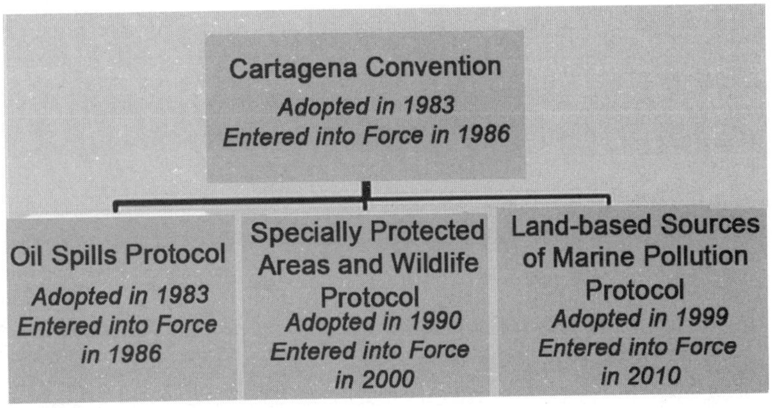

Ans. (D) i.e., Neither 1 nor 2

111. Consider the following animals:

1. Sloth bear 2. Jaguar 3. Hoolock gibbon

Which of the above is/are found in India in their natural habitat?

(a) 1 only (b) 2 and 3 only (c) 1 and 3 only (d) 1, 2 and 3

EXPLANATION

Animals and natural habitat

- Endemic to the Indian subcontinent, the Sloth Bear *(Melursus ursinus)* inhabits tropical and subtropical habitats across India, Nepal, Bhutan and Sri Lanka. Being the most common among the four species of bears in India, it is widely distributed from the foothills of the Himalayas to the southern tip of the Indian peninsula. With sloth bear populations in the Himalayan foothills and northeast India becoming isolated, the Western Ghats and central Indian landscapes now possibly harbor the largest populations.
- The **hoolock gibbons** are three primatespecies of genus ***Hoolock*** in the gibbon family, Hylobatidae, native to eastern Bangladesh, Northeast India and Southwest China.

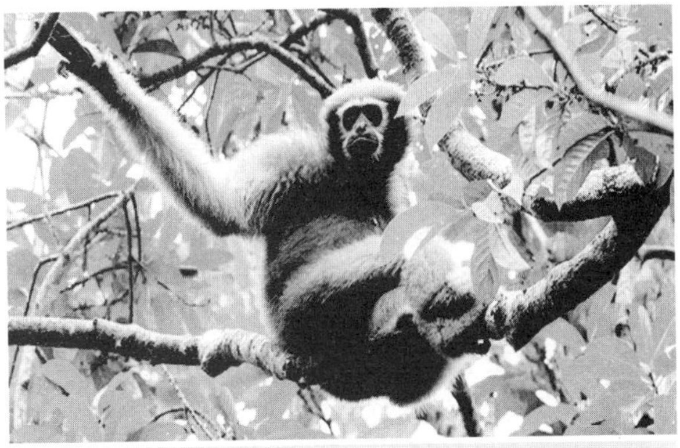

Ans. (C) i.e., 1 and 3 only

112. Consider the following statements:

1. Biodiversity is normally greater in the lower latitude as compared to higher latitudes.
2. Along the mountain gradient, biodiversity is normally greater in the lower altitudes as compared to higher altitudes.

Which of the statements given above is/are correct?

(a) 1 only (b) 2 only (c) Both 1 and 2 (d) Neither 1 nor 2

EXPLANATION

Biodiversity

- Generally, there is an increase in biodiversity from the poles to the tropics. Thus localities at lower latitudes have more species than localities at higher latitudes. This is often referred to as the latitudinal gradient in species diversity.
- Higher you go = colder atmosphere = less biodiversity

Ans. (C) i.e., Both 1 and 2

113. Aflatoxins are formed by:

(a) Aspergillus flavus (b) Candida albicans
(c) Cryptococcus neoformans (d) Coccidioides schenckii

EXPLANATION

Aflatoxins are poisonous carcinogens that are produced by certain molds (*Aspergillus flavus* and *Aspergillus parasiticus*) which grow in soil, decaying vegetation, hay, and grains. They are regularly found in improperly stored staple commodities such as cassava, chili peppers, corn, cotton seed, millet, peanuts, rice, sesame seeds, sorghum, sunflower seeds, tree nuts, wheat, and a variety of spices.

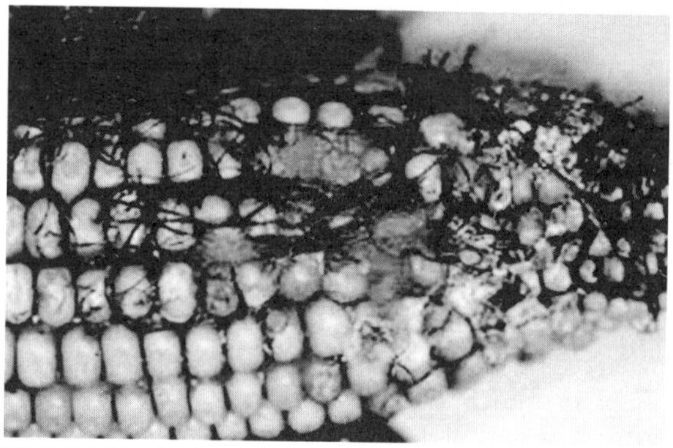

Ans. (A) i.e., Aspergillus flavus

114. Consider the following districts:

1. Munnar **2. Mandi** **3. Krishna**

Which of the above districts is/are well known for tea plantations?

(a) 3 only (b) 2 and 3 only (c) 1 and 2 only (d) 1 only

EXPLANATION

Tea plantation in India

- Kerala is famous for India's first Tea Museum at Nallathanni Estate in Munnar, along with the production of certified organic Green & White Tea, said to be quite rare & exclusive.
- It is on the gentle slopes of the Kangra valley that one finds the organic Tea plantations of the state, producing varieties of green & black Tea, with varieties like Pekoe, Fannings, Hyson etc. with their exquisite flavours in the districts of Mandi & Kangra, surrounded by the majestic Himalayas.

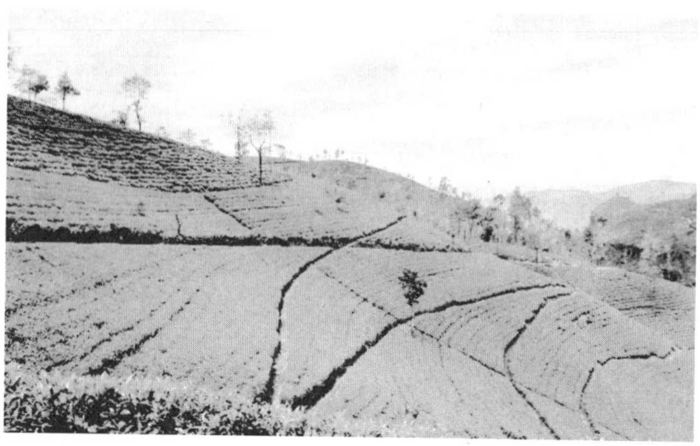

Ans. (C) i.e., **1 and 2 only**

115. 'Fly ash' is emitted from:

(a) Brick kilns

(b) Motor vehicles

(c) Sewage treatment plants

(d) Thermal power plants

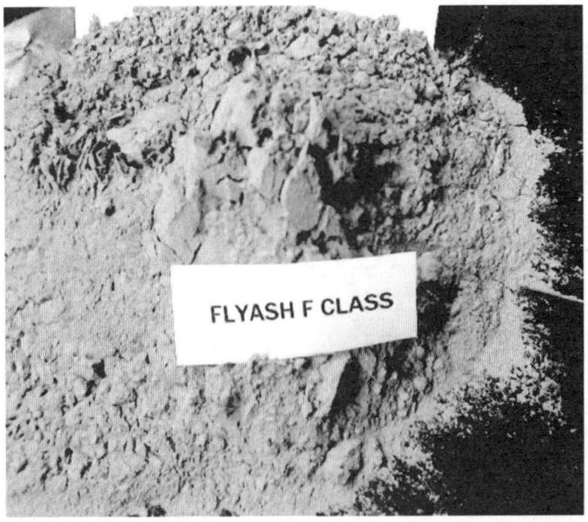

EXPLANATION

Fly ash, also known as "pulverised fuel ash", is a coal combustion product that is composed of the particulates (fine particles of burned fuel) that are driven out of coal fired boilers together with the flue gases. Ash that falls to the bottom of the boiler is called bottom ash. In modern coal fired power plants, fly ash is generally captured by electrostatic precipitators or other particle filtration equipment before the flue gases reach the chimneys.

Ans. (D) i.e., Thermal power plants

116. Calcium carbide is used:

(a) As rodent killer

(b) As insecticide

(c) For fruit ripening

(d) For lowering soil salinity

EXPLANATION

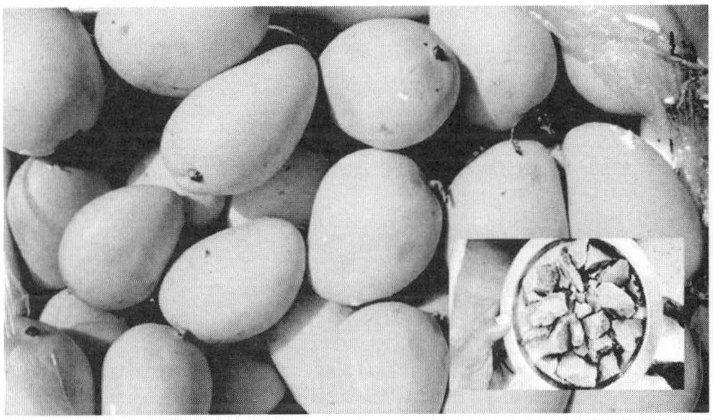

In the artificial ripening of fruit, calcium carbide is sometimes used as source of acetylene gas, which is a ripening agent similar to ethylene. However, this is illegal in some countries because consumption of fruits artificially ripened using calcium carbide can cause serious health problems in those who eat them.

Ans. (C) i.e., For fruit ripening

117. With reference to food additives, consider the following statements:

1. Benzoic acid and sorbic acid function as antimicrobial agents.

2. Citric acid is used to suppress browning of fruits and vegetables.

Which of the statements given above is/are correct?

(a) 1 only

(b) 2 only

(c) Both 1 and 2

(d) Neither 1 nor 2

EXPLANATION

Food additives

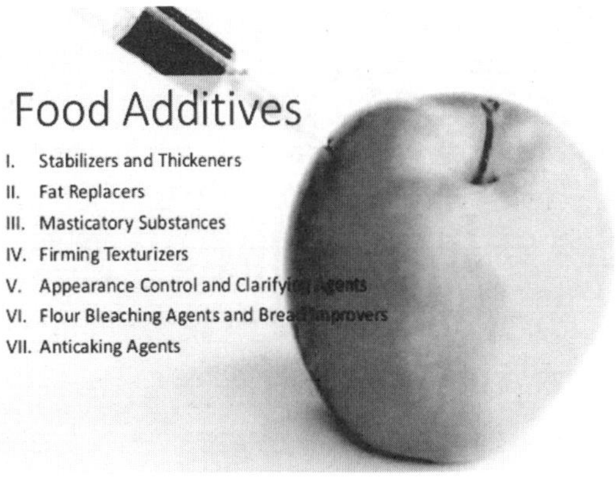

- At low pH, acetic acid (pK 4.75), sorbic acid (pK 4.76), and benzoic acid (pK 4.19) exist substantially in the undissociated state. In this form, these molecules readily cross the cell membrane. However, once in the cytosol, where the pH is kept at 6 to 7, the acid dissociates, generating the conjugate base. This anion accumulates intracellularly to very high levels, since it cannot diffuse back across the membrane. The release of protons in the cytosol can potentially acidify the cytosol, and this mechanism was originally proposed to underlie the physiology of growth inhibition by this class of compounds.

- To keep cut apple slices from ***browning***, dissolve 3 tbsp. of ***citric acid*** in one cup of water.

Ans. (C) i.e., Both 1 and 2

118. With reference to the use of microorganisms in food processing, consider the following statements:

1. Lactic acid bacteria can ferment any monosaccharide or polysaccharide into lactic acid.

2. Baker's yeast is manufactured from single cell isolates of *Saccharomyces* cerevisiae.

Which of the statements given above is/are correct?

(a) 1 only (b) 2 only (c) Both 1 and 2 (d) Neither 1 nor 2

EXPLANATION

Baker's yeast is the common name for the strains of yeast commonly used as a leavening agent in baking bread and bakery products, where it converts the fermentable sugars present in the dough into carbon dioxide and ethanol. Baker's yeast is of the species *Saccharomyces cerevisiae*, which is the same species (but a different strain) commonly used in alcoholic fermentation, which is called brewer's yeast. Baker's yeast is also a single cell microorganism found on and around the human body.

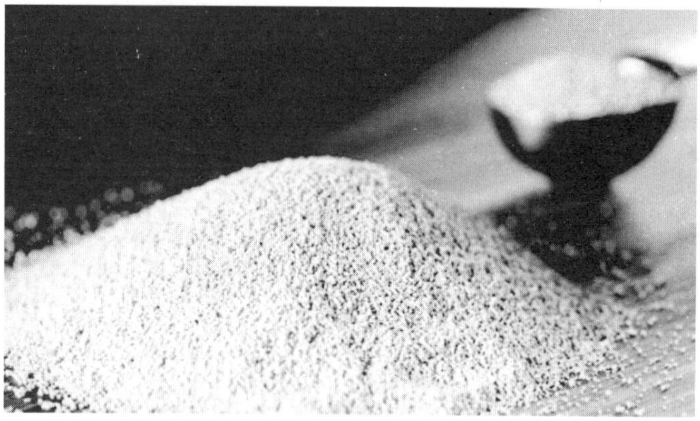

Ans. (B) i.e., 2 only

119. Which of the following chemicals is/are used in food preservation?

1. Calcium propionate 2. Potassium metabisulphite 3. Lecithin

Select the correct answer using the code given below:

(a) 1 and 2 only (b) 3 only

(c) 1, 2 and 3 (d) None of them is used in food preservation

EXPLANATION

Preservative food additives can be *antimicrobial*—which inhibit the growth of bacteria or fungi, including mold—or *antioxidant*, such as oxygen absorbers, which inhibit the oxidation of food constituents. Common antimicrobial preservatives include calcium propionate, sodium nitrate, sodium nitrite, sulfites (sulfur dioxide, sodium bisulfite, potassium hydrogen sulfite, etc.), and EDTA. Antioxidants include butylated hydroxyanisole (BHA) and butylated hydroxytoluene (BHT). Other preservatives include formaldehyde (usually in solution), glutaraldehyde (insecticide), ethanol, and methylchloroisothiazolinone. Lecithin is sold as a food additive and dietary supplement.

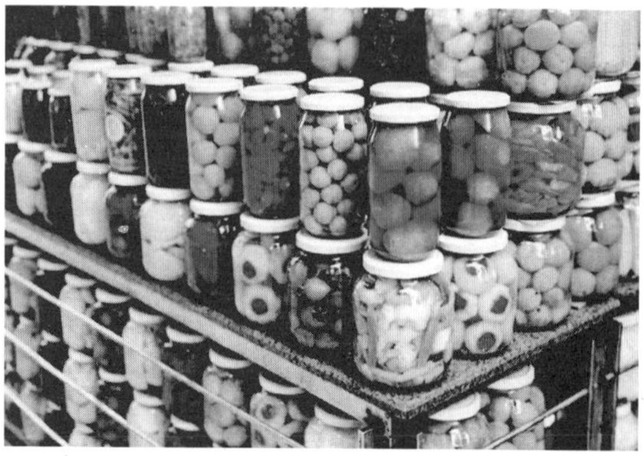

Ans. (C) i.e., 1, 2 and 3

120. What is 'M cessation', sometimes seen in news?

(a) An initiative to help tobacco users to quit tobacco

(b) A mobile phone service that delivers audio messages on pregnancy, child birth and child care

(c) An app to learn all the methods of cashless financial transactions

(d) A government initiative to eradicate the availability of narcotics to general Public

mCessation programme (Quit tobacco for life)

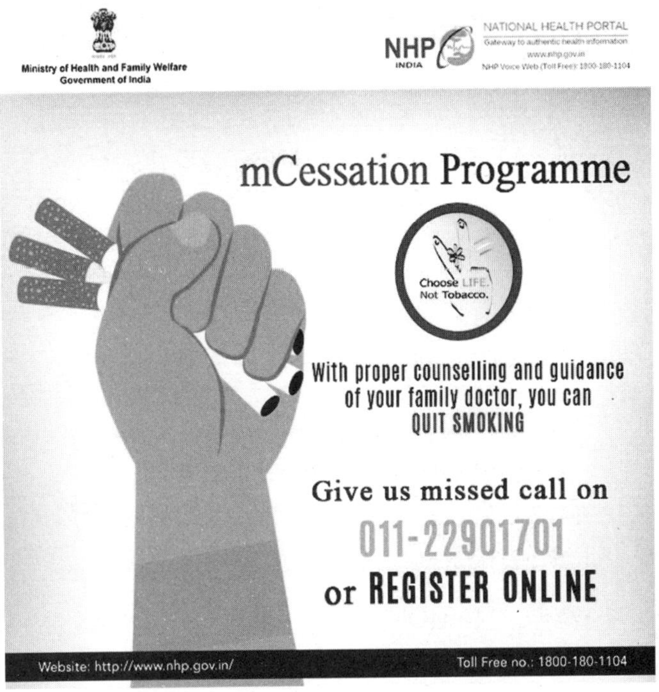

EXPLANATION

Ministry of Health & Family Welfare, in partnership with World Health Organisation and the International Telecommunications Union, has started an initiative for utilising mobile technology for tobacco cessation. WHO-ITU's 'Be Healthy Be Mobile' initiative, aims to reach out to tobacco users of all categories who want to quit tobacco use and support them towards successful quitting through constant text messaging on mobile phones. The initiative is fully supported by the Government of India.

Ans. (A) i.e., An initiative to help tobacco users to quit tobacco

CHAPTER

5 CMS EXAMINATION 2016

PAPER - 2

1. **In a sutured surgical wound, the process of epithelialization is completed within:**

(a) 24 hours (b) 48 hours
(c) 72 hours (d) 96 hours

EXPLANATION

Healing by First Intention

- The wound is closed by routine primary suturing, stapling, or gluing.
- Epithelialization occurs in 24–72 hours.

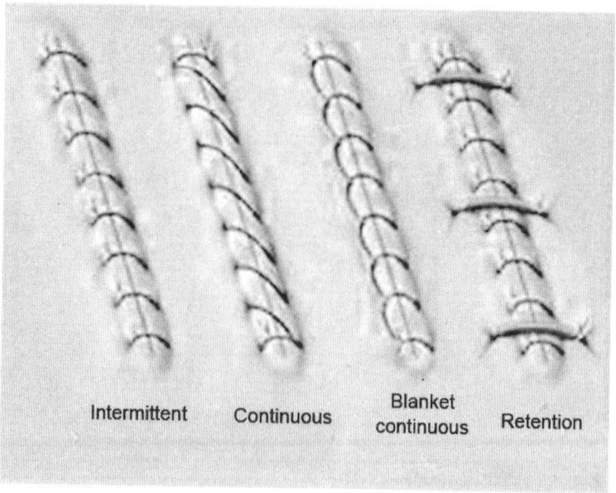

Ans. (C) i.e., 72 hours

2. **Extensive surgical debridement, decompression or amputation may be indicated in all the following clinical settings except:**

(a) Progressive synergistic gangrene
(b) Acute thrombophlebitis
(c) Acute haemolytic streptococcal cellulitis
(d) Acute rhabdomyolysis

EXPLANATION

In general, treatment of thrombophlebitis may include the following:

- Low molecular weight heparin
- Warfarin
- Nonsteroidal anti-inflammatory medications (NSAIDs/ Ibuprofen)
- Support stockings

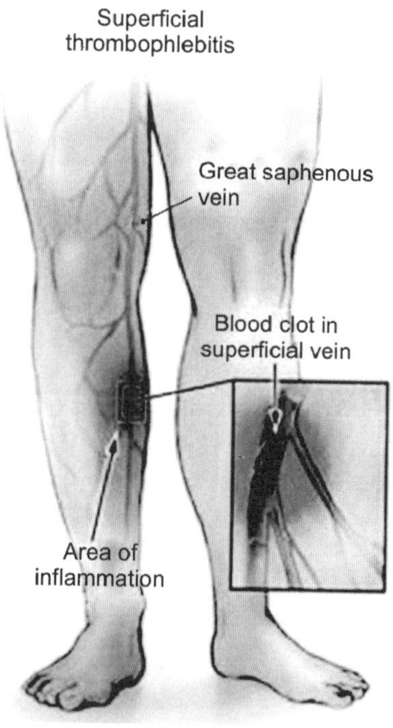

Ans. (B) i.e., Acute thrombophlebitis

3. Which one of the following bacteria is classified as facultative anaerobe?

(a) *Pseudomonas*

(b) *Bacteroides*

(c) *Escherichia*

(d) *Clostridium*

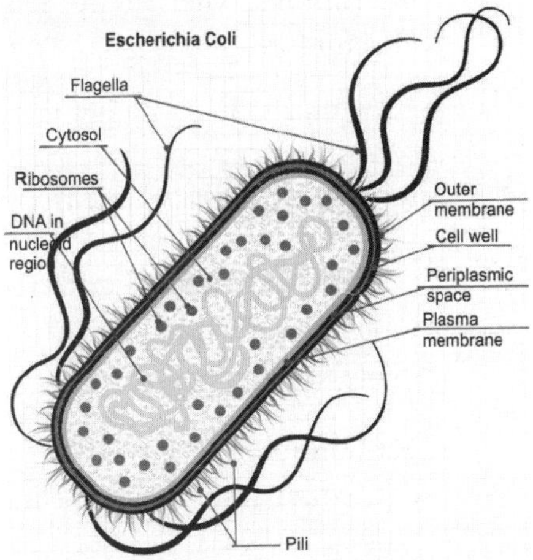

EXPLANATION

Escherichia is a genus of Gram negative, non spore forming, facultatively anaerobic, rod shaped bacteria from the family Enterobacteriaceae. In those species which are inhabitants of the gastrointestinal tracts of warm blooded animals, *Escherichia* species provide a portion of the microbially derived vitamin K for their host.

Ans. (C) i.e., *Escherichia*

4. Which of the following statements is ***not*** correct regarding sebaceous cyst?

(a) It has a punctum

(b) Treatment is incision and drainage

(c) Found on hairy areas of the body

(d) Not found on palms and soles

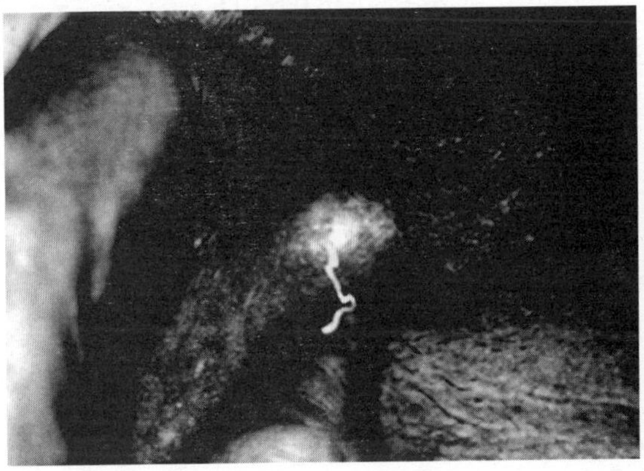

EXPLANATION

Surgical excision of a sebaceous cyst is a simple procedure to completely remove the sac and its contents.

Ans. (B) i.e., Treatment is incision and drainage

5. Match *List I* with *List II* and select the correct answer using the code given below the lists:

List I (Carcinoma)	*List II* (Characteristic)
A. Seminoma testis	1. Hormone dependent
B. Carcinoma prostrate	2. Does not spread by lymphatics
C. Basal cell carcinoma	3. Prognosis depends on thickness
D. Malignant melanoma	4. Highly radiosensitive

Code: A B C D

(a) 4 1 2 3 (b) 4 2 1 3 (c) 3 1 2 4 (d) 3 2 1 4

EXPLANATION

Tumours & Their Features

- Seminoma, 80% of which are diagnosed at stage I, is highly sensitive to both radiotherapy (RT) and chemotherapy (CHT) and, therefore, unlike many malignant neoplasms, cure is an expected outcome in the majority of cases, even with metastatic disease at presentation
- ***Prostate*** cancers are referred to as androgen ***dependent*** or androgen sensitive because treatments that decrease androgen levels or block androgen activity can inhibit their growth.
- ***Basal cell carcinoma*** (BCC) accounts for 80% of all non melanoma ***skin*** cancers. Its ***metastasis is*** extremely rare, ranging between 0.0028 and 0.55 of all BCC cases.

- In a case of malignant melanoma, overall **survival depends** on the **thickness of** the primary **melanoma**, whether the lymph nodes are involved, and whether there is spread **of melanoma** to distant sites.

Ans. (A) i.e., 4 1 2 3

6. **Tumours of anterior mediasternum include the following except:**

(a) Thymoma
(b) Lymphoma
(c) Germ cell tumour
(d) Schwannoma

EXPLANATION

A **schwannoma** is a usually benign nerve sheath tumor composed of Schwann cells, which normally produce the insulating myelin sheath covering peripheral nerves.

Ans. (D) i.e., Schwannoma

7. **In India, the commonest cause of unilateral lymphoedema of lower limb is:**

(a) Lymphoedema tarda
(b) Carcinoma of penis
(c) Filariasis
(d) Tubercular lymphadenopathy

EXPLANATION

The most spectacular symptom of lymphatic filariasis is elephantiasis – edema with thickening of the skin and underlying tissues—which was the first disease discovered to be transmitted by mosquito bites.

Ans. (C) i.e., Filariasis

2016

8. **Nottingham prognostic Index is used for:**

(a) Cancer stomach
(b) Cancer colon
(c) Cancer lung
(d) Cancer breast

EXPLANATION

The **Nottingham prognostic index** (NPI) is used to determine prognosis following surgery for breast cancer. Its value is calculated using three pathological criteria: the size of the lesion; the number of involved lymph nodes; and the grade of the tumour.

Ans. (D) i.e., Cancer breast

9. **A patient has recurrent abdominal pain and jaundice. The blood investigations reveal reticulocytosis and hyperbilirubinemia. What is the clinical diagnosis?**

(a) Hereditary spherocytosis
(b) Mirizzi's syndrome
(c) Choledochal cyst
(d) Sclerosing cholangitis

EXPLANATION

Symptoms of HS include anemia, jaundice, splenomegaly, and fatigue. Furthermore, the detritus of the broken down blood cells – unconjugated or indirect bilirubin – accumulates in the gallbladder, and can cause pigmented gallstones to develop.

Ans. (A) i.e., Hereditary spherocytosis

10. **In gallstone ileus, obstruction most frequently occurs at:**

(a) Duodenum
(b) Jejunum
(c) Proximal ileum
(d) Terminal ileum

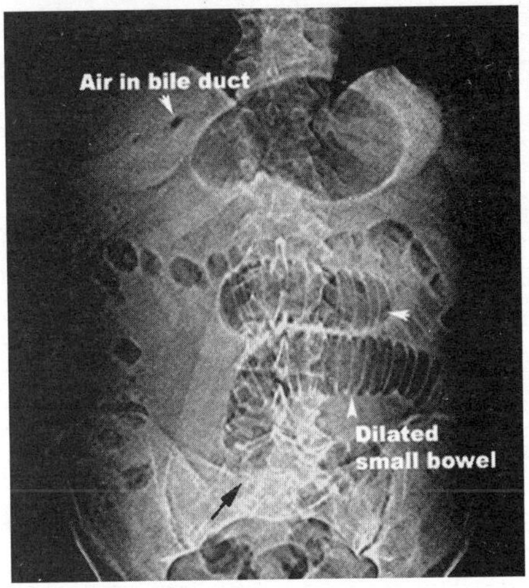

EXPLANATION

First described by Thomas Bartholin in 1654, **gallstone ileus** is a rare form of small bowel obstruction caused by an impaction of a gallstone within the lumen (small opening) of the small intestine. Such a gallstone enters the bowel via a cholecystoenteric fistula. Obstruction occurs most commonly at the near the distal ileum, within 60cm proximally to the ileocecal valve.

Ans. (D) i.e., Terminal ileum

11. **The following conditions are associated with high incidence of pigment gallstones except:**

(a) Cirrhosis
(b) Ileal disease
(c) Thalassemia
(d) Prosthetic heart valve

EXPLANATION

Risk factors for pigment stones include hemolytic anemias [such as from sickle cell disease, hereditary spherocytosis, thalassemia, prosthetic heart valves (Low grade hemolytic anemia occurs in 70% of prosthetic heart valve recipients, and severe hemolytic anemia occurs in 3%)], cirrhosis, and biliary tract infections. People with erythropoietic protoporphyria (EPP) are at increased risk to develop gallstones.

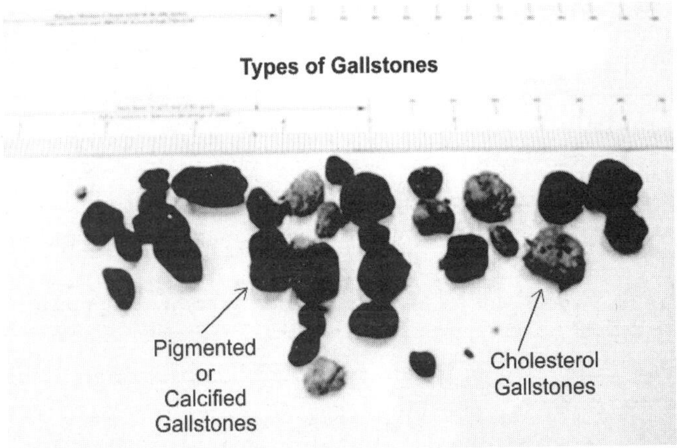

2016

Ans. (B) i.e., Ileal disease

12. **The most common route of spread in a case of pyogenic liver abscess is:**

(a) Haematogenous through portal vein
(b) Ascending infection through biliary duct
(c) Hepatic artery
(d) Local spread

EXPLANATION

In pyogenic liver abscess, the ***infection spreads*** to the ***liver*** via various routes, of which the most identifiable cause is ***biliary***-related

Ans. (B) i.e., Ascending infection through biliary duct

13. **The most common complication of pancreas divisum is:**

(a) Obstructive jaundice
(b) Duodenal obstruction
(c) Recurrent acute pancreatitis
(d) Peptic ulcer

EXPLANATION

A majority of individuals born with pancreas divisum will not have symptoms. In some cases, pancreas divisum is only detected during autopsy. A small group of individuals will develop symptoms which commonly include abdominal pain, nausea, vomiting, and acute and chronic pancreatitis.

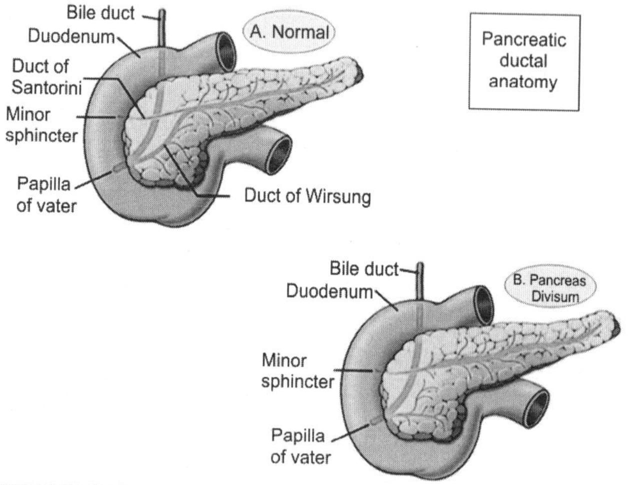

Pancreatic ductal anatomy

Ans. (C) i.e., Recurrent acute pancreatitis

14. The most common major surgical complication following whipple procedure is:

(a) Disruption of pancreatic anastomosis
(b) Biliary peritonitis
(c) Disruption of gastric anastomosis
(d) GI bleeding

EXPLANATION

A **pancreaticoduodenectomy**, **pancreatoduodenectomy**, **Whipple procedure**, or **Kausch Whipple procedure** is a major surgical operation most often performed to remove cancerous tumours off the head of the pancreas. It is also used for the treatment of pancreatic or duodenal trauma, or chronic pancreatitis. Pancreatic anastomotic leakage is the most important complication after pancreaticoduodenectomy. Leakage sometimes causes the development of other abdominal complications, such as intra-abdominal bleeding, intra-abdominal abscess, sepsis and organ failure, and is among the common causes of perioperative morbidity and mortality.

Ans. (A) i.e., Disruption of pancreatic anastomosis

15. A 60-year old male presents with bleeding p/r. Proctoscopy reveals 2nd degree haemorrhoids. The treatment of choice is:

(a) Cryotherapy
(b) Sclerotherapy
(c) Banding
(d) Surgery

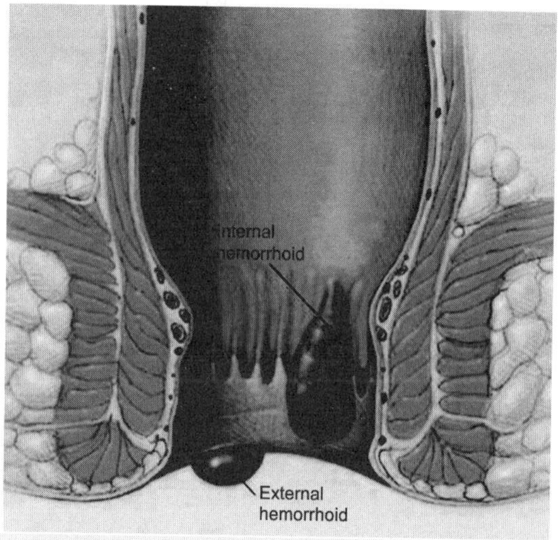

EXPLANATION

Rubber band ligation is typically recommended as the first line treatment in those with grade 1 to 3 disease. It is a procedure in which elastic bands are applied onto an internal hemorrhoid at least 1 cm above the dentate line to cut off its blood supply. Within 5–7 days, the withered hemorrhoid falls off.

Ans. (C) i.e., Banding

16. At present, treatment is recommended for *H. pylori* in association with the following except:

(a) Duodenal ulcer
(b) Early gastric cancer
(c) MALT lymphoma
(d) Benign gastric ulcer

EXPLANATION

Treatment for stomach cancer may include surgery, chemotherapy, and/or radiation therapy. New treatment approaches such as immunotherapy or gene therapy and improved ways of using current methods are being studied in clinical trials.

Ans. (B) i.e., Early gastric cancer

17. **Pott's puffy tumour is a:**

(a) Tuberculosis of the skull bone

(b) Squamous cell cancer of scalp

(c) Subperiosteal abscess associated with osteomyelitis of frontal bone

(d) Fungating scrotal malignancy

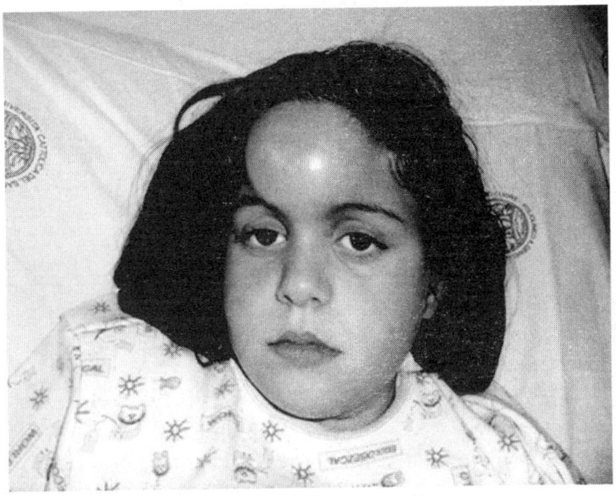

EXPLANATION

Pott's puffy tumor, first described by Sir Percivall Pott in 1760, is a rare clinical entity characterized by subperiosteal abscess associated with osteomyelitis. It is characterized by an osteomyelitis of the frontal bone, either direct or through haematogenic spread. This results in a swelling on the forehead, hence the name.

Ans. (C) i.e., Subperiosteal abscess associated with osteomyelitis of frontal bone

18. **With reference to frozen shoulder, consider the following statements:**

1. It is associated with diabetes and heart disease.

2. It may follow minor trauma.

3. Its differential diagnosis are infection and fractures.

4. Treatment of choice is surgery.

Which of the statements given above are correct?

(a) 1 and 2 only (b) 1, 2 and 3 (c) 2, 3 and 4 (d) 3 and 4 only

EXPLANATION

Frozen Shoulder

- Risk factors for frozen shoulder include tonic seizures, diabetes mellitus, stroke, accidents, lung disease, connective tissue diseases, thyroid disease, and heart disease.
- Differential diagnosis of frozen shoulder include:
  - o Rotator cuff strain/tear/impingement syndrome
  - o GH/Glenohumeral or acromioclavicular joint osteoarthritis (OA)
  - o Subacromial bursitis
  - o Parsonage Turner syndrome: brachial plexus inflammation secondary to a trigger, such as an infection, trauma, or autoimmune condition
  - o Fracture, posterior dislocation

Ans. (B) i.e., 1, 2 and 3

19. **The prognosis in reduced or unreduced fractures involving epiphyseal plate is very poor if the fracture line:**

(a) Runs along the epiphyseal plate
(b) Extends into epiphysis
(c) Crushes the epiphyseal plate
(d) Crosses the epiphyseal plate

EXPLANATION

The physis is crushed in type V epiphyseal injuries as per Salter Harris classification.

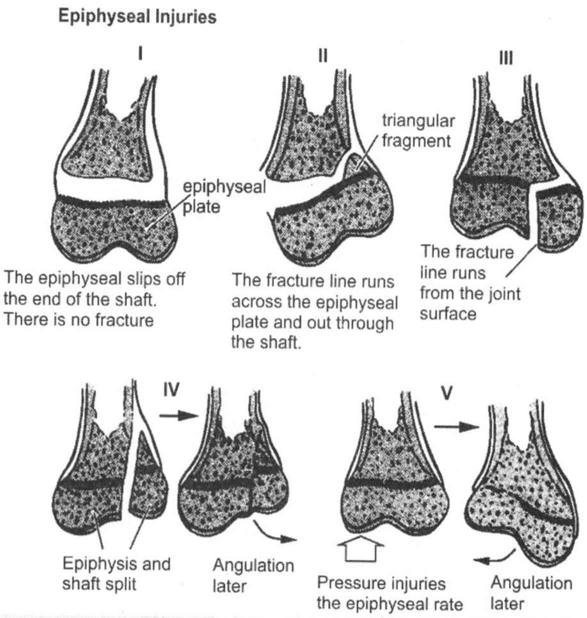

Ans. (C) i.e., Crushes the epiphyseal plate

20. A 30-year old man met with an accident and presented with multiple fractures of ribs and paradoxical movement with severe respiratory distress. X-ray shows pulmonary contusion on right side without pneumothorax or haemothorax. Which one of the following is the initial choice of treatment?

(a) Immediate internal fixation
(b) Endotracheal intubation and mechanical ventilation
(c) Thoracic epidural analgesia and O2 therapy
(d) Stabilization with towel clips

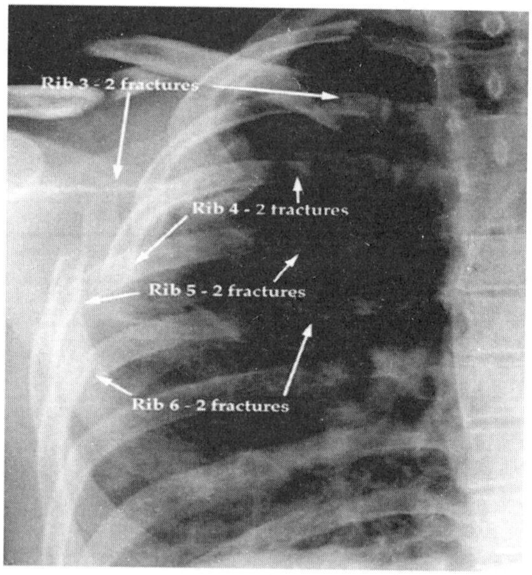

EXPLANATION

A person with flail chest (paradoxical respiration) may be intubated with a double lumen tracheal tube. In a double lumen endotracheal tube, each lumen may be connected to a different ventilator. Usually one side of the chest is affected more than the other, so each lung may require drastically different pressures and flows to adequately ventilate.

Ans. (B) i.e., Endotracheal intubation and mechanical ventilation

21. Which of the following is *not* a clinical feature of tetanus?

(a) Risus sardonicus
(b) Opisthotonus
(c) Loss of consciousness
(d) Respiratory failure

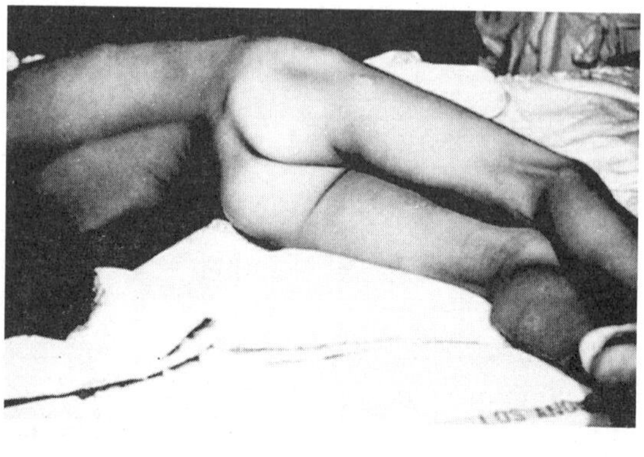

EXPLANATION

Tetanus often begins with mild spasms in the jaw muscles—also known as lockjaw or trismus. The spasms can also affect the facial muscles resulting in an appearance called *risus sardonicus*. Chest, neck, back, abdominal muscles, and buttocks may be affected. Back muscle spasms often cause arching, called opisthotonos (see figure). Sometimes the spasms affect muscles that help with breathing, which can lead to breathing problems.

Ans. (C) i.e., Loss of consciousness

22. **Hyperchloremic acidosis is a common complication of:**

(a) Ureterosigmoidostomy (b) Diarrhoea
(c) Vomiting (d) Ileostomy

EXPLANATION

A **ureterosigmoidostomy** is a surgical procedure where the ureters which carry urine from the kidneys, are diverted into the sigmoid colon. It is done as a treatment for bladder cancer, where the urinary bladder had to be removed. In the large intestine, sodium is swapped for potassium, and chloride for bicarbonate, this causes an hyperchloremic acidosis and hypokalaemia.

Ans. (A) i.e., Ureterosigmoidostomy

23. **Endoluminal probe for transrectal ultrasonography operates at the frequency of:**

(a) 2.5 MHz (b) 5.0 MHz
(c) 7.5 MHz (d) 15.0 MHz

EXPLANATION

Transrectal USG imaging usually employs a higher frequency 8–10 MHz probe with a long transducer length, similar to a transvaginal probe.

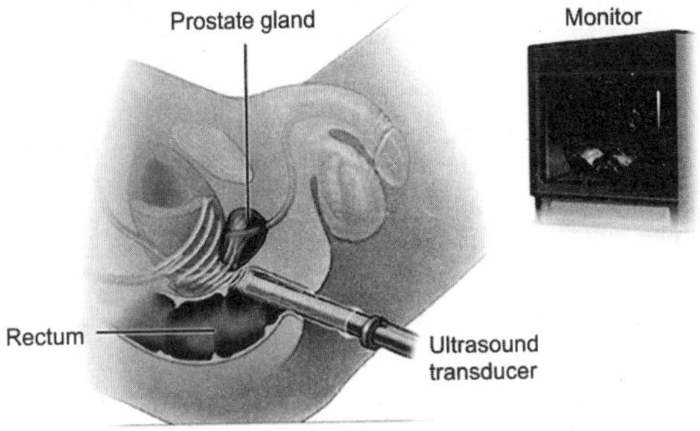

Ans. (C) i.e., 7.5 MHz

24. **A Seldinger needle is used for:**

(a) Liver biopsy (b) Breast biopsy
(c) Lymphangiography (d) Arteriography

EXPLANATION

The Seldinger technique, using Sldinger needle is used for angiography, insertion of chest drains and central venous catheters, insertion of PEG tubes using the push technique, insertion of the leads for an artificial pacemaker or implantable cardioverter defibrillator, and numerous other interventional medical procedures.

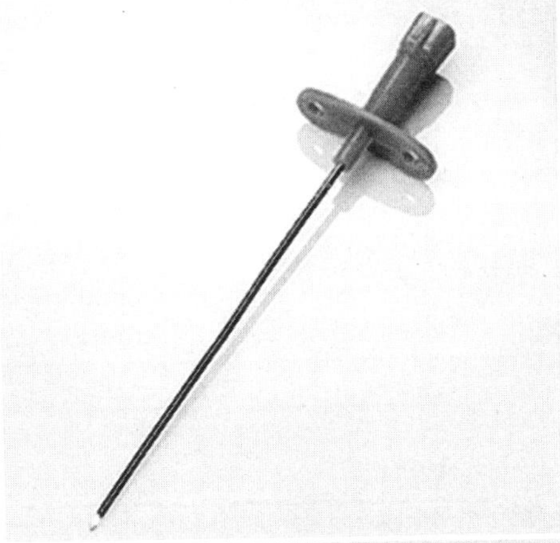

Ans. (D) i.e., Arteriography

25. **The ideal temperature to store the whole blood in blood bank is**

(a) -4 degree C (b) 0 degree C (c) 4 degree C (d) 8 degree C

EXPLANATION

More than 70% of red cells should remain viable in circulation 24 hours after transfusion of stored blood in CPDA-1 for 35 days. The blood is stored at 2–6°C to maintain the optimal viability.

Ans. (C) i.e., 4 degree C

2016

26. **Bisgaard treatment refers to that of:**

(a) Ruptured tendo achillis
(b) Venous ulcer
(c) An ischaemic ulcer
(d) An ingrowing toe nail

EXPLANATION

Most venous ulcers respond to patient education, elevation of foot, elastic compression, and evaluation (known as the Bisgaard regimen).

Ans. (B) i.e., Venous ulcer

27. **Glasgow coma scale (GCS) score ranges between:**

(a) 0 and 15 (b) 1 and 15 (c) 2 and 15 (d) 3 and 15

EXPLANATION

The **Glasgow Coma Scale** (GCS) is a neurological scale which aims to give a reliable and objective way of recording the conscious state of a person for initial as well as subsequent assessment. A patient is assessed against the criteria of the scale, and the resulting points give a patient score between 3 (indicating deep unconsciousness) and either 14 (original scale) or 15 (more widely used modified or revised scale).

Glasgow Coma Scale

Eye opening (E)	
• Spontaneous	4
• To speech	3
• To pain	2
• Nil	1
Best motor response (M)	
• Obeys	6
• Localises	5
• Withdraws	4
• Abnormal flexion	3
• Extensor response	2
• Nil	1
Verbal response (V)	
• Orientated	5
• Confused conversation	4
• Inappropriate words	3
• Incomprehensible sounds	2
• Nil	1
Coma score = E + M + V	
• Minimum	3
• Maximum	15

Ans. (D) i.e., Respiratory failure

28. **The most common cause of intestinal obstruction is:**

(a) Obstructed hernia
(b) Inflammatory abdominal conditions
(c) Gastrointestinal malignancy
(d) Bands and adhesions

EXPLANATION

Small bowel obstructions are most often due to adhesions and hernias while large bowel obstructions are most often due to tumors and volvulus.

Ans. (D) i.e., Bands and adhesions

2016

29. **The most common site for nosocomial (hospital acquired) infection is:**

(a) Respiratory tract
(b) Urinary tract
(c) Surgical site
(d) Blood stream

EXPLANATION

Indwelling catheters have recently been identified with hospital acquired infections. Procedures using Intravascular Antimicrobial Lock Therapy can reduce infections that are unexposed to blood borne antibiotics. Introducing antibiotics, including ethanol, into the catheter (without flushing it into the bloodstream) reduces the formation of biofilms.

Ans. (B) i.e., Urinary tract

30. **A patient has carcinoid tumour of appendix of size more than 2.5 cm. The management of choice is:**

(a) Appendecectomy
(b) Appendecectomy and 24 hour urinary HIAA
(c) Appendecectomy and abdominal CT scan
(d) Right hemicolectomy

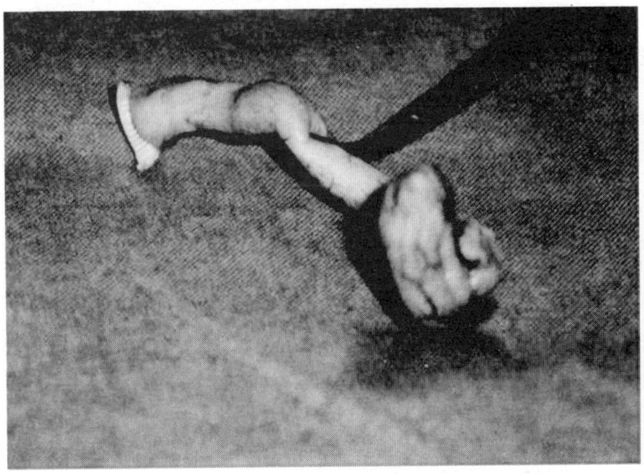

EXPLANATION

Open ***right hemicolectomy*** (open ***right colectomy***) is a procedure that involves removing the cecum, the ascending colon, the hepatic flexure (where the ascending colon joins the transverse colon), the first third of the transverse colon, and part of the terminal ileum, along with fat and lymph nodes.

Ans. (D) i.e., Right hemicolectomy

2016

31. **What is the most common cause of intestinal obstruction in neonates?**

(a) Meconium ileus
(b) Duodenal atresia
(c) Volvulus neonatorium
(d) Hirschsprung's disease

EXPLANATION

Duodenal atresia is the congenital absence or complete closure of a portion of the lumen of the duodenum. It causes increased levels of amniotic fluid during pregnancy (polyhydramnios) and intestinal obstruction in newborn babies.

Ans. (B) i.e., Duodenal atresia

32. **Match *List I* with *List II* and select the correct answer using the code given below the lists:**

***List I* (Drug)**	***List II* (Complications)**
A. Cisplatinum	1. Haemorrhagic cystitis
B. Adriamycin	2. Pulmonary fibrosis
C. Bleomycin	3. Cardiomyopathy
D. Cyclophosphamide	4. Tubular necrosis

Code: A B C D

(a) 3 4 2 1
(b) 4 3 1 2
(c) 3 4 1 2
(d) 4 3 2 1

EXPLANATION

Chemotherapeutic Agents and Their Complications

- The pathophysiology of cisplatin induced AKI (acute kidney injury) involves proximal tubular injury, oxidative stress, inflammation, and vascular injury in the kidney. There is predominantly acute tubular necrosis and also apoptosis in the proximal tubules.
- Established ***doxorubicin cardiomyopathy*** is a lethal disease. When congestive heart failure develops, mortality is approximately 50%.
- The major limitation of ***bleomycin*** therapy is ***pulmonary toxicity***, which can be life threatening in up to 10% of patients receiving the drug.
- *Cyclophosphamide* is an alkylating agent used intravenously or orally in the treatment of both malignant and nonneoplastic diseases. A known adverse effect of such treatment is ***hemorrhagic cystitis.***

Ans. (D) i.e., 4 3 2 1

33. **Consider the following statements:**

Haemophilia A (haemophilia) and Haemophilia B (christmas disease)

1. **Are variants of the same disease process**
2. **Are due to congenital deficiency of factor VIII and factor IX respectively**
3. **Both are sex linked characteristics and transmitted by asymptomatic females**
4. **Can occur both in males and females**

Select the correct answer using the code given below:

(a) 2 and 3 (b) 1, 2 and 4 (c) 2 only (d) 3 only

EXPLANATION

Hemophilia

- There are two main types of haemophilia: haemophilia A, which occurs due to not enough clotting factor VIII, and haemophilia B, which occurs due to not enough clotting factor IX.
- They are typically inherited from one's parents through an X chromosome with a nonfunctional gene.
- Since the mutations causing the disease are X-linked recessive, a female carrying the defect on one of her X chromosomes may not be affected by it, as the equivalent allele on her other chromosome should express itself to produce the necessary clotting factors, due to X-inactivation.

Ans. (A) i.e., 2 and 3

34. **A 30-year old lady sustained chest injury in an accident and presented with massive haemothorax on right side. Tube thoracostomy drained 1800 ml of blood. What is the most appropriate treatment?**

(a) Correction of hypovolemic shock
(b) Put one more chest tube
(c) Clamp the chest tube to cause the tamponade
(d) Resuscitation and prepare for urgent thoracotomy

EXPLANATION

In some cases of hemothorax, bleeding continues and surgery is necessary to stop the source of bleeding. For example, if the hemothorax was caused by aortic rupture in high energy trauma, surgical intervention (thoracotomy) is mandatory.

Ans. (D) i.e., Resuscitation and prepare for urgent thoracotomy

2016

35. In a case of obstructed hernia, strangulation is suggested by which of the following?

1. Presence of shock
2. Pain is never completely absent
3. Localised tenderness is associated with rebound tenderness
4. Pain persists despite conservative management
5. An external hernia becomes tense, tender, irreducible, with recent increase in size

Select the correct answer using the code given below:

(a) 1, 2, 3, and 4 only
(b) 1, 2, 4 and 5 only
(c) 1, 3 and 5 only
(d) 1, 2, 3, 4 and 5

EXPLANATION

Strangulated hernias

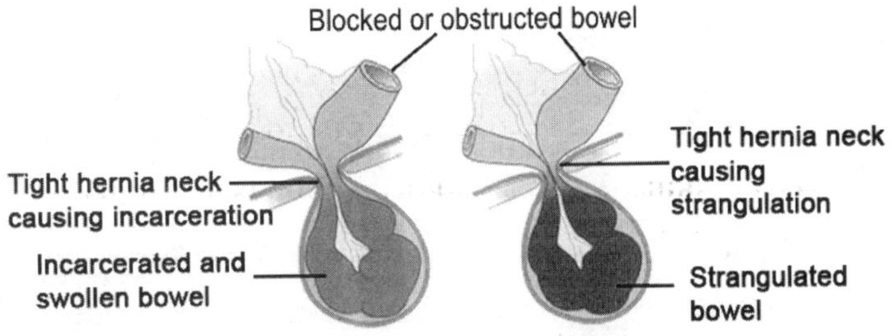

- They are always painful and pain is followed by tenderness. Nausea, vomiting, or fever may occur in these cases due to bowel obstruction. Also, there may be recent increase in size.
- An incarcerated **hernia** can become **strangulated**, which cuts off the blood flow to the tissue that's trapped and can lead to life threatening complications. Excruciating pain due to ischaemic changes in entrapped gastrointestinal tissue may endanger life causing neurogenic **shock**.

Ans. (D) i.e., 1, 2, 3, 4 and 5

2016

36. Regarding haemorrhagic shock, which one of the following statements is correct?

(a) Clinically manifested when > 10% of loss of total blood volume occurs
(b) Tachycardia presents in 100% of hypovolemic patients
(c) Loss of 40% of circulating volume is life threatening
(d) In acute stage of shock, systemic vasodilation becomes evident

Hemorrhage classes

Class	Blood loss	Response	Treatment
I	<15% (0.75 Litre)	Minimum fast heart rate, normal blood pressure	Minimal
II	15–30% (0.75–1.5 Litre)	Fast heart rate, min. low blood pressure	Intravenous fluids
III	30–40% (1.5–2 Litre)	Very fast heart rate, low blood pressure, confusion	Fluids and packed RBCs
IV	>40% (>2 Litre)	Critical blood pressure and heart rate	Aggressive interventions

Ans. (C) i.e., Loss of 40% of circulating volume is life threatening

37. Consider the following statements:

Poor prognostic indicators in advanced germ cell tumours show

1. primary sites in mediastinum
2. non pulmonary metastasis
3. lactate dehydrogenase more than 10 times of normal value

Which of the statements given above are correct?

(a) 1, 2 and 3 (b) 2 and 3 only (c) 1 and 3 only (d) 1 and 2 only

EXPLANATION

A nonseminoma extragonadal germ cell tumor is in the good prognosis group if:

- The tumor is in the back of the abdomen; and
- The tumor has not spread to organs other than the lungs; and
- The levels of tumor markers AFP and β-hCG are normal and LDH is slightly above normal.

Ans. (A) i.e., 1, 2 and 3

38. Which one of the following structures is *not* removed during a classical radical neck dissection?

(a) Trapezius
(b) Sternocleidomastoid/SCM
(c) Internal jugular vein/IJV
(d) Spinal Accessory nerve/SAN

EXPLANATION

Radical Neck Dissection (RND) - Removal of all ipsilateral cervical lymph node groups from levels I through V, together with SAN, SCM and IJV.

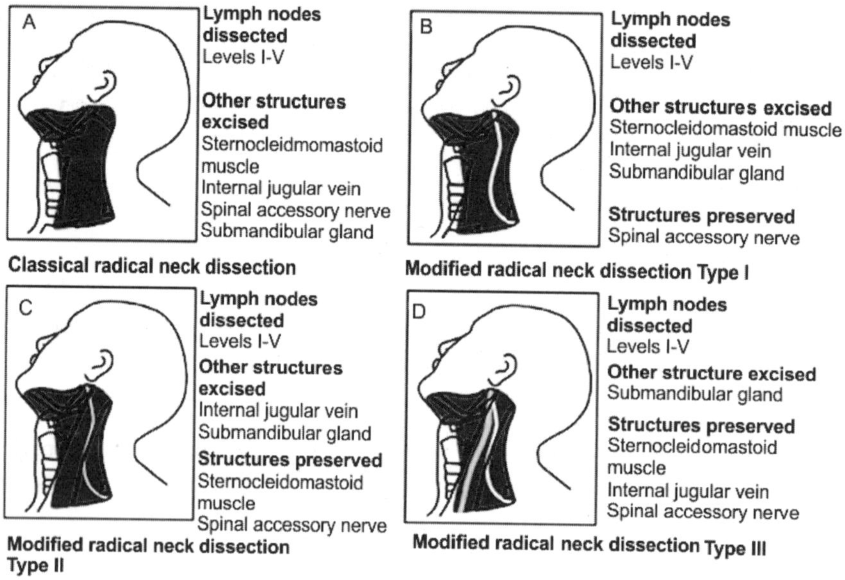

Ans. (A) i.e., Trapezius

39. Mousseau Barbin Tube (M.B.Tube) is used for:

(a) Advance cancer stomach
(b) Advance cancer oesophagus
(c) Advance cancer oropharynx
(d) All of these

EXPLANATION

Oesophageal Cancer is a lethal malignancy with propensity for early spread, and late presentation. Quite a number of patients present late; necessitating palliation as the main aim of treatment. Palliation involves the restoration of luminal continuity. This may be achieved by dilatation, tumour fulguration, and or stent insertion or intubation. Mousseau Barbin tube is one of the oesophageal traction tubes developed for use in these patients.

Ans. (B) i.e., Advance cancer oesophagus

40. Which one of the following is the investigation of choice in a patient with haematemesis?

(a) Flexible upper gastrointestinal endoscopy
(b) Barium meal for stomach and duodenum

(c) Contrast enhanced CT scan

(d) Selective left gastric angiography

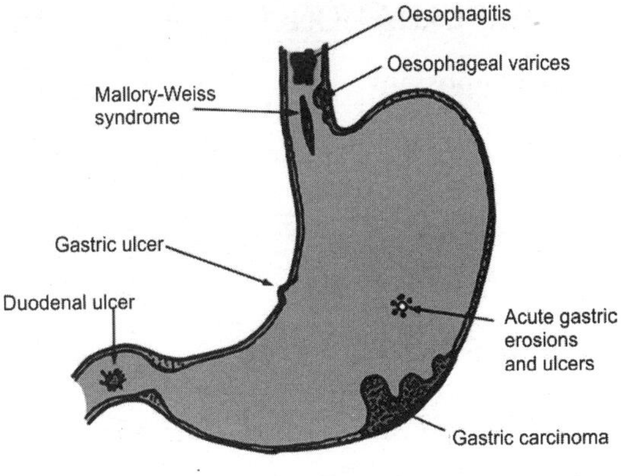

EXPLANATION

Upper gastrointestinal endoscopy is recommended as first choice in acute digestive bleeding which is assumed to originate in the upper gastrointestinal tract (haematemesis or melaena)

Ans. (A) i.e., Flexible upper gastrointestinal endoscopy

41. **The two important values necessary for describing the variation in a series of observations are:**

(a) Mean and standard deviation
(b) Mean and range
(c) Median and range
(d) Median and standard deviation

EXPLANATION

Variation in a series of observations

- The sample mean is the average and is computed as the sum of all the observed outcomes from the sample divided by the total number of events.
- The ***standard deviation*** is a summary measure of the differences of each observation from the ***mean***.

Ans. (A) i.e., Mean and standard deviation

42. **The time period between entry of infective agent in a host and maximal infectivity of that host is:**

(a) Incubation period
(b) Serial interval
(c) Generation time
(d) Period of communicability

EXPLANATION

Generation time

- It is the time interval between entry of an infectious agent and maximal infectivity of the host.
- Lesser the generation time of a specific pathogen means lesser the incubation period and vice versa.

Ans. (C) i.e., Generation time

43. **Consider the following statements:**

Symposium is a method of health education characterised by

1. **a series of speeches on a selected topic**
2. **presentation of different aspects of a topic by 3 or 4 experts.**
3. **a discussion among the symposium members**
4. **the chairperson making a comprehensive summary at the end of the session**

Which of these statements are correct?

(a) 2 and 3 only
(b) 1, 3 and 4
(c) 1, 2 and 4
(d) 1, 2 and 3

2016

EXPLANATION

Symposium

- A symposium is generally defined as a meeting organized so that experts in a given field can meet, present papers, and discuss issues and trends or make recommendations for a certain course of action.
- A keynote speaker who will deliver remarks on the overall theme of the symposium.

Ans. (C) i.e., 1, 2 and 4

44. Match *List I* with *List II* and select the correct answer using the code given below the lists:

List I (Major Group of Insecticides)	*List II* (Name of Insecticide)
A. Stomach poison	1. Temephos
B. Organochlorine compound	2. Propoxur
C. Organophosphorous compound	3. Sodium fluoride
D. Carbamates	4. Dieldrin

Code: A B C D

(a) 4 3 1 2 (b) 4 3 2 1 (c) 3 4 1 2 (d) 3 4 2 1

EXPLANATION

Insecticide Group and Their Members

- ***Sodium fluoride*** is used as a ***stomach poison*** for plant feeding insects.
- ***Dieldrin*** is an organochloride originally produced in 1948 by J. Hyman and Co, Denver, as an insecticide.
- Temefos or **temephos** (trade name Abate) is an **organophosphate** larvicide used to treat water infested with disease carrying insects including mosquitoes, midges, and black fly larvae.
- ***Propoxur*** (Baygon) is a carbamate insecticide and was introduced in 1959.

Ans. (C) i.e., 3 4 1 2

45. Consider the following diseases:

1. Rift valley fever
2. Yellow Fever
3. Chickungunya fever
4. West Nile fever

Which of the above diseases are transmitted by *Aedes* mosquito?

(a) 1, 2 and 3 (b) 2, 3 and 4

(c) 1, 2 and 4 (d) 1, 3 and 4

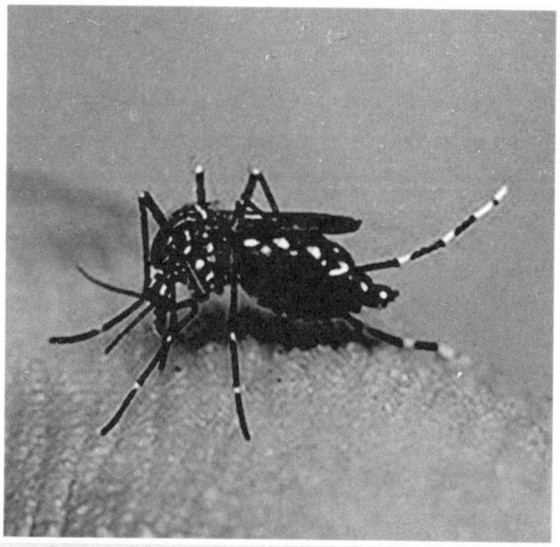

EXPLANATION

Aedes aegypti, the **yellow fever mosquito**, is a mosquito that can spread dengue fever, chikungunya, Zika fever, Mayaro and yellow fever viruses, and other disease agents.

Two species—*Culex tritaeniorhynchus* and *Aedes vexans*—are known to transmit the virus responsible for causing Rift valley fever.

Ans. (A) i.e., 1, 2 and 3

46. Consider the following statements:

Prophylactic disinfection includes:

1. disinfection of urine specimen of patient with enteric fever
2. pasteurization of milk
3. disinfection of contaminated linen
4. disinfection of water by chlorine

Which of these statements are correct?

(a) 1, 2, 3 and 4 (b) 2 and 4 only (c) 1, 2 and 4 only (d) 1 and 3 only

EXPLANATION

Recurrent (***prophylactic***) ***disinfection***: It is prevention of an infection by chlorination of water, pasteurization of milk, hand washing etc.

Ans. (B) i.e., 2 and 4 only

47. Consider the following statements:

1. Registration of birth, even if the child is born in a hospital, is essentially the responsibility of parents only.
2. At present, the registration of birth has to be done not more than 15 days after the birth.

Which of these statements is/are correct?

(a) 1 only (b) 2 only (c) Both 1 and 2 (d) Neither 1 nor 2

EXPLANATION

Persons required to register births and deaths.

It shall be the duty of the persons specified below to give or cause to be given, either orally or in writing, according to the best of their knowledge and belief, within such time as may be prescribed (within 21 days), information to the Registrar of the several particulars required to be entered in the forms prescribed by the State Government under subsection (1) of section 16,—

(a) In respect of births and deaths in a house, whether residential or non residential, not being any place referred to in clauses (b) to (e), the head of the house or, in case more than one household live in the house, the head of the household, the person, who is so recognised by the house or the household, and if he is not present in the house at any time during the period within which the birth or death has to be reported, the nearest relative of the head present in the house, and in the absence of any such person, the oldest adult male person present therein during the said period;

(b) In respect of births and deaths in a hospital, health centre, maternity or nursing home or other like institution, the medical officer in charge or any person authorised by him in this behalf;

(c) In respect of births and deaths in a jail, the jailor in charge;

(d) In respect of births and deaths in a choultry, chattram, hostel, dharmasala, boarding house, lodging house, tavern, barrack, toddy shop or place of public resort, the person in charge thereof;

(e) In respect of any new born child or dead body found deserted in a public place, the headman or other corresponding officer of the village in the case of a village and the officer in charge of the local police station elsewhere: Provided that any person who finds such child or dead body, or in whose charge such child or dead body may be placed, shall notify such fact to the headman or officer aforesaid;

(f) In any other place, such person as may be prescribed.

Ans. (D) i.e., 2 and 4 only

48. Sullivan Index is the measure of which of the following?

(a) Disability rate (b) Pregnancy rate (c) Literacy rate (d) Quality of life

EXPLANATION

Health expectancy calculated by **Sullivan's** method is the number of remaining years, at a particular age, that an individual can expect to live in a healthy state. It is computed by subtracting the probable duration of bed disability and inability to perform major activities from the life expectancy.

Ans. (A) i.e., Disability rate

49. Consider the following statements:

The strategy to eradicate poliomyelitis in India comprised of:

1. **Conducting national immunisation days**
2. **Mopping up rounds with OPV**
3. **Acute flaccid paralysis surveillance**
4. **Public awareness through multimedia**

Which of these statements are correct?

(a) 1 and 3 only (b) 2 and 4 only (c) 1, 2 and 3 only (d) 1, 2, 3 and 4

EXPLANATION

Key Factors in Polio Eradication

- OPV is included in National Immunization Schedule
- The supplementary immunization activities were initiated as National Immunization Days in 1995. These were the mainstay of polio immunization activities for rapidly enhancing population immunity against WPV against a backdrop of low routine immunization rates. House to house vaccination drives were held to vaccinate those children who were not covered by the fixed sites vaccination during supplementary immunization activities
- Acute flaccid paralysis surveillance in India was strengthened, and it achieved a desired non polio acute flaccid paralysis rate of >2 per 100000 in almost all the states.
- Public awareness through radio and television.

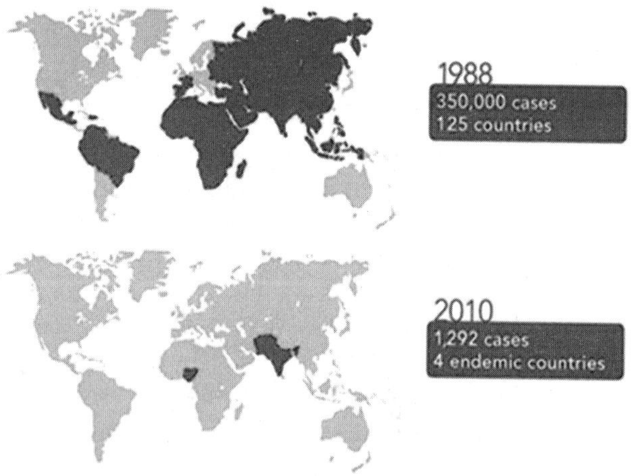

Ans. (D) i.e., 1, 2, 3 and 4

50. In the estimation of statistical probability, Z score is applicable to:

(a) Normal distribution

(b) Skewed distribution

(c) Binomial distribution

(d) Poisson distribution

EXPLANATION

Simply put, a **Z score** is the number of standard deviations from the mean a data point is. But more technically it's

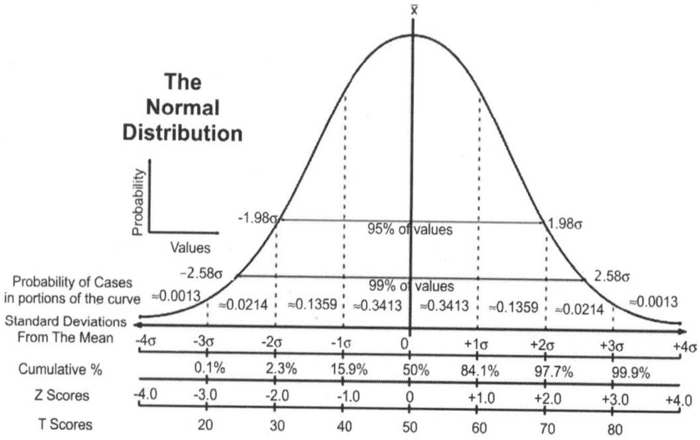

a measure of how many standard deviations below or above the population mean a raw **score** is. A **z scoreis** also known as a standard **score** and it can be placed on a normal distribution curve.

Ans. (A) i.e., Normal distribution

51. **Consider the following vectors:**

1. **Aedes mosquito** 2. **Flea** 3. **Ticks** 4. **Itchmite**

Transovarian transmission is demonstrated in

(a) 1 and 2 (b) 2 and 4 (c) 1 and 3 (d) 3 and 4

EXPLANATION

Transovarial or **transovarian transmission** occurs in certain arthropod vectors as they transmit disease causing pathogens from parent arthropod to offspring arthropod. For instance, *Rickettsia rickettsii*, carried within ticks, is passed on from parent to offspring tick by transovarial transmission. This is the mechanism by which many Rickettsiae are maintained in their arthropod hosts through generations, which occurs also in aedes mosquito vector of the yellow fever virus and in phlebotomine sandflies that transmit pappataci fever.

Ans. (C) i.e., 1 and 3

52. **The most sensitive indicator of the health status of a community is the:**

(a) Crude death rate (b) Maternal mortality rate

(c) Infant mortality rate (d) Child mortality rate

EXPLANATION

The **infant mortality** rate (IMR), defined as the number of deaths in children under 1 year of **age** per 1000 live births in the same year, has in the past been regarded as a highly sensitive (proxy) measure of **population** health.

Ans. (C) i.e., Infant mortality rate

2016

53. **Chemoprophylaxis is an example of:**

(a) Specific protection (b) Health promotion (c) Early detection (d) Rehabilitation

EXPLANATION

Level	Definition
Primal and primordial prevention	Any measure aimed at helping future parents provide their upcoming child with adequate attention, as well as secure physical and affective environments from conception to first birthday (i.e., over the child's *primal period* of life). Primordial prevention refers to measures designed to avoid the development of risk factors in the first place, early in life.
Primary prevention	Methods to avoid occurrence of disease either through eliminating disease agents or increasing resistance to disease. Examples include immunization against disease, maintaining a healthy diet and exercise regimen, and avoiding smoking.
Secondary prevention	Methods to detect and address an existing disease prior to the appearance of symptoms. Examples include treatment of hypertension (a risk factor for many cardiovascular diseases), cancer screenings.
Tertiary prevention	Methods to reduce the harm of symptomatic disease, such as disability or death, through rehabilitation and treatment. Examples include surgical procedures that halt the spread or progression of disease.
Quaternary prevention	Methods to mitigate or avoid results of unnecessary or excessive interventions in the health system.

Ans. (A) i.e., Specific protection

54. **A rapid mass screening method that can be employed by a paramedical worker for detecting malnutrition in preschool (age: 1 to 5 years) children is:**

(a) Weight for age
(b) Height for age
(c) Mid arm circumference
(d) Body Mass Index

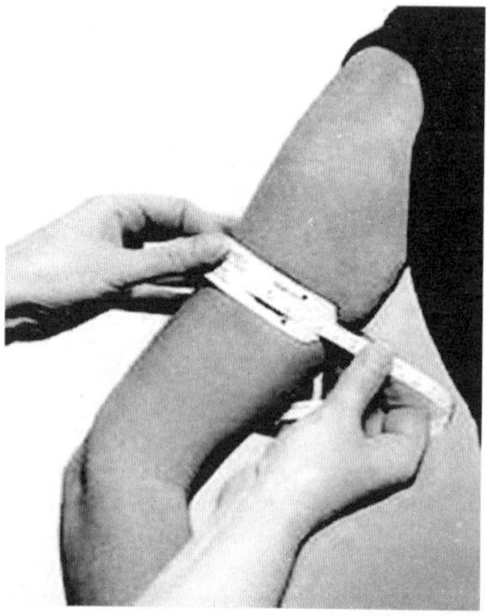

EXPLANATION

Mid Upper **Arm Circumference** (MUAC) is the **circumference** of the left upper **arm**, measured at the **mid** point between the tip of the shoulder and the tip of the elbow (olecranon process and the acromium). MUAC is used for the assessment of nutritional status.

Ans. (C) i.e., Mid arm circumference

55. **The most important single determinant of infant mortality is:**

(a) Birth weight
(b) Age of the mother
(c) Order of birth
(d) Inteval between births

EXPLANATION

Preterm ***birth*** (born before 37 weeks of pregnancy) and being small for gestational age, which are the reasons for ***low birth weight*** (LBW), are also important indirect causes of neonatal ***deaths.*** LBW contributes to 60% to 80% of all neonatal ***deaths.***

Ans. (A) i.e., Birth weight

2016

56. **The immunoglobulins that can be transported across the placenta include:**

(a) IgG only
(b) IgA only
(c) Both IgG and IgA
(d) Neither IgG nor IgA

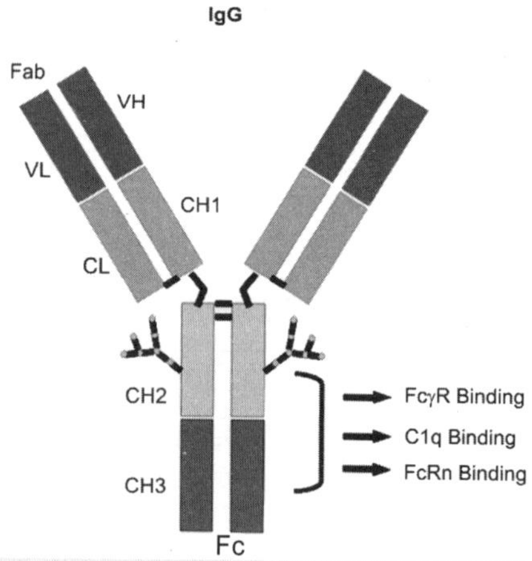

EXPLANATION

IgG is secreted as a monomer that is small in size allowing it to easily perfuse tissues. It is the only antibody isotype that has receptors to facilitate passage through the human placenta, thereby providing protection to the fetus *in utero.*

Ans. (A) i.e., IgG only

57. **Consider the following statements:**

1. **The duration of immunity is longer when live vaccine is administered as compared to the administration of killed vaccine.**
2. **In the case of killed vaccine, single dose is sufficient whereas multiple doses are always required in the case of live vaccines.**

Which of these statements is/are correct?

(a) 1 only
(b) 2 only
(c) Both 1 and 2
(d) Neither 1 nor 2

EXPLANATION

Live vaccines use a weakened (or attenuated) form of the microorganism that causes a disease. Because these vaccines are so similar to the natural infection that they help prevent, they create a strong and long lasting immune response. Just 1 or 2 doses of most live vaccines can give a lifetime of protection against a microorganism and the disease it causes.

Mnemonics – Live Vaccines

ROME Is My Best Place To go Yet	• BOYs Love The CRIME
• Rubella	• B = BCG
• Oral Polio vaccine	O = OPV
• Measles	Y = YELLOW FEVER
• Epidemic typhus	
• Influenza	• Love = LIVE ATTENUATED
• Mumps	
• BCG	The = TYPHOID
• Plague	C = CHICKEN POX
• Typhoid oral vaccine	R = RUBELLA
• Yellow fever	I = INFLUENZA
	M = MUMPS, MEASLES
	E = EPIDEMIC TYPHUS

Ans. (A) i.e., 1 only

58. Match *List I* with *List II* and select the correct answer using the code given below the lists:

List I (Disease)	*List II* (Incubation Period)
A. Measles	1. 6 weeks to 6 months
B. Diphtheria	2. 15 to 50 days
C. Hepatitis A	3. 10 to 14 days
D. Hepatitis B	4. 2 to 6 days

Code: A B C D

(a) 3 4 1 2 (b) 4 3 2 1 (c) 4 3 1 2 (d) 3 4 2 1

EXPLANATION

Diseases and Incubation Period

- **Measles** is a highly contagious infectious disease caused by the measles virus. Symptoms usually develop 10–12 days after exposure to an infected person and last 7–10 days.
- **Diphtheria** is an infection caused by the bacterium *Corynebacterium diphtheriae*. Signs and symptoms may vary from mild to severe. They usually start two to five days after exposure.
- **Hepatitis A** is an infectious disease of the liver caused by the hepatitis A virus (HAV). Many cases have few or no symptoms, especially in the young. The time between infection and symptoms, in those who develop them, is between two and six weeks.
- **Hepatitis B** is an infectious disease caused by the hepatitis B virus (HBV) that affects the liver. It may take 30 to 180 days for symptoms to begin.

Ans. (D) i.e., 3 4 2 1

59. **Throat swab positive and Schick test negative indicate that the person is:**

(a) Suffering from diphtheria

(b) Susceptible to diphtheria

(c) Hypersensitive to diphtheria

(d) Immune to diphtheria

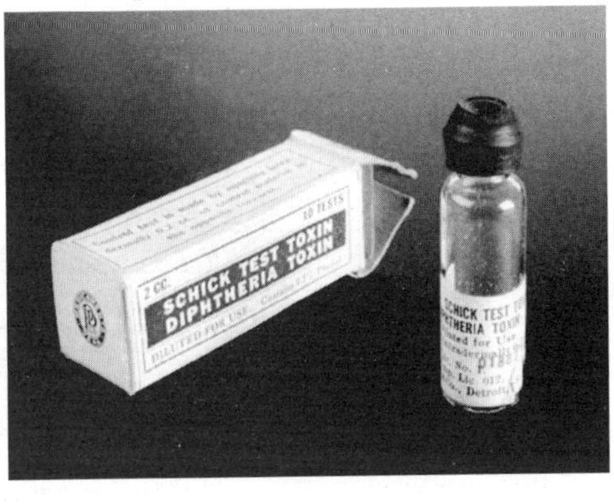

EXPLANATION

Diphtheria

- Isolation of *C. diphtheriae* from a Gram stain or throat culture from a clinical specimen support the diagnosis of diphtheria.

- The **Schick test**, invented between 1910 and 1911, is a test used to determine whether or not a person is susceptible to diphtheria.

Ans. (A) i.e., Suffering from diphtheria

60. **The following are manifestations of psychosis except:**

(a) Psycho-neurosis (b) Schizophrenia
(c) Manic depressive psychosis (d) Paranoia

EXPLANATION

Psycho-Neurosis is a class of functional mental disorders involving chronic distress but neither delusions nor hallucinations. The term is no longer used by the professional psychiatric community in the United States, having been eliminated from the *Diagnostic and Statistical Manual of Mental Disorders* in 1980 with the publication of DSM III. It is still used in the ICD-10 Chapter V F40–48.

Ans. (A) i.e., Psychoneurosis

61. **Consider the following definitions:**

'Effectiveness measures the extent to which predetermined objectives are achieved. Efficiency measures how well the resources are utilized.'

In view of these definitions, which of the following assertions are *true*?

1. **Percentage of bed occupancy measures effectiveness**
2. **Immunization coverage rate measures efficiency**
3. **Cost per patient treated measures efficiency**
4. **Reduction in mortality measures effectiveness**

Select the correct answer using the code given below:

(a) 1 and 2 (b) 2 and 3 only (c) 3 and 4 only (d) 2, 3 and 4

EXPLANATION

Vaccine

- Vaccine efficacy and vaccine effectiveness measure the proportionate reduction in cases among vaccinated persons. Vaccine efficacy is used when a study is carried out under ideal conditions, for example, during a clinical trial.
- Vaccine effectiveness is used when a study is carried out under typical field (that is, less than perfectly controlled) conditions.
- Vaccine efficacy/effectiveness (VE) is measured by calculating the risk of disease among vaccinated and unvaccinated persons and determining the percentage reduction in risk of disease among vaccinated persons relative to unvaccinated persons.
- The greater the percentage reduction of illness in the vaccinated group, the greater the vaccine efficacy/effectiveness.

Ans. (D) i.e., 2, 3 and 4

62. **With reference to the Revised National Tuberculosis Control Programme, consider the following statements:**

1. **Active case finding is pursued under this Programme.**
2. **Microscopy centres are established in the districts for every one lakh population and in hilly and tribal areas for every 50,000 population.**

Which of these statements is/are correct?

(a) 1 only (b) 2 only (c) Both 1 and 2 (d) Neither 1 nor 2

2016

EXPLANATION

Under RNTCP, diagnosis and treatment facilities are provided free of cost to all TB patients. For quality diagnosis, designated microscopy centers have been established for every one lac population in the general areas and for every 50,000 population in the tribal, hilly and difficult areas. More than 13000 microscopy centers have been established in the country. Free treatment services are available for TB at all Government hospitals, Community Health Centers (CHC), Primary Health Centers (PHCs). DOT centers have been established near to residence of patients to the extent possible. All public heatlh facilties, subs centres, Community Volunteers, ASHA, Women Self Groups etc. also function as DOT Providers/DOT Centers.

Ans. (B) i.e., 2 only

63. **Districts are classified into different categories regarding neonatal tetanus/NT risk. Which one of the following correctly describes 'Neonatal Tetanus Elimination' status?**

(a) Incidence rate more than 2/1000 births, two doses of TT vaccine coverage less than 70%, attended deliveries between 60% and 70%.

(b) Incidence rate between 1 to 2/1000 births, three doses of TT vaccine coverage 70%, attended deliveries more than 75%.

(c) Incidence rate 0.5 to 1/1000 births, three doses of TT vaccine coverage between 70% and 80%, attended deliveries between 65% and 70%.

(d) Incidence rate less than 0.1/1000 births, two doses of TT vaccine coverage more than 90%, attended deliveries more than 75%.

EXPLANATION

Classification of Districts

Category	NT incidence rates	Immunization coverage levels	Proportion of clean deliveries by trained professionals
NT High risk	>1/1000 live births	TT2 coverage <70%	Attended deliveries <50%
NT Control	<1/1000 live births	TT2 coverage >70%	Attended deliveries >50%
NT elimination	<0.1/1000 live births	TT2 coverage >90%	Attended deliveries >75%

Ans. (D) i.e., Incidence rate less than 0.1/1000 births, two doses of TT vaccine coverage more than 90%, attended deliveries more than 75%

64. **Influenza vaccine is recommended for:**

1. Elderly
2. Persons with underlying chronic diseases
3. HIV infected
4. General population

Select the correct answer using the code given below:

(a) 1 and 2 only (b) 4 (c) 2 and 3 only (d) 1, 2 and 3

EXPLANATION

When vaccine supply is limited, vaccination efforts should focus on delivering vaccination to the following people (no hierarchy is implied by order of listing):

- Children aged 6 months through 4 years (59 months);
- People aged 50 years and older;
- People with chronic pulmonary (including asthma), cardiovascular (except hypertension), renal, hepatic, neurologic, hematologic, or metabolic disorders (including diabetes mellitus);

- People who are immunosuppressed (including immunosuppression caused by medications or by Human Immunodeficiency Virus).

Ans. (D) i.e., 1, 2 and 3

65. **With reference to mumps, consider the following statements:**
    1. **The average age of incidence of mumps is higher than that of measles and chicken pox.**
    2. **The mumps disease tends to be more severe in adults than in children. Which of the statements given above is/are correct?**

    (a) 1 only (b) 2 only
    (c) Both 1 and 2 (d) Neither 1 nor 2

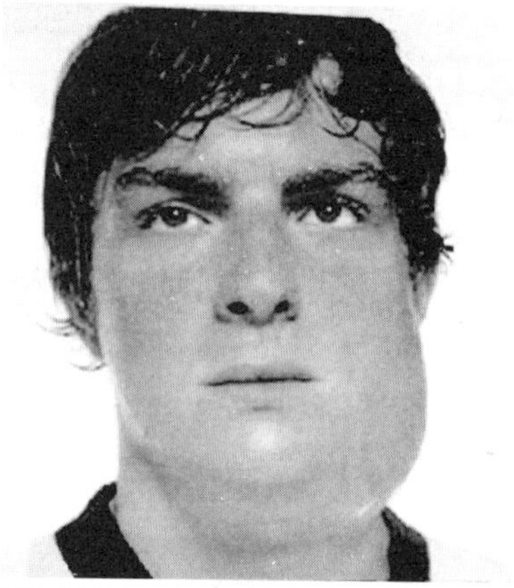

EXPLANATION

Symptoms of mumps typically occur 16 to 18 days after exposure and resolve after seven to ten days. Symptoms in adults are often more severe than in children.

Ans. (C) i.e., Both 1 and 2

66. Consider the following statements about content/yield of 100gm of some foodstuffs:
    1. Fat content of Bengal gram is less than that of maize
    2. Protein content of maize is more than that of rice
    3. Calorie yield of fish and egg is same

    Which of the statements given above is/are correct?

    (a) 1 only (b) 2 only (c) 1 and 2 (d) 2 and 3

EXPLANATION

Nutrient component	Maize/Corn	Rice (white)	Rice (brown)
Water (g)	10	12	10
Energy (kJ)	1528	1528	**1549**
Protein (g)	9.4	7.1	7.9

Ans. (B) i.e., 2 only

67. Consider the following statements:
    1. Protein content of soyabean is more than that of meat (per 100 gm)
    2. Fat content of fish is more than that of soyabean (per 100 gm)
    3. Calorie yield for each 100 gm of fish is almost the same as for 100 gm of banana
    4. Fat content of soyabean is more than that of eggs (per 100 gm)

    Which of the above statements are correct?

    (a) 1 and 2 (b) 1 and 4 only (c) 2 and 3 (d) 1, 3 and 4

EXPLANATION

Protein content (per 100 gram)

Soyabean	43.2
Meat	20–22

2016

Calorie yield (per 100 gram)

Fish	84
Banana	89

Fat content (per 100 gram)

Soyabean	19.5
Egg	6.0

Ans. (B) i.e., 2 only

68. Consider the following features of food poisoning:

'Incubation period less than 24 hours, source of infection is milk products, and symptoms include diarrhoea and vomiting.'

To which of the following does the above description apply?

1. Staphylococcal food poisoning

2. Salmonella food poisoning

3. Botulism

Select the correct answer using the code given below:

(a) 1 only (b) 1 and 2 (c) 1 and 3 (d) 2 only

EXPLANATION

Common Food Poisoning

- *S. aureus* is responsible for food poisoning. It is capable of generating toxins that produce food poisoning in the human body particularly after consumption of dairy products. Its incubation period lasts one to six hours, with the illness itself lasting from 30 minutes to 3 days.
- **Salmonellosis** is a symptomatic infection caused by bacteria of the *Salmonella* type. The most common symptoms are diarrhea, fever, abdominal cramps, and vomiting. This typically occurs between 12 hours and 36 hours after exposure with symptoms lasting from two to seven days. Infection is usually spread by eating contaminated meat, eggs, or milk.

Ans. (B) i.e., 1 and 2

69. For adolescents, what is the weekly iron and folic acid supplementation dose?

(a) 60mg elemental iron and 400 microgram folic acid

(b) 100mg elemental iron and 500 microgram folic acid

(c) 120mg elemental iron and 400 microgram folic acid

(d) 150mg elemental iron and 500 microgram folic acid

EXPLANATION

WIFS (Weekly Iron – Folic acid Supplementation) programme covers the adolescent population studying in Govt Schools in Classes VI to XII all over the State. Under this programme weekly dose of IFA Tablet (100mg Elemental Iron + 500μgm Folic Acid) is provided to beneficiaries in Schools under supervision of teachers. This will go a long way in prevention of Anemia and also control of mild Anemia.

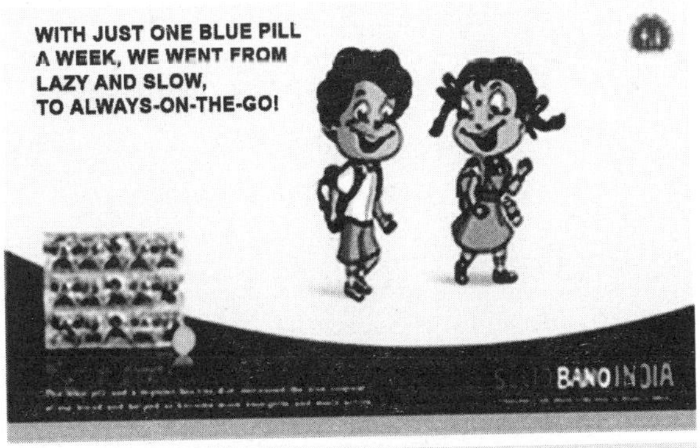
WITH JUST ONE BLUE PILL
A WEEK, WE WENT FROM
LAZY AND SLOW,
TO ALWAYS-ON-THE-GO!

Ans. (B) i.e., 100mg elemental iron and 500 microgram folic acid

70. Which of the following statements is/are *true* about proportional case rate of malaria?

1. This indicator is used since morbidity rate is difficult to determine.
2. This is defined as the number of cases of malaria for every 100 patients seen in hospital OPDs.
3. It is a crude index since cases are not related to their time and space distribution.

Select the correct answer using the code given below:

(a) 2 only (b) 2 and 3 only (c) 3 only (d) 1, 2 and 3

EXPLANATION

Proportional case rate

- The number of cases diagnosed as clinical malaria for every 100 patients attending hospitals and dispensaries [used in India].
- It is a crude indicator because the cases are not related to their time and place of distribution.

Ans. (D) i.e., 1, 2 and 3

71. Consider the following statements:

1. Type 2 poliovirus was eliminated in India in 2005.
2. Main cause of vaccine derived polioviruses (VDPV) is Type 2 component of OPV.

Which of the statements given above is/are correct?

(a) 1 only (b) 2 only
(c) Both 1 and 2 (d) Neither 1 nor 2

EXPLANATION

Until 2015, over 90% of circulating VDPV cases were due to the type 2 component in OPV. With the transmission of wild poliovirus type 2 already successfully interrupted since 1999, in April 2016 a switch was implemented from trivalent OPV to bivalent OPV in routine immunization programmes. The removal of the type 2 component of OPV is associated with significant public health benefits, including a reduction of the risk of cases of circulating VDPV2.

Structure of Polio

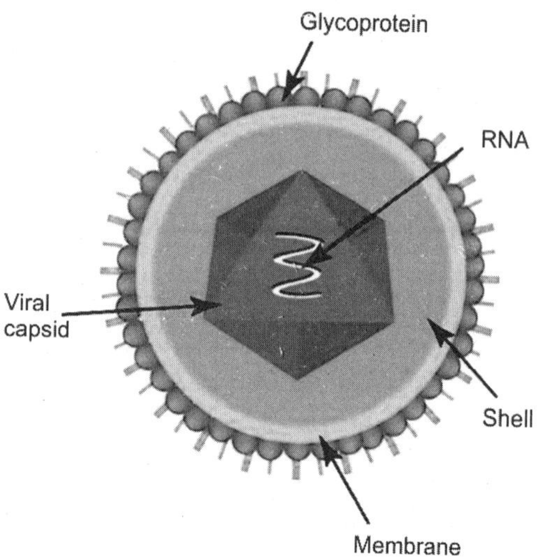

Ans. (B) i.e., 2 only

72. Which of the following statements is *true* about hydatid disease?

(a) It is a zoonosis
(b) It is rare in sheep rearing countries
(c) It is a protozoal disease
(d) Man is the definitive host

EXPLANATION

Zoonoses are infectious diseases that can be naturally transmitted between non human animals (usually vertebrates) and humans.

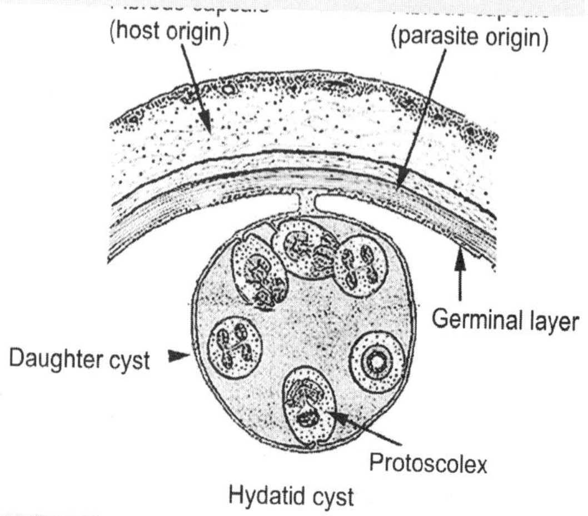

Hydatid cyst

Ans. (A) i.e., It is a zoonosis

73. Which of the following statements is *true* about direct age standardization?

(a) Standardized mortality ratio is used
(b) A standard population is used
(c) Age specific death rates are not known
(d) Number of people in each age group is not known

EXPLANATION

There are two methods of standardisation commonly used in epidemiological studies, and these are characterized by whether the standard used is a population distribution (**direct method**) or a set of specific rates (**indirect method**). Both direct and indirect standardisation involves the calculation of numbers of expected events (e.g. deaths), which are compared to the number of observed events.

Ans. (B) i.e., A standard population is used

74. **Match *List I* with *List II* and select the correct answer using the codes given below the lists:**

List I (Disease)	*List II* (Example)
A. Nosocomial	1. Cytomegaloviral infection
B. Opportunistic	2. Hepatitis B viral infection
C. Iatrogenic	3. Aplastic anemia
D. Epornithic	4. Influenza

Code*:* A B C D

(a) 2 1 3 4 (b) 2 1 4 3 (c) 1 2 4 3 (d) 1 2 3 4

EXPLANATION

Types of infections

- A **hospital acquired infection** (HAI), also known as a **nosocomial infection**, is an infection that is acquired in a hospital or other health care facility. Hepatitis B viral infection can be acquired by contaminated needles.
- An **opportunistic infection** is an infection caused by pathogens (bacteria, viruses, fungi, or protozoa) that take advantage of an opportunity not normally available, such as a host with a weakened immune system, an altered microbiota (such as a disrupted gut microbiota), or breached integumentary barriers. CMV infection occurs in AIDS patients.
- Exposure to ionizing radiation from radioactive materials or radiation producing devices is also associated with the development of aplastic anemia. Marie Curie, famous for her pioneering work in the field of radioactivity, died of aplastic anemia after working unprotected with radioactive materials for a long period of time; the damaging effects of ionizing radiation were not then known.
- Epornithic is an outbreak (epidemic) of disease in a bird population. Influenza may also affect other animals, including pigs, horses, and birds.

Ans. (A) i.e., 2 1 3 4

75. **With reference to International Certificate of Vaccination for Yellow Fever, the validity of the certificate begins how many days after the vaccination?**

(a) 5 days
(b) 10 days
(c) 14 days
(d) 20 days

2016

EXPLANATION

Protective efficacy of yellow fever vaccine starts from 10th day of vaccination and lasts for 10 years.

Countries at risk for yellow fever and having reported at least one outbreak, 1985-1997

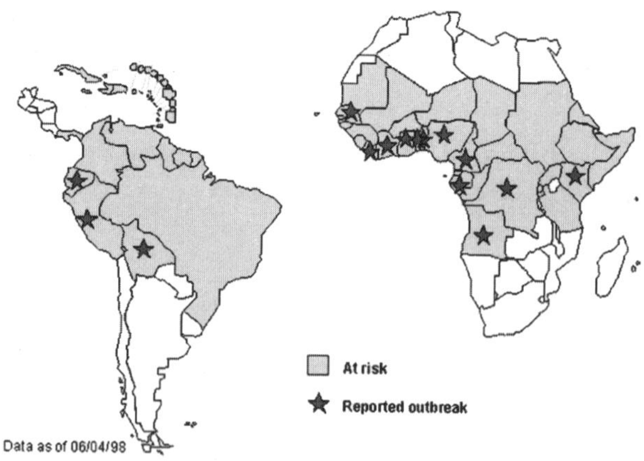

Ans. (B) i.e., 10 days

76. **With reference to dengue virus, consider the following statements:**

1. **In India, all the four serotypes are found.**
2. **The reservoir of infection is both man and mosquito.**
3. **Adults usually have a milder disease than children.**
4. **Dengue hemorrhagic fever is caused by infection with more than one dengue virus.**

Which of the statements given above is/are correct?

(a) 1 and 2 only (b) 1, 2 and 4 (c) 4 only (d) 2, 3 and 4

EXPLANATION

Dengue virus

- Delhi, the capital of **India** is endemic for **dengue viruses** because**all the four serotypes** are reported from here.
- The **dengue virus** is spread through a human to **mosquito** to human cycle of **transmission**
- Dengue Hemorrhagic Fever/DHF without shock is a severe form of dengue fever, proposed to be the result of two sequential infections with different dengue serotypes, the first infection with type I or II sensitizing the patient to the second infection with type III or IV, resulting in immunological catastrophe.

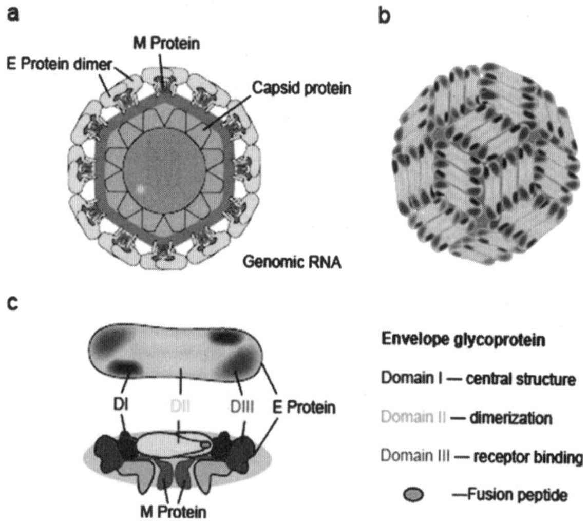

Ans. (B) i.e., 1, 2 and 4

77. **What is the window period for HIV infection?**

(a) 3–15 days (b) 6–24 weeks
(c) 6–8 months (d) None of these

EXPLANATION

The window period is time between potential exposure to HIV infection and the point when the test will give an accurate result. During the window period a person can be infected with HIV and be very infectious

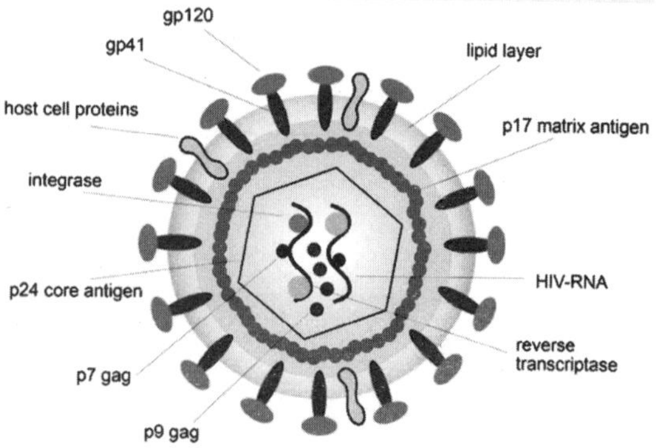

but still test HIV negative. The window period can be from ***10 days to 3*** months, depending on the person's body and on the HIV test that's used.

Ans. (B) i.e., 6–24 weeks

78. Among the following foodstuffs, which one has the highest protein content per 100gm?

(a) Black gram (b) Egg (c) Ragi (d) Wheat

EXPLANATION

Protein content (per 100 gram)

Black gram	17.1 g
Egg	6.0 g
Ragi	7.3 g
Wheat	6.8 g

Ans. (A) i.e., Black gram

79. Smoking is associated with all the following diseases except:

(a) Emphysema
(b) Cardiovascular disease
(c) Sarcoidosis
(d) Lung cancer

EXPLANATION

The cause of sarcoidosis is unknown. Some believe it may be due to an immune reaction to a trigger such as an infection or chemicals in those who are genetically predisposed. Those with affected family members are at greater risk.

Ans. (C) i.e., Sarcoidosis

80. Consider the following:

1. Skin
2. Water
3. Faeces
4. Urine

Bleaching powder can be used for disinfection of which of the above?

(a) 1 and 2 only
(b) 1, 2 and 3
(c) 2 and 3 only
(d) 2, 3 and 4

EXPLANATION

Disinfection

- For feces and urine, 8 percent of bleaching powder solution is used.
- Sodium hypochlorite solution, 3–6%, (common household bleach) is typically diluted for safe use when disinfecting surfaces and when used to treat drinking water.

Ans. (D) i.e., 2, 3 and 4

81. A 35-year old nulliparous woman complains of menorrhagia and mass per abdomen. On examination, the positive findings are: she is anaemic, has a pelvic mass of 16–18 weeks size, firm in consistency which moves with the movement of cervix. What is the most likely clinical diagnosis?

(a) Leiomyoma
(b) Adenomyosis
(c) Endometrial carcinoma
(d) Ovarian tumour

EXPLANATION

Uterine fibroids are leiomyomata of the uterine smooth muscle. As other leiomyomata, they are benign, but may lead to excessive menstrual bleeding (menorrhagia), often cause anemia and may lead to infertility.

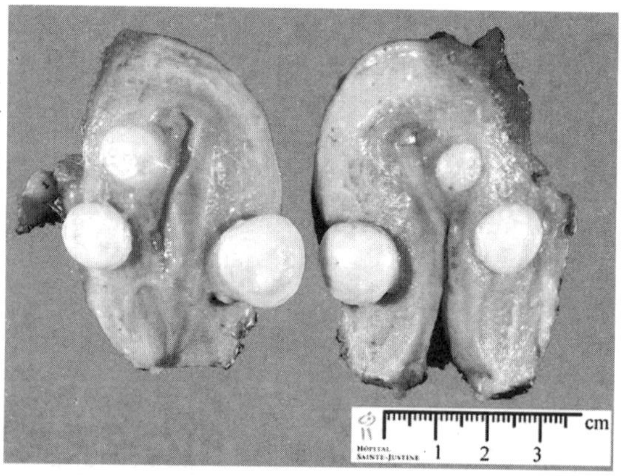

Ans. (A) i.e., Leiomyoma

82. **Abundant cornified cells in vaginal exfoliative cytology indicate:**

(a) Early proliferative phase
(b) Late proliferative phase
(c) Early secretory phase
(d) Late secretory phase

EXPLANATION

During the early follicular/proliferative phase, exfoliated vaginal epithelial cells have vesicular nuclei and are basophilic. During the late follicular phase, and the influence of the rising estradiol level, the vaginal epithelial cells display pyknotic nuclei and are acidophilic. Superficial ***cells*** without nuclei are often referred to as being "fully ***cornified***".

Ans. (B) i.e., Late proliferative phase

2016

83. **Consider the following statements:**

1. Carbon dioxide is the safest gas for creating pneumoperitoneum in operative laparoscopy.

2. Laparoscopic sterilization is not recommended during the period of immediate postpartum.

Which of the statements given above is/are correct?

(a) 1 only
(b) 2 only
(c) Both 1 and 2
(d) Neither 1 nor 2

EXPLANATION

Laparoscopy

- **Laparoscopic** surgery is now widely performed to treat various abdominal diseases. Currently, carbon dioxide is the most frequently used gas for insufflation of the abdominal cavity (pneumoperitoneum).
- The puerperal laparoscopic sterilization procedure compares favorably with the other open tubal ligation and mini laparotomy procedures; however, it is cautioned that the postpartum (within 72 hours) procedure has greater technical difficulties compared with interval methods, and only highly trained professionals with abundant experience should attempt puerperal procedures.

Ans. (C) i.e., Both 1 and 2

84. **Polyhydramnios at term is diagnosed when AFI is more than:**

(a) 10cm
(b) 15cm
(c) 20cm
(d) 25cm

EXPLANATION

Polyhydramnios (polyhydramnion, hydramnios, **polyhydramnios**) is a medical condition describing an excess of amniotic fluid in the amniotic sac. It is seen in about 1% of pregnancies. It is typically diagnosed when the amniotic fluid index (AFI) is greater than 24 cm.

Ans. (D) i.e., 25 cm

85. **Which of the following is *not* a potentially teratogenic infection if contracted in pregnancy?**

(a) Rubella (b) Cytomegalovirus
(c) Influenza virus (d) Chicken pox

EXPLANATION

Teratogenic infections

- TORCH group **infections** (toxoplasmosis, others, rubella, cytomegalovirus, herpes) are the most serious **infectious** diseases during pregnancy due to the seriousness of possible embryofetal lesions.
- Neonatal ***chickenpox*** may occur by transplacental transmission, ascending ***infection*** or via the neonatal respiratory tract.

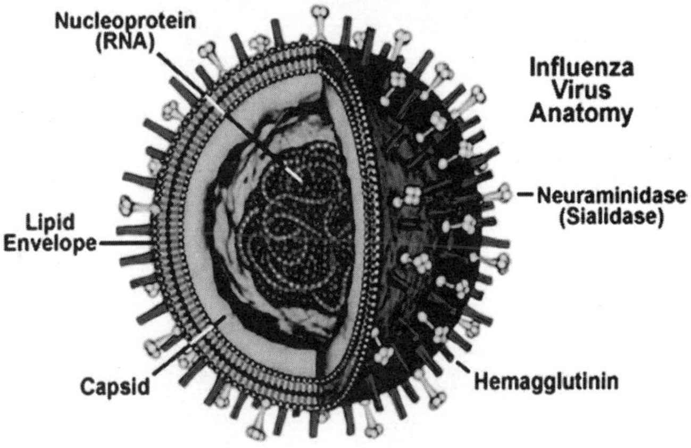

Ans. (C) i.e., Influenza virus

86. **Active management of 3rd stage of labour includes the following except:**

(a) Injection oxytocin 10 IU intramuscularly
(b) Controlled cord traction
(c) Uterine massage
(d) Injection oxytocin 10 IU intravenously

EXPLANATION

1 mL (10 units) of Oxytocin can be given as I/M injection after the delivery of the placenta.

Ans. (D) i.e., Injection oxytocin 10 IU intravenously

2016

87. **Regarding hypertensive disorders of pregnancy, the following are true except:**

(a) Significant proteinuria is more than/equal to 0.3g/24hr
(b) Eclampsia may present in the absence of hypertension
(c) A protein : creatinine ratio more than 30mg/mmol is considered significant
(d) Urinary dipstick result of +1 is equivalent to urinary protein concentration of 300mg/dl

EXPLANATION

Eclampsia is the onset of seizures (convulsions) in a woman with preeclampsia. Preeclampsia is a disorder of pregnancy in which there is high blood pressure and either large amounts of protein in the urine or other organ dysfunction.

Ans. (B) i.e., Eclampsia may present in the absence of hypertension

88. **Which of the following is *not* a characteristic of Mayer Rokitansky Kuster Hauser syndrome?**

(a) Cardiac anomalies (b) Mullerian duct aplasia
(c) Renal abnormalities (d) Skeletal abnormalities

EXPLANATION

Mayer Rokitansky Kuster Hauser syndrome

- Typical MRKH – Isolated uterovaginal aplasia/hypoplasia: Prevalence – 64%.

- Atypical MRKH – Uterovaginal aplasia/hypoplasia with renal malformation or uterovaginal aplasia/hypoplasia with ovarian dysfunction: Prevalence – 24%.

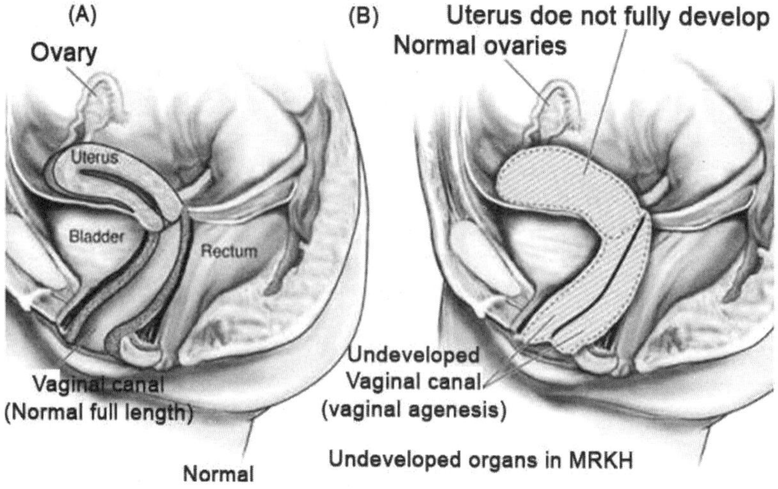

Ans. (A) i.e., Cardiac anomalies

89. Which one of the following is *not* a contraindication for prescribing combined oral contraceptive pills?

(a) Thromboembolic disease
(b) Viral hepatitis
(c) Rheumatic heart disease
(d) Pelvic inflammatory disease

EXPLANATION

Oral contraceptive use has been shown to protect against gonococcal ***pelvic inflammatory disease*** (*PID*), but the effect on chlamydial *PID* is uncertain.

Ans. (D) i.e., Pelvic inflammatory disease

90. The following are used in the staging of carcinoma of the cervix except:

(a) Pelvic lymph node involvement
(b) Vaginal involvement
(c) Hydroureter
(d) Parametrial involvement

EXPLANATION

Stage 0

- The carcinoma is confined to the surface layer (cells lining) of the cervix. Also called carcinoma *in situ* (CIS).

Stage I

- The carcinoma has grown deeper into the cervix, but has not spread beyond it (extension to the corpus would be disregarded). Stage One is subdivided as follows:
  - o IA Invasive carcinoma which can be diagnosed only by microscopy, with deepest invasion <5 mm and the largest extension <7 mm.
    - – IA-1 Measured stromal invasion of <3.0mm in depth and extension of <7.0mm
    - – IA-2 Measured stromal invasion of >3.0mm and not >5.0mm with an extension of not >7.0mm
  - o IB Clinically visible lesions limited to the cervix uteri or preclinical cancers greater than stage IA
    - – IB-1 Clinically visible lesion <4.0cm in greatest dimension.

– IB-2 Clinically visible lesion >4.0cm in greatest dimension.

Stage II

- Cervical carcinoma invades beyond the uterus, but not to the pelvic wall or to the lower third of the vagina
  - o **IIA** Without parametrial invasion
    - – **IIA-1** Clinically visible lesion <4.0cm in greatest dimension
    - – **IIA-2** Clinically visible lesion >4.0cm in greatest dimension
  - o **IIB** With obvious parametrial invasion

Stage III

- The tumour extends to the pelvic wall and/or involves lower third of the vagina and/or causes hydronephrosis or non functioning kidney
  - o **IIIA** Tumour involves lower third of the vagina, with no extension to the pelvic wall
  - o **IIIB** Extension to the pelvic wall and/or hydronephrosis or non functioning kidney

Stage IV

- The carcinoma has extended beyond the true pelvis or has involved (biopsy proven) the mucosa of the bladder or rectum. A bullous oedema, as such, does not permit a case to be allotted to Stage IV
  - o **IVA** Spread of the growth to adjacent organs
  - o **IVB** Spread to distant organs

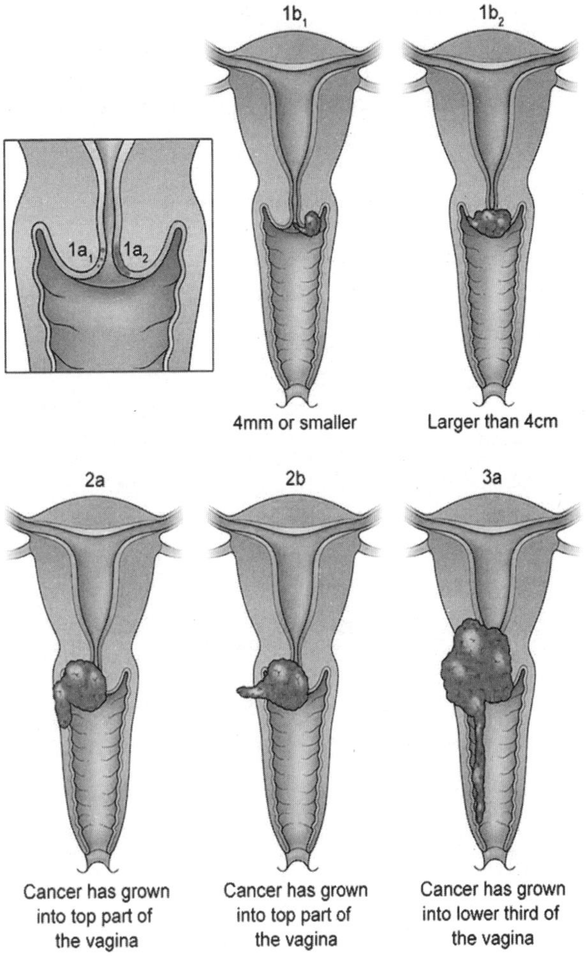

Ans. (A) i.e., Pelvic lymph node involvement

91. **Presence of signet ring cells in a cellular or myxomatous stroma is diagnostic of:**

(a) Gynandroblastoma (b) Hilus cell tumour
(c) Struma ovarii (d) Krukenberg tumour

EXPLANATION

Microscopically, Krukenberg tumors are often characterized by mucin secreting signet ring cells in the tissue of the ovary; when the primary tumor is discovered, the same signet ring cells are typically found. However, other microscopic features can predominate. Krukenberg tumors are most commonly metastases from gastric cancer, particularly adenocarcinoma, or breast cancer particularly invasive lobular breast carcinoma.

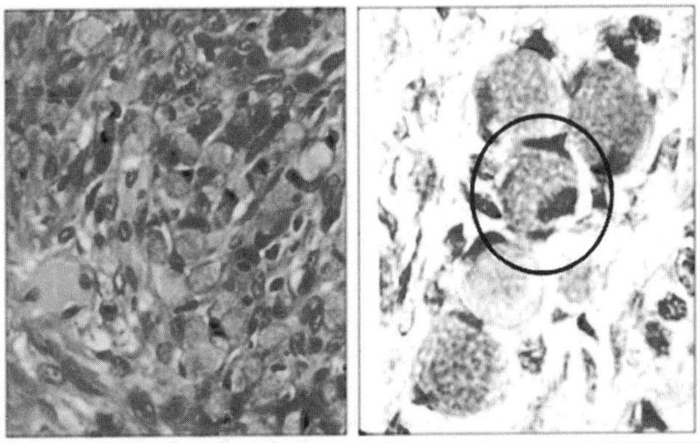

Ans. (D) i.e., Krukenberg tumour

92. A 58-year old woman, post menopausal for last 8 years comes with history of spotting per vaginum. What is the most likely cause?

(a) Endometrial hyperplasia
(b) Endometrial carcinoma
(c) Atrophic endometritis
(d) Estrogen replacement therapy

EXPLANATION

Atrophic endometritis is the most common cause of postmenopausal bleeding (66.67%), followed by endometrial carcinoma (13.6%) and endometrial polyp (11.6%).

Ans. (C) i.e., Atrophic endometritis

93. A diabetic obese patient comes with history of post menopausal bleeding. On examination, there is a supra pubic mass and per vagina there is purulent discharge. The probable diagnosis is:

(a) Carcinoma cervix
(b) Carcinoma endometrium
(c) Uterine myoma
(d) Ovarian carcinoma

EXPLANATION

Approximately 40% of cases of endometrial carcinoma are related to obesity. Endometrial cancer is also associated with excessive estrogen exposure, high blood pressure and diabetes. Whereas taking estrogen alone increases the risk of endometrial cancer, taking both estrogen and a progestogen in combination, as in most birth control pills, decreases the risk.

Ans. (B) i.e., Carcinoma endometrium

2016

94. An adolescent girl with stage 1a dysgerminoma is managed by:

(a) Unilateral salpingo-oophorectomy alone
(b) Total abdominal hysterectomy with unilateral salpingo-oophorectomy
(c) Bilateral salpingo-oophorectomy alone
(d) Chemotherapy

EXPLANATION

A preponderance (75–80%) of ***dysgerminomas*** present as ***stage*** I cancers and, therefore, can be treated by ***surgical*** resection alone with a unilateral salpingo-oophorectomy.

Ans. (A) i.e., Unilateral salpingo-oophorectomy alone

95. Which of the following conditions is best treated by a posterior colpotomy?

(a) Pelvic abscess
(b) Pyometra
(c) Pyosalpinx
(d) Pelvic haematocele

EXPLANATION

Culdocentesis is a medical procedure involving the extraction of fluid from the pouch of Douglas (a rectouterine pouch posterior to the vagina) through a needle. It can be one diagnostic technique used in identifying pelvic inflammatory disease (in which case purulent fluid will be extracted) and ruptured ectopic pregnancies that cause hemoperitoneum.

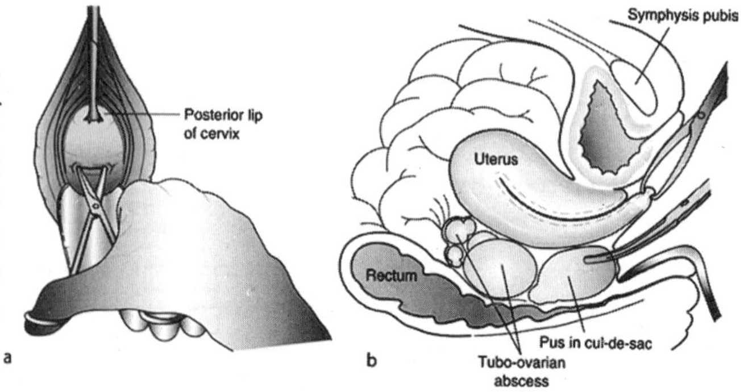

In the procedure, the rectouterine pouch is often reached through the posterior fornix of the vagina. The process of creating the hole is called "colpotomy" if a scalpel incision is made to drain the fluid rather than using a needle.

Ans. (A) i.e., Pelvic abscess

96. **Which of the following suture materials has the least tissue reaction?**

(a) Cotton/Linen (b) Stainless steel (c) Chromic catgut (d) Silk

EXPLANATION

Stainless steel wire is quite inert and has the ***least tissue reaction*** of any ***suture.***

Ans. (B) i.e., Stainless steel

97. **Menopause is associated with the following except:**

(a) Osteoporosis (b) Ischemic heart disease (c) Loss of libido (d) Delusion

EXPLANATION

A **delusion** is a mistaken belief that is held with strong conviction even in the presence of superior evidence to the contrary. As a pathology, it is distinct from a belief based on false or incomplete information, confabulation, dogma, illusion, or some other misleading effects of perception.

Ans. (D) i.e., Delusion

98. **Which one of the following conditions simulates the menstrual pattern of pain?**

(a) Intramural fibroid (b) Adenomyosis
(c) Haematometra (d) Granulosa cell tumour of ovary

EXPLANATION

Hematometra typically presents as cyclic, cramping pain in the midline of the pelvis or lower abdomen. Patients may also report urinary frequency and urinary retention. Premenopausal women with hematometra often experience abnormal vaginal bleeding, including dysmenorrhea (pain during menstruation) or amenorrhea (lack of menstruation), while postmenopausal women are more likely to be asymptomatic.

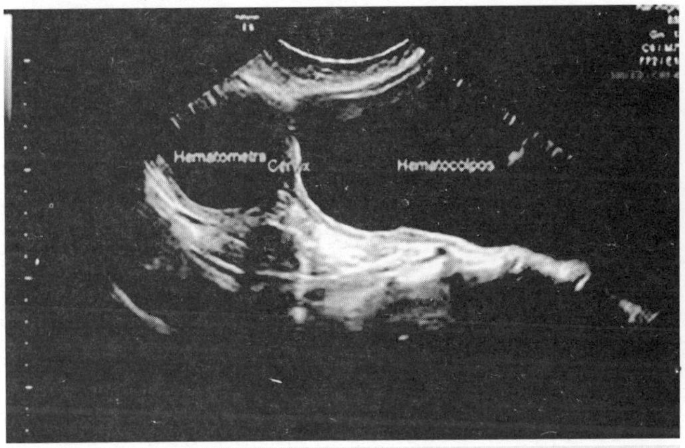

Ans. (C) i.e., Haematometra

99. **Which of the undermentioned conditions does *not* cause postmenopausal vaginal bleeding?**

(a) Benign cystic teratoma of ovary
(b) Senile vaginitis
(c) Carcinoma of cervix
(d) Prolapse of uterus with decubitus ulcer

EXPLANATION

A **teratoma** is a tumor made up of several different types of tissue, such as hair, muscle, or bone. They typically form in the ovaries, testicles, or tailbone/coccyx and less commonly in other areas. Symptoms may be minimal if the tumor is small.

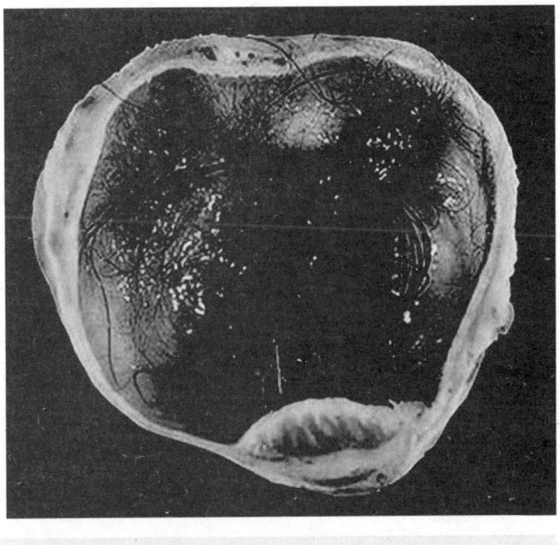

Ans. (A) i.e., Benign cystic teratoma of ovary

100. Defective fusion of the Mullerian ducts may give rise to which of the following?

(a) Uterus bicornis unicollis

(b) Imperforate anus

(c) Imperforate hymen

(d) Absence of the ovaries

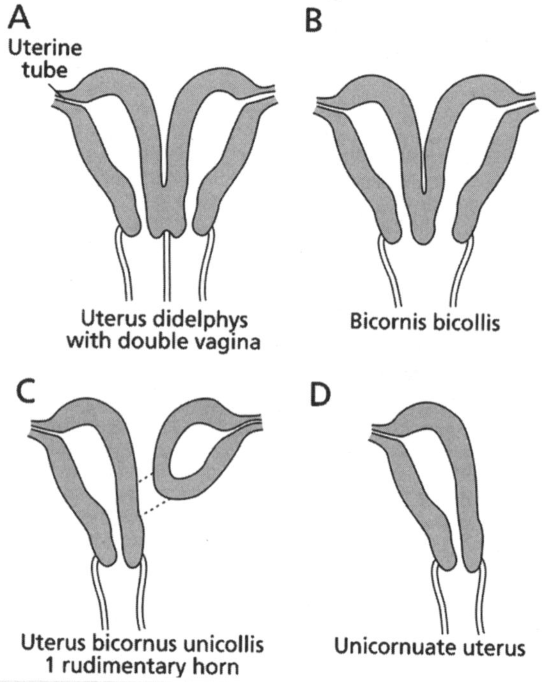

EXPLANATION

More extensive fusion of the Mullerian ducts results in the uterus bicornis unicollis which is characterised by:

- Single vagina
- Single cervix
- Double, single horned uteruses which are partially fused.

Ans. (A) i.e., Uterus bicornis unicollis

101. For a woman who has had unprotected intercourse two days ago, which one of the following emergency contraceptive methods *cannot* be suggested?

(a) LNG IUD (LNg IUD)

(b) Ulipristal acetate

(c) Levonorgestrel 150 mg

(d) Yuzpe regimen

EXPLANATION

Intrauterine device (IUD) with progestogen, sold under the brand name **Mirena** among others, is a intrauterine device that releases the hormone levonorgestrel. It is used for birth control/contraception, heavy menstrual periods, and to prevent excessive build of the lining of the uterus in those on estrogen replacement therapy.

Ans. (A) i.e., LNG IUD (LNg IUD)

102. Deep transverse arrest of head in labour occurs in:

(a) Android pelvis (b) Anthropoid pelvis (c) Platypelloid pelvis (d) Gynaecoid pelvis

EXPLANATION

The ***android pelvis*** is identified by a funnel shape. It is found in approximately 20% of women. The ***android pelvis*** has characteristics of male pelvis.

Four Pelvic Types

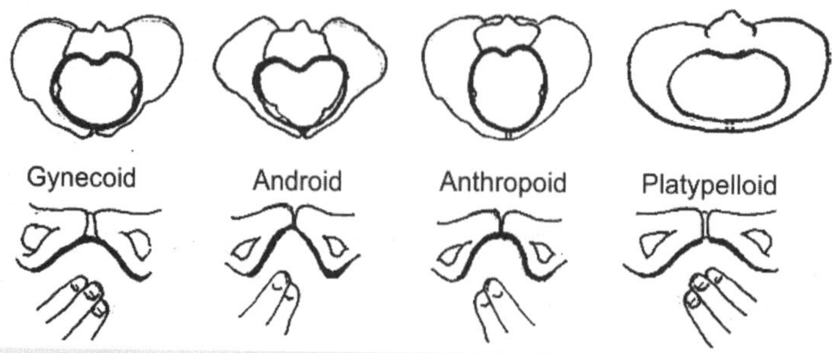

Ans. (A) i.e., Android pelvis

103. Early deceleration of foetal heart rate in labour is due to:

(a) Congenital heart block

(b) Umbilical cord compression

(c) Foetal head compression

(d) Hyperpyrexia

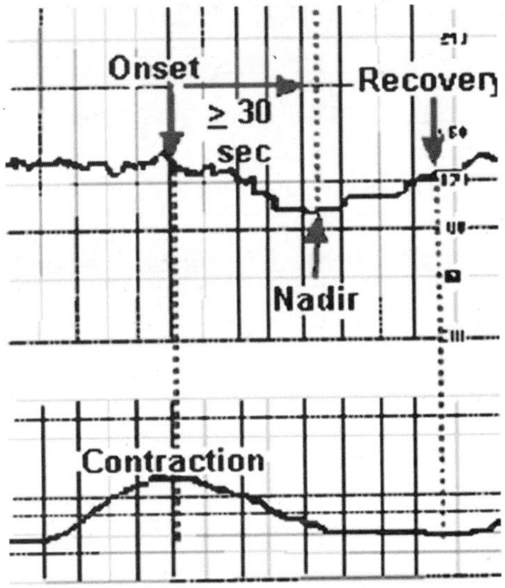

EXPLANATION

Early decelerations appear to be caused by vagal discharge produced when the head is compressed by uterine contractions. The onset and depth of early decelerations mirror the shape of the contraction, and tend to be proportional to the strength of the contraction.

Ans. (C) i.e., Foetal head compression

104. McRoberts manoeuvre is used during labour for management of:

(a) Normal labour to assist extension of head

(b) Extended arms of breech during assisted breech delivery

(c) Shoulder dystocia

(d) Delivery of after coming head of breech

EXPLANATION

The **McRoberts maneuver** is an obstetrical maneuver used to assist in childbirth. It is named after William A. McRoberts, Jr. It is employed in case of shoulder dystocia during childbirth and involves hyperflexing the mother's legs tightly to her abdomen. It is effective due to the increased mobility at the sacroiliac joint during pregnancy, allowing rotation of the pelvis and facilitating the release of the fetal shoulder.

Ans. (C) i.e., Shoulder dystocia

105. Which one of the following is *not* a suitable condition for outlet forceps application?

(a) Cervix fully dilated

(b) Membranes absent

(c) Vertex presentation

(d) Head is above ischial spine level

EXPLANATION

Type of Procedure	Criteria
Outlet forceps	1. Scalp is visible at the introitus without separating labia 2. Fetal skull has reached pelvic floor 3. Sagittal suture is in anteroposterior diameter or right or left occiput anterior or posterior position 4. Fetal head is at or on perineum 5. Rotation does not exceed 45°

Ans. (D) i.e., Head is above ischial spine level

106. Polyhydramnios is *not* caused by which one of the following?

(a) Anencephaly

(b) Spina bifida

(c) Single kidney

(d) Oesophageal atresia

EXPLANATION

Renal agenesis or obstruction of the urinary tract of the fetus preventing micturition such as posterior urethral valves in males, leads to oligohydramnions.

Ans. (C) i.e., Single kidney

107. Which of the following is the type of antepartum haemorrhage where blood loss is foetal?

(a) Abruptio placenta
(b) Placenta previa
(c) Vasa previa
(d) Cirumvallate placenta

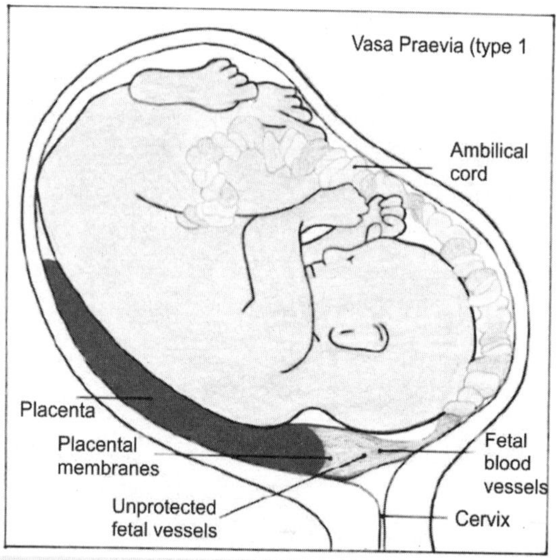

EXPLANATION

Vasa praevia, is a condition in which fetal blood vessels cross or run near the internal opening of the uterus. These vessels are at risk of rupture when the supporting membranes rupture, as they are unsupported by the umbilical cord or placental tissue.

Ans. (C) i.e., Vasa previa

108. Which one of the following conditions is *not* associated with oligohydramnios during pregnancy?

(a) Post term pregnancy
(b) Ruptured membrane
(c) Intra uterine growth restriction
(d) Oesophageal atresia

EXPLANATION

Gastrointestinal abnormalities such as esophageal atresia and duodenal atresia (causing inability to swallow amniotic fluid), anencephaly, facial cleft, neck masses, tracheoesophageal fistula, and diaphragmatic hernias can cause polyhydramnios.

Ans. (D) i.e., Oesophageal atresia

109. A 23-year old presents with recurrent abortions at 16 weeks gestation. She should be investigated for:

(a) TORCH infection
(b) Hepatitis B infection
(c) Incompetent cervix
(d) Balanced paternal translocation

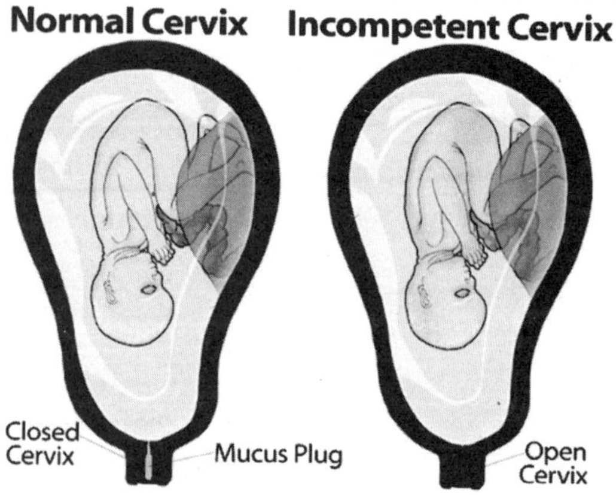

EXPLANATION

Cervical weakness/incompetent cervix may cause miscarriage or preterm birth during the second and third trimesters.

Ans. (C) i.e., Incompetent cervix

110. Which of the following is the most common cause of abortion during first trimester?

(a) Cervical incompetence
(b) Progesterone deficiency
(c) Antiphospholipid antibody syndrome
(d) Chromosomal anomalies of foetus

2016

EXPLANATION

About 80% of miscarriages occur in the **first** 12 weeks of pregnancy (the **first trimester**). The underlying **cause** in about half of cases involves chromosomal abnormalities.

Ans. (D) i.e., Chromosomal anomalies of foetus

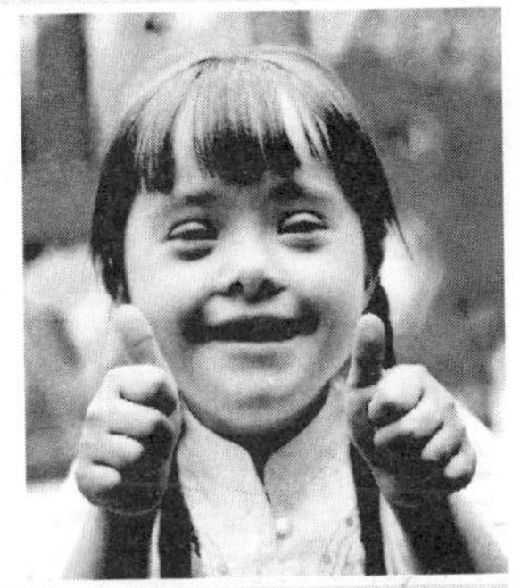

111. Abnormally low alpha-fetoprotein in maternal serum indicates:

(a) Down's syndrome (b) Anencephaly

(c) Encephalocele (d) Meningocele

EXPLANATION

AFP	UE_3	hCG	Associated condition
Low	Low	High	Down syndrome

Ans. (A) i.e., Down's syndrome

112. Umbilical cord blood stem cells are used to treat all the following diseases except:

(a) Parkinsonism (b) Leukemia (c) Diabetes (d) Osteoporosis

EXPLANATION

Management of Osteoporosis

- Bisphosphonates are useful in decreasing the risk of future fractures in those who have already sustained a fracture due to osteoporosis. This benefit is present when taken for three to four years.
- Teriparatide (a recombinant parathyroid hormone) has been shown to be effective in treatment of women with postmenopausal osteoporosis.

Ans. (D) i.e., Osteoporosis

113. A patient of ectopic pregnancy had beta-hCG less than 6000 IU/ml. Medical management was done by single dose methotrexate. Beta-hCG repeated after 48 hours was found 7000 IU/ml. What will you do further?

(a) Repeat the injection of methotrexate

(b) Operate the patient

(c) Follow up with Beta-hCG after one week

(d) Follow up with Beta-hCG after 72 hours

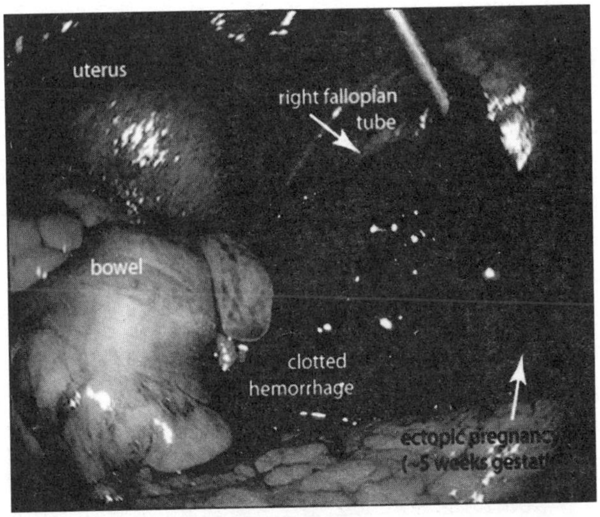

EXPLANATION

Early treatment of an ectopic pregnancy with methotrexate is a viable alternative to surgical treatment which was developed in the 1980s. If administered early in the pregnancy, methotrexate terminates the growth of the developing embryo; this may cause an abortion, or the developing embryo may then be either resorbed by the woman's body or pass with a menstrual period. Also, it may lead to the inadvertent termination of an undetected intrauterine pregnancy, or severe abnormality in any surviving pregnancy. Therefore, it is recommended that methotrexate should only be administered when hCG has been serially monitored with a rise less than 35% over 48 hours, which practically excludes a viable intrauterine pregnancy.

Ans. (D) i.e., Follow up with Beta-hCG after 72 hours

2016

114. A 35-year old married woman with no risk factors for cervical cancer is having Pap smear showing 'atypical squamous cells of undermined significance (ASCUS)' for the first time. What is the further step in the management?

(a) Repeat Pap immediately
(b) Cryotherapy
(c) Large loop excision of the transformation zone
(d) To follow up with Pap test at 6 months

EXPLANATION

Atypical ***squamous cells*** of undetermined significance (ASCUS): ***Squamous cells*** are thin and flat and grow on the surface of a healthy cervix. In the case of ASCUS, the Pap smear reveals slightly abnormal ***squamous cells***, but the changes don't clearly suggest that precancerous ***cells*** are present.

Ans. (D) i.e., To follow up with Pap test at 6 months

115. For a primary amenorrhoea individual having an XY karyotype, normal infantile female external and internal genitalia fibrous bands in place of gonad, lack of development of secondary sexual characters, what is the most probable diagnosis?

(a) Testicular ferminization syndrome
(b) Mixed gonadal dysgenesis
(c) Swyer syndrome
(d) Defective antimullerian harmone

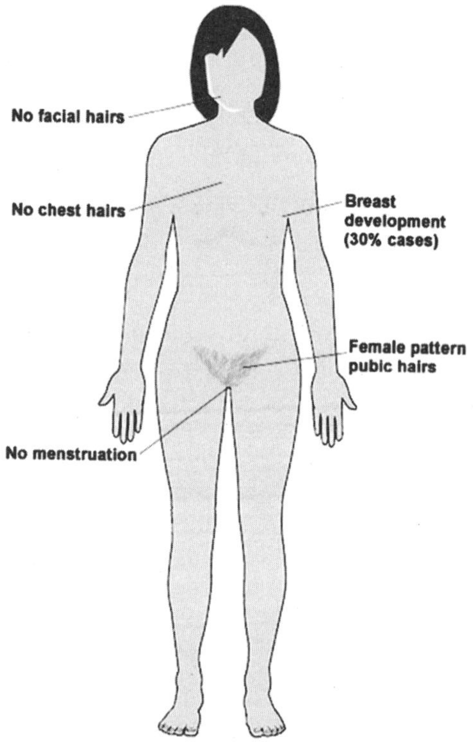

EXPLANATION

Swyer syndrome, or **XY gonadal dysgenesis**, is a type of hypogonadism in a person whose karyotype is 46, XY. The person is externally female with streak gonads, and if left untreated, will not experience puberty. Such gonads are typically surgically removed (as they have a significant risk of developing tumors) and a typical medical treatment would include hormone replacement therapy.

Ans. (C) i.e., Swyer syndrome

116. A lady who is using oral contraceptive pills comes with a complaint of vaginal discharge and pruritus vulvae. On local examination, there is curdy white discharge from the vagina. What is the most likely clinical diagnosis?

(a) Trichomonal vaginitis
(b) Monilial vaginitis
(c) Gardnerella vaginalis
(d) Atrophic vaginitis

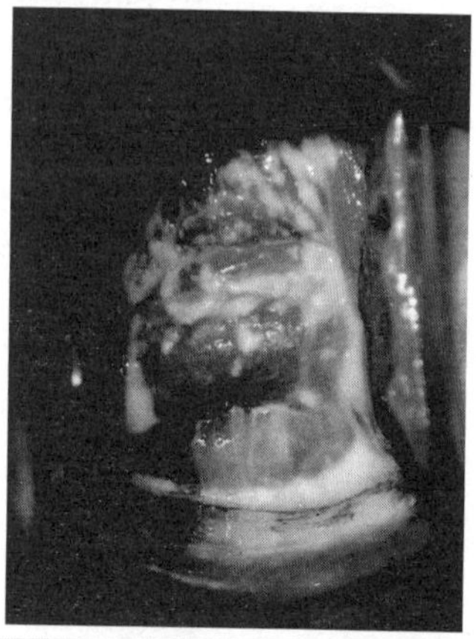

EXPLANATION

Candidial infection of the vagina or vulva may cause severe itching, burning, soreness, irritation, and a whitish or whitish gray cottage cheese like discharge.

Ans. (B) i.e., Monilial vaginitis

117. Antisperm antibodies are usually present in:

(a) Cervix (b) Vagina
(c) Uterus (d) Fallopian tube

EXPLANATION

Antisperm antibodies (ASA) are immunoglobulins of IgG, IgA, and/or IgM, which are directed against sperm antigens. ASA can be detected in ejaculate, cervical mucus, follicular fluid, and blood serum.

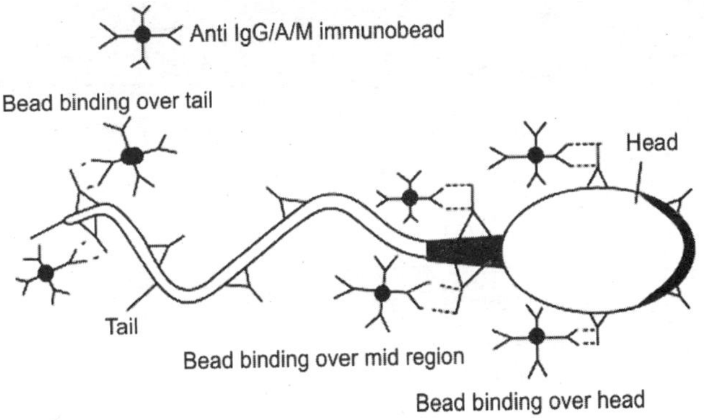

Ans. (A) i.e., Cervix

118. For a woman who has been operated for chocolate cyst with normal menstrual cycle, any of the following may be prescribed except:

(a) Injection leuprolide (b) Tranexamic acid (c) Tablet dienogest (d) Oral progestogens

EXPLANATION

Tranexamic acid (TXA) is a medication used to treat or prevent excessive blood loss from major trauma, postpartum bleeding, surgery, tooth removal, nosebleeds, and heavy menstruation.

Ans. (B) i.e., Tranexamic acid

119. For a 40-year old hypertensive woman, which one of the following is *not* recommended for contraception?

(a) NuvaRing (b) Minipill (c) IUCD (d) LNG IUD (LNg IUD)

EXPLANATION

Women who have any of the following conditions should not use the Nuvaring: abnormal blood fat levels, clotting disorders, diabetes, heart disease, high blood pressure, migraine headaches with vision problems or "constant stomach pain caused by pancreatic dysfunction along with high levels of fats in the blood".

Ans. (A) i.e., NuvaRing

2016

120. A 30-year old female has severe dysmenorrhoea and dyspareunia. On examination, uterus is 8 weeks size, uniformly enlarged and there is tenderness in posterior fornix. What is the most probable diagnosis?

(a) Fibroid uterus
(b) Dysfunctional uterine bleeding
(c) Adenomyosis
(d) Endometrial carcinoma

EXPLANATION

Patients with adenomyosis ofen present with painful menses (dysmenorrhea), profuse menses (menorrhagia), or both. Other possible symptoms are pain during sexual intercourse, chronic pelvic pain and irritation of the urinary bladder.

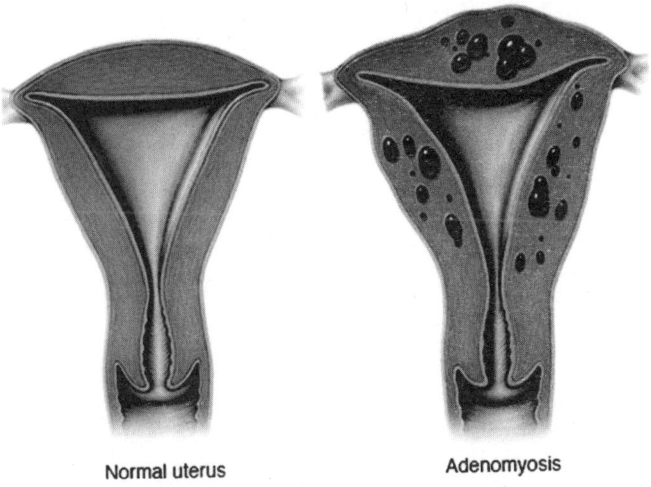

Ans. (C) i.e., Adenomyosis

CHAPTER

6 CMS EXAMINATION 2016

PAPER - 1

2016

1. A 40-year old male is admitted with acute inferior wall myocardial infarction. Half an hour later his B.P. is 80/50mm Hg and heart rate is 40/minute with sinus rhythm. The *most appropriate* step in the management of this patient would be:

(a) Administration of normal saline 300ml over 15 minutes

(b) Immediate insertion of temporary pacemaker

(c) Intravenous administration of atropine sulfate

(d) Intravenous administration of isoprenaline 50 μg/minute

EXPLANATION

Bradycardia is defined as any rhythm disorder with a heart rate less than 60 beats per minute. There are 3 medications that are used in the Bradycardia ACLS Algorithm. They are atropine, dopamine (infusion), and epinephrine (infusion).

ECG Changes during Myocardial Infarction (MI)

Location of MI	Leads affected	Vessel involved	ECG changes
Anterior wall	V_2 to V_4	• Left Anterior Descending artery (LAD) — Diagonal branch	• Poor R-wave progression • ST-segment elevation • T-wave inversion
Septal wall	V_1 to V_2	• Left Anterior Descending artery (LAD) — Septal branch	• R-wave disappears • ST-segment rises • T-wave inverts
Lateral wall	I, aV_L, V_5, V_6	• Left Coronary Artery (LCA) — Circumflex branch	• ST-segment elevation
Inferior wall	II, III, aV_F	• Right Coronary Artery (RCA) — Posterior descending branch	• T-wave inversion • ST-segment elevation
Posterior wall	V_1 to V_4	• Left Coronary Artery (LCA) — Circumflex branch • Right Coronary Artery (RCA) — Posterior descending branch	• Tall R-waves • ST-segment depression • Upright T-waves

Ans. (C) i.e., Intravenous administration of atropine sulfate

2. The characteristic feature of tricuspid insufficiency in the jugular venous pulse is:

(a) Prominent 'A' wave
(b) Exaggerated 'X' and 'Y' descents
(c) Cannon waves
(d) Obliteration of the 'X' descent and prominent 'CV' wave

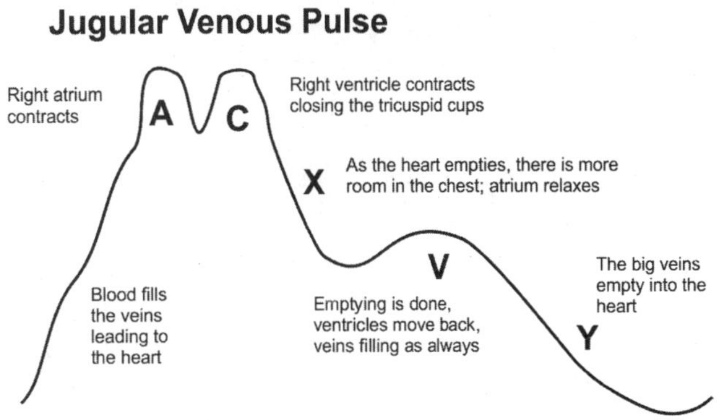

EXPLANATION

There may be giant CV waves in the jugular pulse and a palpably (and sometimes visibly) pulsatile liver on abdominal exam in tricuspid insufficiency.

Ans. (D) i.e., Obliteration of the 'X' descent and prominent 'CV' wave

3. Match *List I* with *List II* and select the correct answer using the code given below the lists:

List I (Clinical Features)	*List II (Diagnosis)*
A. Osler's node	1. Patent ductus arteriosus with reversal of shunt
B. Differential cyanosis	2. Aortic stenosis with aortic regurgitation
C. Bisferiens pulse	3. Pulmonary hypertension
D. Graham Steell murmur	4. Subacute bacterial endocarditis

Code: A B C D

(a) 4 1 2 3 (b) 4 1 3 2 (c) 1 4 2 3 (d) 1 4 3 2

EXPLANATION

Terms and conditions

- **Osler's nodes** are painful, red, raised lesions found on the hands and feet. They are associated with a number of conditions, including infective endocarditis
- **Differential cyanosis** is defined as a difference in oxygen saturation (O_2 sat) of at least 5% or a difference in partial pressure of oxygen (PaO_2) of at least 20mmHg between the arms and legs associated with congenital heart disease or persistent pulmonary hypertension of the newborn (PPHN).
- Pulsus **bisferiens**, also known as biphasic **pulse**, is an aortic waveform with two peaks per cardiac cycle, a small one followed by a strong and broad one. It is a sign of problems with the aortic valve, including aortic stenosis and aortic regurgitation, as well as hypertrophic cardiomyopathy causing subaortic stenosis.
- A **Graham Steell murmur** is a heart murmur typically associated with pulmonary regurgitation. It is a high pitched early diastolic

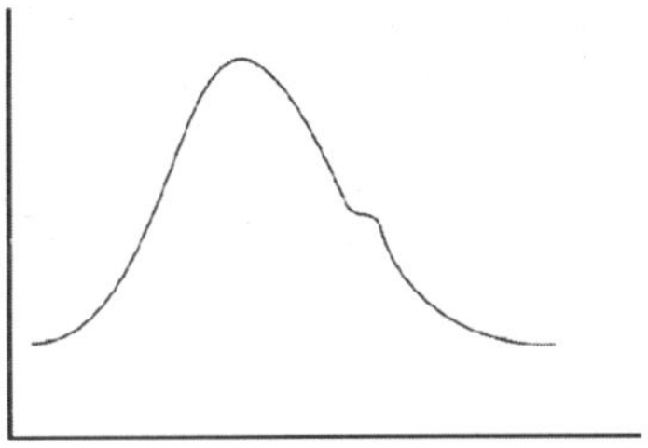
Normal

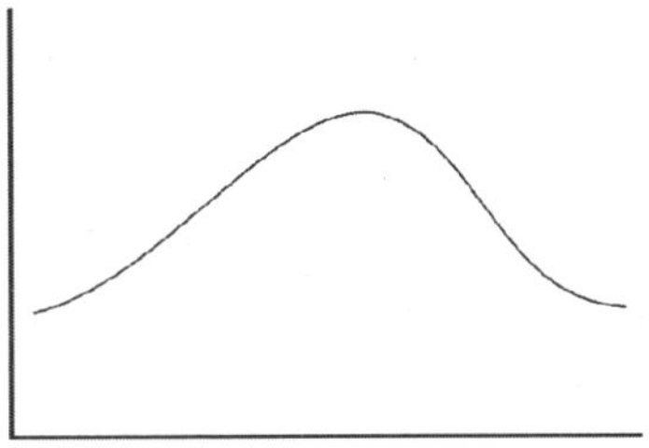
Show rising
e.g. aortic stenosis

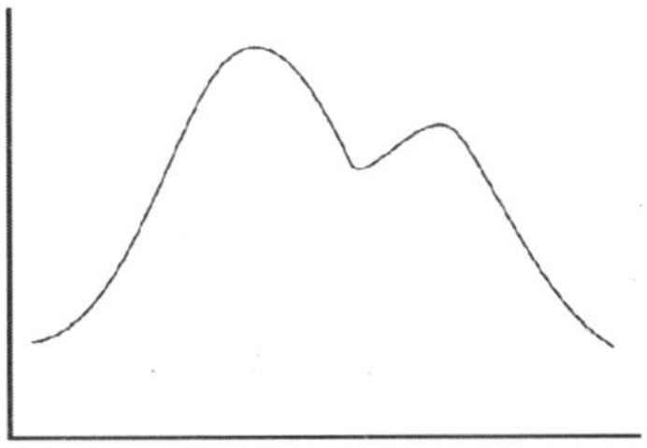
Bisiferiens
e.g. aortic stenosis mixed with aortic regurgitation

murmur heard best at the left sternal edge in the second intercostal space with the patient in full inspiration, originally described in 1888.

Ans. (A) i.e., 4 1 2 3

4. **Acute aortic regurgitation occurs in:**

(a) Infective endocarditis
(b) Ankylosing spondylitis
(c) Marfan's syndrome
(d) Rheumatoid arthritis

EXPLANATION

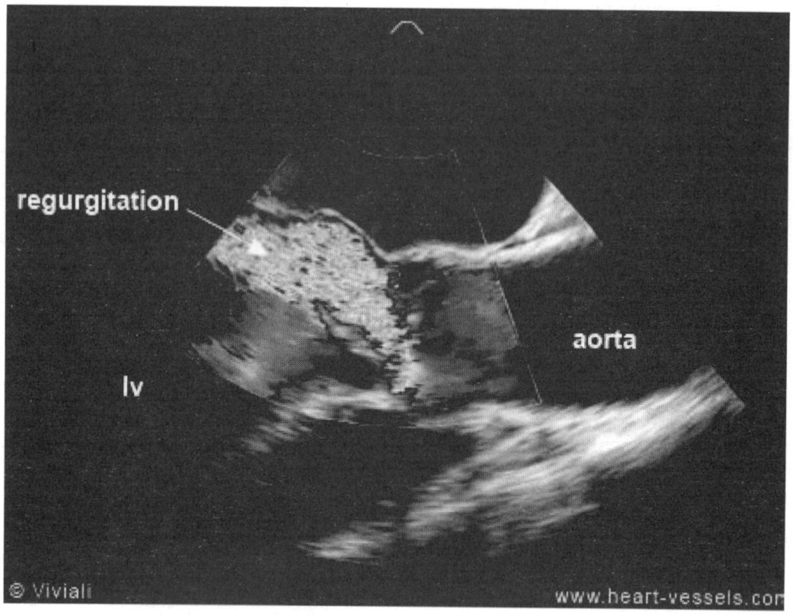

In acute cases of aortic insufficiency, the main causes are infective endocarditis, aortic dissection or trauma. In terms of the cause of aortic insufficiency, is often due to the aortic root dilation (*annuloaortic ectasia*), which is idiopathic in over 80% of cases, but otherwise may result from aging, syphilitic aortitis, osteogenesis imperfecta, aortic dissection, Behcet's disease, reactive arthritis and systemic hypertension.

Ans. (A) i.e., Infective endocarditis

2016

5. **The following are early complications of acute myocardial infarction except:**

(a) Papillary muscle dysfunction
(b) Ventricular septal defect
(c) Ventricular free wall rupture
(d) Dressler's syndrome

EXPLANATION

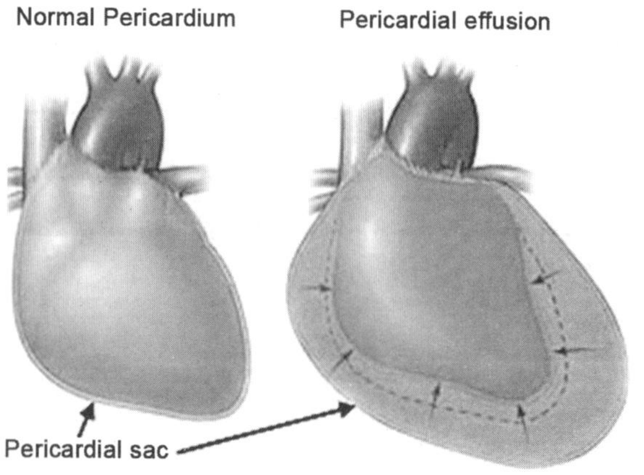

Dressler syndrome was, historically, a phenomenon complicating about 7% of myocardial infarctions; however, in the era of percutaneous coronary intervention, it is very uncommon. The disease consists of a persistent low grade fever, chest pain (usually pleuritic in nature), pericarditis (usually evidenced by a pericardial friction rub), and/or a pericardial effusion. The symptoms tend to occur 2–3 weeks after myocardial infarction, but can also be delayed for a few months.

Ans. (D) i.e., Dressler's syndrome

6. **For which one of the following serum proteins, the levels of protein do not decrease in nephrotic syndrome?**

(a) Albumin
(b) Transferrin
(c) Fibrinogen
(d) Ceruloplasmin

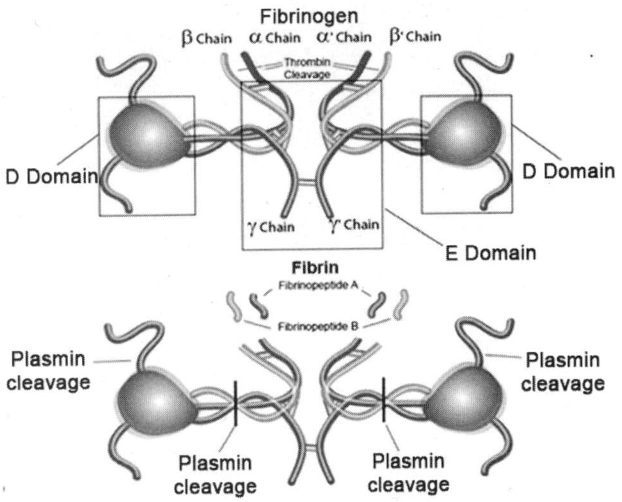

EXPLANATION

Nephrotic syndrome is a platelet hyper-aggregability state. Nephrotic syndrome is characterized by hypoalbuminemia and hyperlipidemia and is associated with an increased incidence of thromboembolism and increased platelet hyperaggregability. Fibrinogen is consistently elevated in nephrotic syndrome.

Ans. (C) i.e., Fibrinogen

7. **Following are the causes of high anion gap acidosis except:**

(a) Renal tubular acidosis
(b) Acute renal failure
(c) Chronic renal failure
(d) Diabetic ketoacidosis

EXPLANATION

Anion Gap

- $Na^+ - (Cl^- + HCO_3^-)$
- The Anion Gap (AG) is a derived variable primarily used for the evaluation of metabolic acidosis to determine the presence of unmeasured anions
- The normal anion gap depends on serum phosphate and serum albumin concentrations
- An elevated anion gap strongly suggests the presence of a metabolic acidosis
- RTA causes NAGMA (normal anion gap metabolic acidosis).

The Differential Diagnosis of a Wide-Gap Metabolic Acidosis: The "MUDPILES" Mnemonic

M	Methanol
U	Uremia
D	Diabetic ketoacidosis
P	Phenformin (metformin)
I	Iron, isoniazid
L	Lactic acidosis (shock, cellular toxins such as cyanide or carbon monoxide)
E	Ethylene glycol, ethanol (alcoholic ketoacidosis)
S	Salicylates

Ans. (A) i.e., Renal tubular acidosis

8. **A patient of cirrhosis develops oliguria and worsening azotemia. Urinary sediment is normal. Urinary sodium concentration is 5mEq/L. The most likely cause could be:**

(a) Interstitial nephritis
(b) Acute tubular necrosis
(c) Acute glomerulonephritis
(d) Hepatorenal syndrome

EXPLANATION

Hepatorenal syndrome (often abbreviated **HRS**) is a life threatening medical condition that consists of rapid deterioration in kidney functions in individuals with cirrhosis or fulminant liver failure. HRS is usually fatal unless a liver transplant is performed, although various treatments, such as dialysis, can prevent advancement of the condition.

Type 2 HRS is slower in onset and progression. It is defined by an increase in serum creatinine level to >133μmol/L (1.5mg/dL) or a creatinine clearance of less than 40mL/min, and a urine sodium < 10μmol/L

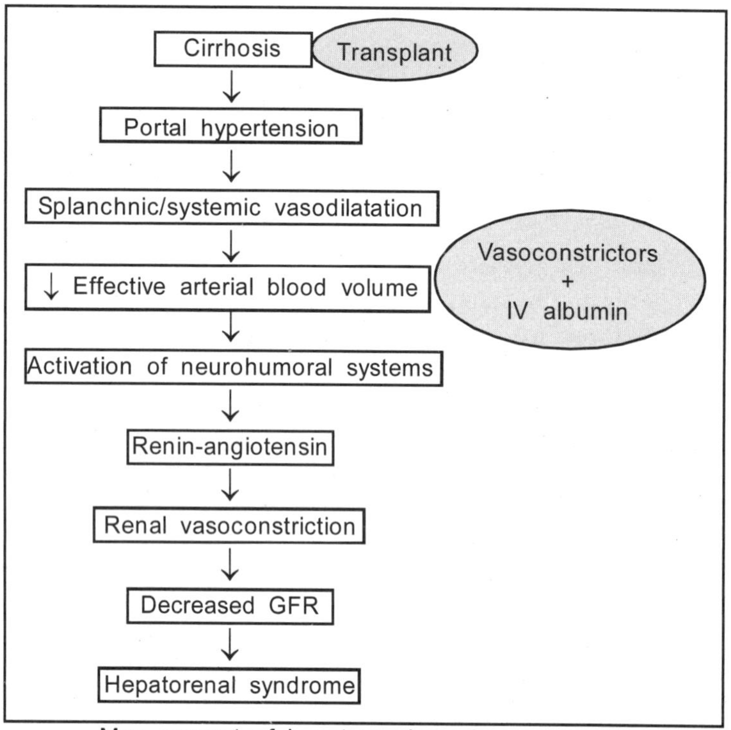

Management of hepatorenal syndrome based on reversing the main pathophysiologic mechanisms

Ans. (D) i.e., Hepatorenal syndrome

9. **Which one of the following infections is related to subacute sclerosing panencephalitis (SSPE)?**
   (a) HIV
   (b) Measles virus
   (c) Japanese B encephalitis virus
   (d) JC virus

EXPLANATION

Subacute sclerosing panencephalitis (SSPE) is a rare and chronic form of progressive brain inflammation caused by a persistent infection with measles virus (which can be a result of a mutation of the virus itself). The condition primarily affects children and young adults. It has been estimated that about 1 in 10,000 people infected with measles will eventually develop SSPE.

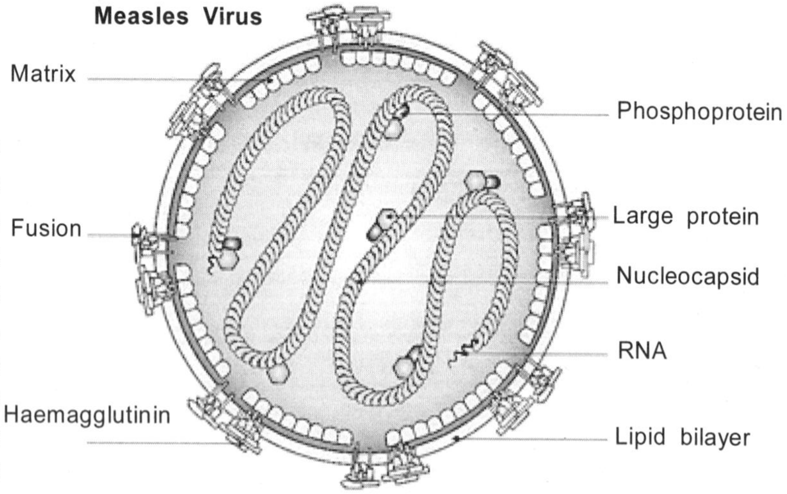

Ans. (B) i.e., Measles virus

10. **Consider the following:**

    1. Failure to swing the arms while walking
    2. Nystagmus
    3. Cogwheel rigidity
    4. Festinant gait

    Typical features of Parkinsonism include which of the above?

    (a) 2, 3 and 4 (b) 1, 2 and 4 (c) 1 and 3 only (d) 1, 3 and 4

EXPLANATION

Features of Parkinsonism

- Rigidity is stiffness and resistance to limb movement caused by increased muscle tone, an excessive and continuous contraction of muscles. In parkinsonism the rigidity can be uniform ("lead pipe rigidity") or ratchety ("cogwheel rigidity").
- Other recognized motor signs and symptoms include gait and posture disturbances such as festination (rapid shuffling steps and a forward flexed posture when walking with no flexed arm swing).

Typical appearance of Parkinson's disease

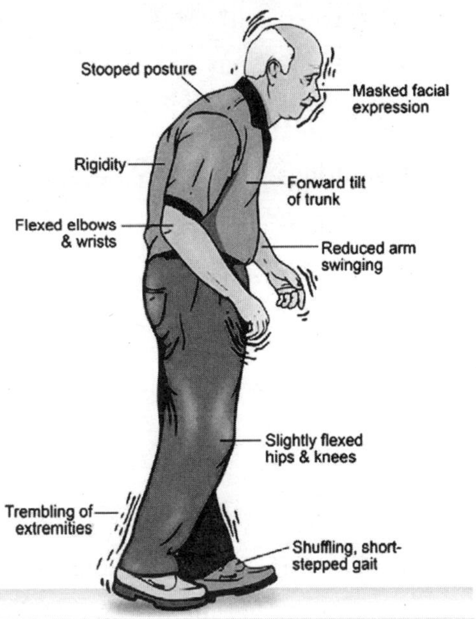

Ans. (D) i.e., 1, 3 and 4

11. **Consider the following sites of lesion:**

1. Left optic tract
2. Left optic radiation
3. Optic chiasma
4. Left lateral geniculate body

Right homonymous hemianopia will result from lesions at which of the above?

(a) 1 and 3 only (b) 1, 2 and 4 (c) 2, 3 and 4 (d) 1, 2 and 3

EXPLANATION

Homonymous hemianopsia (or **homonymous hemianopia**) is hemianopic visual field loss on the same side of both eyes. Homonymous hemianopsia occurs because the right half of the brain has visual pathways for the left hemifield of both eyes, and the left half of the brain has visual pathways for the right hemifield of both eyes. When one of these pathways is damaged, the corresponding visual field is lost

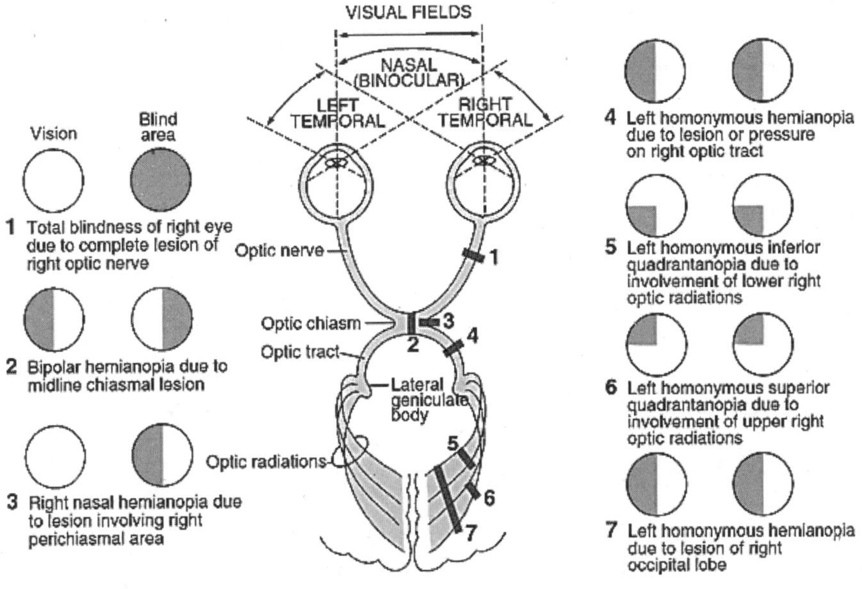

Ans. (B) i.e., 1, 2 and 4

2016

12. **Raised alkaline phosphatase is seen in the following except:**

(a) Hyperparathyroidism (b) Obstructive jaundice

(c) Osteomalacia (d) Multiple myeloma

EXPLANATION

Conditions in which ALP is raised:

- Biliary obstruction
- Osteoblastic bone tumors
- Osteomalacia
- Osteoporosis
- Hepatitis
- Cirrhosis
- Myelofibrosis
- Paget's diseae
- Sarcoidosis
- Hyperparathyroidism

Ans. (D) i.e., Multiple myeloma

13. **Consider the following statements about acromegaly:**

1. **Fibroma molluscum and acanthosis nigricans are common findings.**
2. **Growth hormone secretion is increased by TRH in 50 to 80% of acromegalics.**
3. **Acroosteolysis is a common radiological finding**
4. **Diabetes mellitus may be associated in nearly 25% of acromegalics**

Which of the statements given above are correct?

(a) 1, 2 and 3 (b) 1, 3 and 4 (c) 1, 2 and 4 (d) 2, 3 and 4

EXPLANATION

Features of acromegaly:

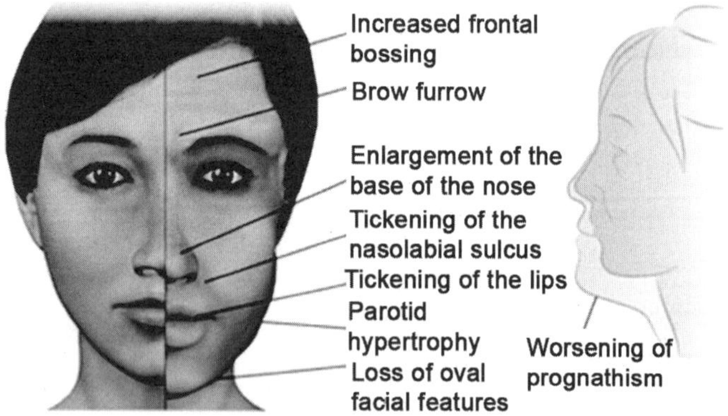

- A **skin tag/fibroma molluscum**, or **acrochordon** (pl. acrochorda), is a small benign tumour that forms primarily in areas where the skin forms creases, such as the neck, armpit and groin.
- **Acanthosis nigricans** is a brown to black, poorly defined, velvety hyperpigmentation of the skin. It is usually found in body folds, such as the posterior and lateral folds of the neck, the armpits, groin, navel, forehead, and other areas.
- Abnormal responsiveness of growth hormone- (GH-) producing pituitary adenomas to hypothalamic hormones is well known. This paradoxical response of GH to thyrotropin releasing hormone (TRH) in GH producing pituitary adenomas was first reported in 1972 and observed in 50–75% of untreated acromegalic patients.
- Diabetes mellitus (excess of GH leads to insulin resistance) occurs in acromegaly.

Ans. (C) i.e., 1, 2 and 4

14. **Causes of hypomagnesemia include all of the following except:**

(a) Beta blocker (b) Chronic pancreatic insufficiency

(c) Poorly controlled diabetes mellitus (d) Alcoholism

2016

EXPLANATION

Causes of hypomagnesemia

- Acute pancreatitis
- Hypomagnesemia occurs in 30% of alcohol abusers and in 85% of delirium tremens inpatients, due to malnutrition and chronic diarrhea. Alcohol stimulates the kidneys' excretion of magnesium, which is also increased because of alcoholic and diabetic ketoacidosis, low blood phosphate levels, and hyperaldosteronism resulting from liver disease.

Ans. (A) i.e., β blocker

15. **Which of the following conditions are associated with secondary diabetes mellitus?**

    1. **Thyrotoxicosis, pheochromocytoma and acromegaly**
    2. **Haemochromatosis**
    3. **Pancreatic carcinoma**

    Select the correct answer using the code given below:

    (a) 2 and 3 only
    (b) 1, 2 and 3
    (c) 1 and 3 only
    (d) 1 and 2 only

EXPLANATION

Conditions associated with DM

- Endocrinopathies
  - o Growth hormone excess (acromegaly)
  - o Cushing syndrome
  - o Hyperthyroidism
  - o Pheochromocytoma
  - o Glucagonoma
- Drugs
  - o Glucocorticoids
  - o Thyroid hormone
  - o Beta adrenergic agonists
- Genetic defects in insulin processing or insulin action
  - o Defects in proinsulin conversion
  - o Insulin gene mutations
  - o Insulin receptor mutations
- Exocrine pancreatic defects
  - o Chronic pancreatitis
  - o Pancreatectomy
  - o Pancreatic neoplasia
  - o Cystic fibrosis
- Genetic defects of β cell function
  - o Maturity onset diabetes of the young
  - o Mitochondrial DNA mutations
  - o Hemochromatosis

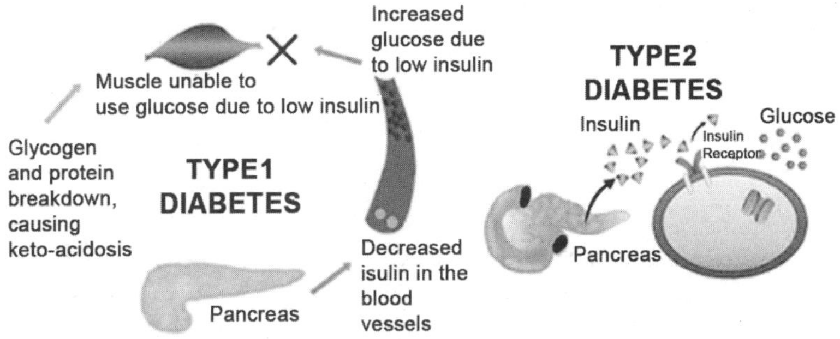

Ans. (B) i.e., 1, 2 and 3

2016

16. Consider the following statements:

1. Boils/suppurative lesions around the nose must be promptly treated with antibiotics.
2. Suppurative lesions around the nose lead to cavernous sinus thrombosis.

Which of the statements given above is/are correct?

(a) 1 only (b) 2 only
(c) Both 1 and 2 (d) Neither 1 nor 2

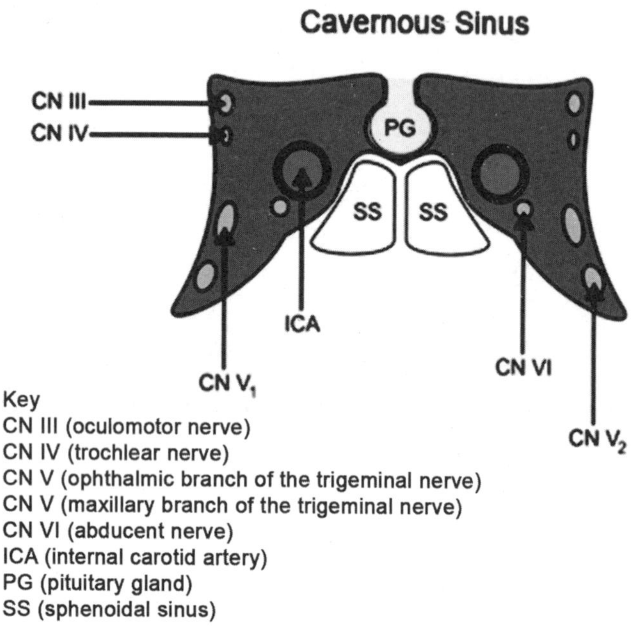

EXPLANATION

The relationship between dangerous area of face (area around nose) and a risk of cavernous sinus thrombosis was described as early as 1852. In 1937 a study found that 61% of the cases of cavernous sinus thrombosis were the result of furuncles on the upper part of the face. While the disorder has become extremely uncommon with the development of antibiotics, it still carries a very small chance to develop a high risk of death and needs to be treated aggressively with antibiotics.

Ans. (C) i.e., Both 1 and 2

17. Which one of the following is *not* the ECG change of hyperkalemia?

(a) Tall T wave
(b) Tall P wave
(c) Prolonged PR interval
(d) QRS widening

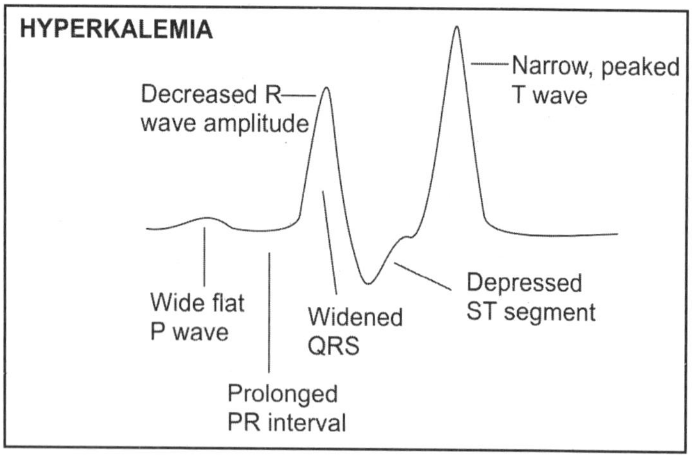

EXPLANATION

Classic teaching of the chronological ECG changes of hyperkalemia include:

1. Peaked T waves
2. Prolongation of PR interval
3. Widening QRS Complex
4. Loss of P wave
5. "Sine Wave"
6. Asystole

Ans. (B) i.e., Tall P wave

18. Which one of the following tests has the highest chance of detecting HIV infection in a blood donor during the window period?

(a) Demonstration of antibody to HIV by ELISA
(b) CD4 count
(c) p24 antigen detection
(d) Western blot test

EXPLANATION

p24 antigen is a viral protein that makes up most of the viral core of HIV. Serum concentrations of **p24 antigen** are high in the first few weeks after infection; tests sensitive to **p24 antigen** are therefore useful for diagnosing very early HIV infection when antibody levels are still low.

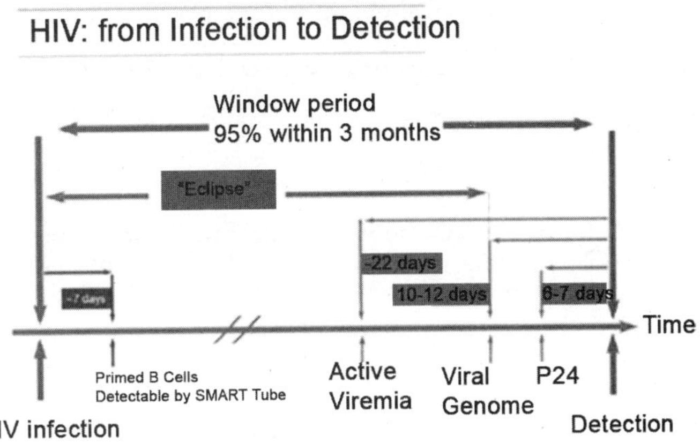

Ans. (C) i.e., p24 antigen detection

19. **Which of the following features are characteristic of tuberculoid leprosy?**

1. **Type 2 lepra reaction**
2. **A few lesions with well demarcated edges**
3. **Early and marked nerve damage**
4. **Tendency to heal spontaneously**

Select the correct answer using the code given below:

(a) 1, 2 and 3 (b) 2, 3 and 4

(c) 1 and 4 (d) 2 and 3 only

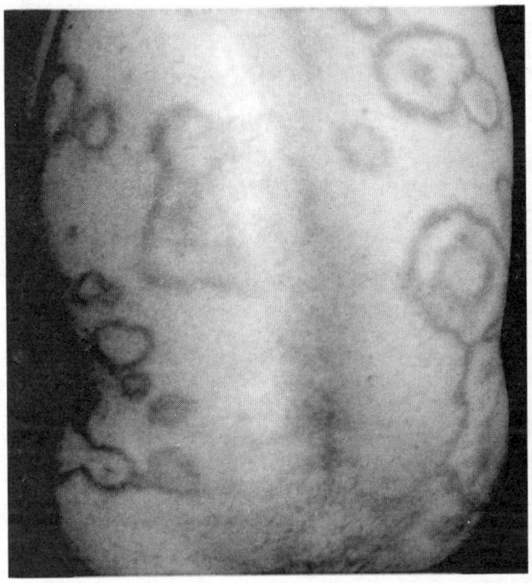

EXPLANATION

Tuberculoid leprosy is a form of leprosy characterized by solitary skin lesions that are asymmetrically distributed with few lesions and well demarcated edges. There is also early and marked nerve damage. It tends to heal spontaneously.

Ans. (B) i.e., 2, 3 and 4

20. **Which one of the following immunological reactions occurs in Goodpasture's syndrome?**

(a) Type I Atopy

(b) Type II cytotoxicity

(c) Type III immune complex

(d) Type IV cell mediation

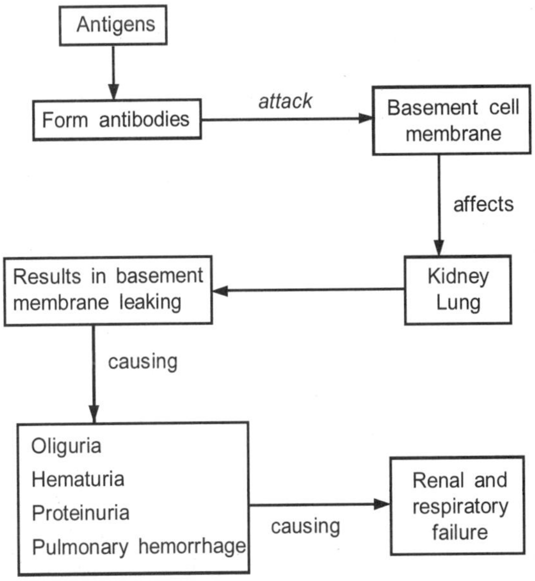

EXPLANATION

A type II reaction involves interaction of immunoglobulins with foreign or autoantigens closely associated with cell membranes. Cell lysis may result from complement activation (and development of membrane attack complexes) and from recruitment of leukocytes, including neutrophils, lymphocytes, and macrophages. So called killer lymphocytes may be involved in antibody dependent, cell mediated cytotoxicity (ADCC).

Ans. (B) i.e., Type II cytotoxicity

21. Consider the following statements about leptospirosis:

1. It is a ubiquitous enzootic disease.
2. Its incubation period ranges from 2 to 20 days.
3. The intensity of jaundice is directly related to prognosis.
4. Urine may show microscopic haematuria.

Which of the statements given above are correct?

(a) 1, 2 and 4 (b) 1, 2 and 3 (c) 1, 3 and 4 (d) 2, 3 and 4

EXPLANATION

Leptospirosis

- It is transmitted by both wild and domestic animals. The most common animals that spread the disease are rodents. It is often transmitted by animal urine or by water or soil containing animal urine coming into contact with breaks in the skin, eyes, mouth, or nose.
- The symptoms appear after an incubation period of 7–12 days. The first phase (acute or septic phase) ends after 3–7 days of illness. The patient is asymptomatic for 3–4 days until the second phase begins with another episode of fever.
- ***Urinalysis shows*** proteinuria, pyuria, and often ***microscopic hematuria***.

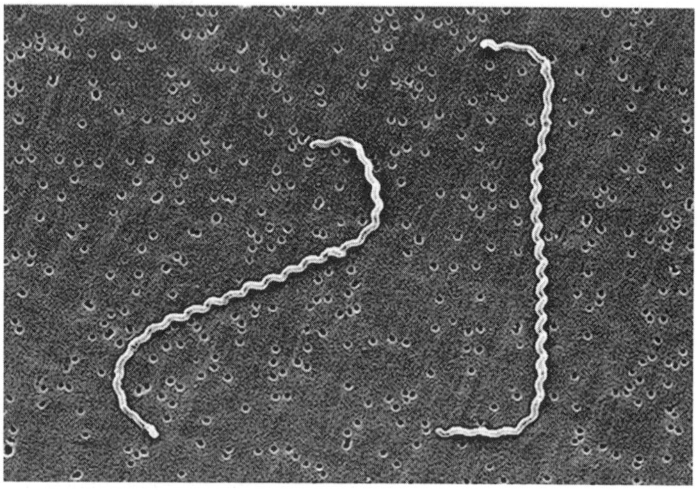

Ans. (A) i.e., 1, 2 and 4

22. SVC syndrome can occur in the following except:

(a) Pneumomediastinum
(b) Goitre
(c) Bronchogenic carcinoma
(d) Lymphoma

EXPLANATION

Pneumomediastinum (from Greek *pneuma*– "air", also known as **mediastinal emphysema**) is pneumatosis (abnormal presence of air or other gas) in the mediastinum. First described in 1819 by Rene Laennec, the condition can result from physical trauma or other situations that lead to air escaping from the lungs, airways, or bowel into the chest cavity.

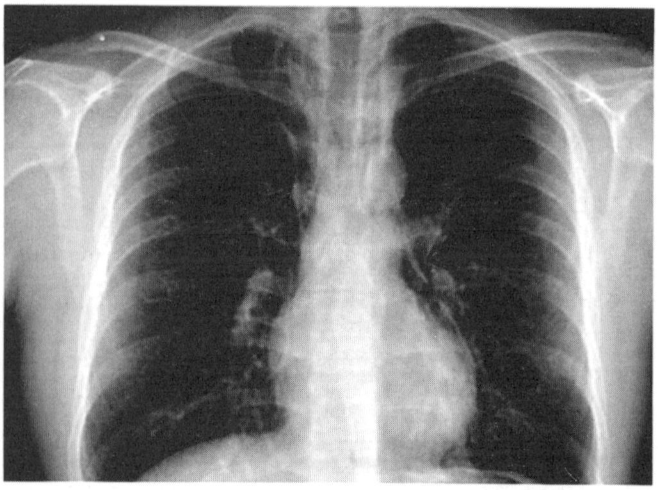

Ans. (A) i.e., Pneumomediastinum

23. Match *List I* with *List II* and select the correct answer using the code given below the lists:

List I (Physical Sign)	*List II* (Medical Condition)
A. Koebner phenomenon	1. Lepra reaction
B. Erythema nodosum	2. Pemphigus vulgaris
C. Erythema multiforme	3. Stevens Johnson syndrome
D. Nikolsky's sign	4. Psoriasis

Code: A B C D

(a) 1 4 3 2 (b) 4 1 2 3 (c) 1 4 2 3 (d) 4 1 3 2

EXPLANATION

Terms and conditions

- The **Koebner phenomenon** or **Köbner phenomenon**, also called the **Koebner response** or the **isomorphic response**, attributed to Heinrich Köbner, is the appearance of skin lesions on lines of trauma. Causes of the Koebner phenomenon that are secondary to scratching rather than an infective or chemical cause include vitiligo, psoriasis, lichen planus, lichen nitidus, pityriasis rubra pilaris, and keratosis follicularis (Darier disease).
- **Erythema nodosum** (EN), also known as **subacute migratory panniculitis of Vilanova and Piñol**, is an inflammatory condition characterized by inflammation of the fat cells under the skin, resulting in tender red nodules or lumps that are usually seen on both shins. EN may also be due to excessive antibody production in lepromatous leprosy leading to deposition of immune complexes.
- **Erythema multiforme** (EM) is a skin condition of unknown cause; it is a type of erythema possibly mediated by deposition of immune complexes (mostly IgM bound complexes) in the superficial microvasculature of the skin and oral mucous membrane that usually follows an infection or drug exposure. Erythema multiforme major" (Stevens–Johnson syndrome) resembles "erythema multiforme".
- **Nikolsky's sign** is a clinical dermatological sign, named after Pyotr Nikolsky (1858–1940), a Russian physician who trained and worked in the Russian Empire. The sign is present when slight rubbing of the skin results in exfoliation of the outermost layer. It is also associated with pemphigus vulgaris and pemphigus foliaceus.

Ans. (D) i.e., 4 1 3 2

24. **Which one of the following is the major site of absorption of Vitamin B_{12}?**

(a) Stomach

(b) Terminal ileum

(c) Duodenum

(d) Mid Jejunum

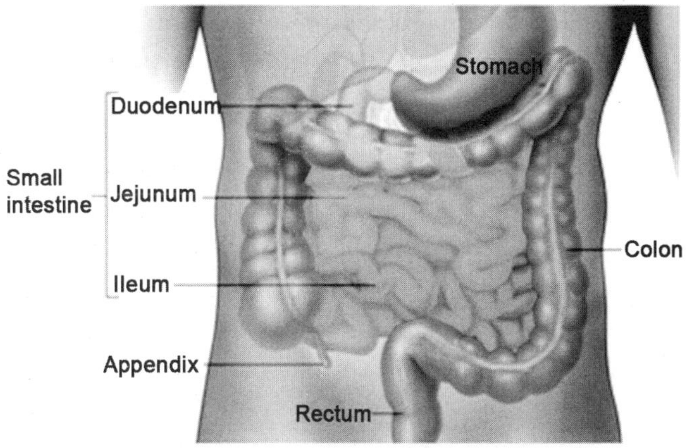

EXPLANATION

B_{12} must be attached to IF (intrinsic factor) for it to be efficiently absorbed, as receptors on the enterocytes in the terminal ileum of the small bowel only recognize the B_{12} IF complex; in addition, intrinsic factor protects the vitamin from catabolism by intestinal bacteria.

Ans. (B) i.e., Terminal ileum

25. **The following features regarding polymyositis are true except:**

(a) Progressive proximal muscle involvement
(b) 25% patients may present with dysphagia
(c) Ocular muscle involvement is common
(d) Elevated levels of serum creatine kinase

EXPLANATION

The hallmark of polymyositis is weakness and/or loss of muscle mass in the proximal musculature, as well as flexion of the neck and torso. Dysphagia (difficulty swallowing) or other problems with esophageal motility occur in as many as 1/3 of patients. Diagnosis is fourfold: History and physical examination, elevation of creatine kinase, electromyograph (EMG) alteration, and a positive muscle biopsy.

Ans. (C) i.e., Ocular muscle involvement is common

26. **Match *List I* with *List II* and select the correct answer using the code given below the lists:**

***List I* (Inflammatory Joint Disease)**	***List II* (Clinical Finding)**
A. Reiter's Syndrome	1. Onycholysis
B. Rheumatoid arthritis	2. Keratoderma blenorrhagica
C. Psoriatic arthritis	3. Xerostomia
D. Sjogren's syndrome	4. Baker's cysts

Code: A B C D

(a) 4 2 3 1
(b) 2 4 1 3
(c) 2 4 3 1
(d) 4 2 1 3

EXPLANATION

Terms and conditions

- **Onycholysis** is a common medical condition characterized by the painless detachment of the nail from the nail bed, usually starting at the tip and/or sides. Onycholysis can occur in many conditions, including psoriasis.
- **Keratoderma blennorrhagicum** etymologically meaning keratinized (kerato-) skin (derma-) mucousy (blenno-) discharge (-rrhagia) (also called **keratoderma blennorrhagica**) are skin lesions commonly found on the palms and soles but which may spread to the scrotum, scalp and trunk. The lesions may resemble psoriasis. Keratoderma blennorrhagicum is commonly seen as an additional feature of reactive arthritis in almost 15% of male patients.

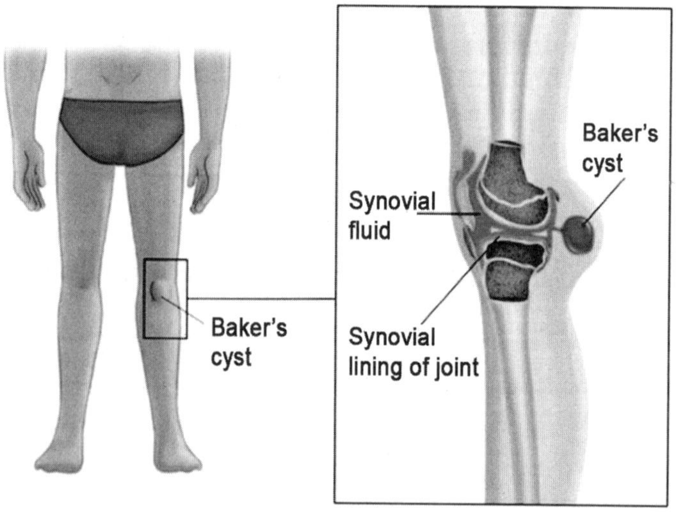

- **Xerostomia**, also known as **dry mouth** and **dry mouth syndrome**, is dryness in the mouth, which may be associated with a change in the composition of saliva, or reduced salivary flow, or have no identifiable cause. Xerostomia may be caused by autoimmune conditions which damage saliva producing cells. Sjögren's syndrome is one such disease, and it is associated with symptoms including fatigue, myalgia and arthralgia.
- A **Baker's cyst**, also known as a **popliteal cyst**, is a type of non serious fluid collection behind the knee. Often there are no symptoms. If symptoms do occur these may include swelling and pain

behind the knee, or knee stiffness. Risk factors include other knee problems such as osteoarthritis, meniscal tears, or rheumatoid arthritis.

Ans. (B) i.e., 2 4 1 3

27. **The following drugs are useful in generalized anxiety disorders except:**

(a) Risperidone (b) Amitryptiline (c) Buspirone (d) Venlafaxine

EXPLANATION

Risperidone, sold under the trade name **Risperdal** among others, is an antipsychotic medication. It is mainly used to treat schizophrenia, bipolar disorder, and irritability in people with autism.

Ans. (A) i.e., Risperidone

28. **Systemic inflammatory response syndrome (SIRS) can have the following features except:**

(a) Hypothermia (b) Bradycardia
(c) Tachypnea (d) Leucopenia (WBC < 4000)

EXPLANATION

Heart rate in SIRS is more than 90 beats/minute.

Ans. (B) i.e., Bradycardia

29. **Which of the following is *not* a complication of malaria?**

(a) ARDS (b) Acidosis (c) Hyperglycaemia (d) Coma

EXPLANATION

Hypoglycemia is a frequently encountered complication in falciparum **malaria** that is usually ascribed to increased glucose use and impaired glucose production caused by the inhibition of gluconeogenesis.

Ans. (C) i.e., Hyperglycaemia

30. **Cardiac troponin may be elevated in:**

(a) Muscular dystrophy
(b) Chronic kidney failure
(c) Acute liver failure
(d) Epilepsy

The troponin complex:

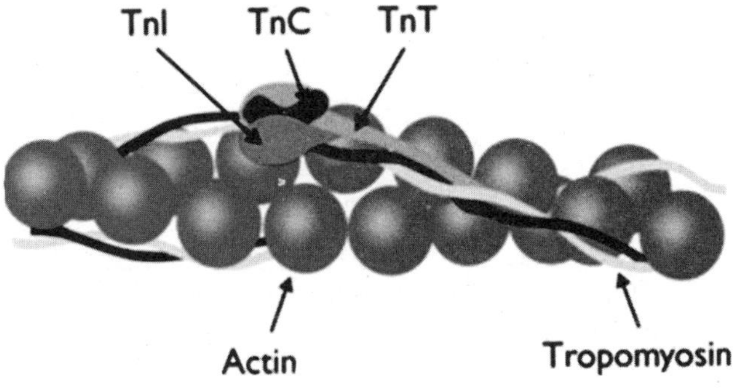

EXPLANATION

Patients with end stage renal disease can have chronically elevated troponin T levels, which are linked to a poorer prognosis. Troponin I is less likely to be falsely elevated.

Ans. (B) i.e., Chronic kidney failure

31. **Which of the following are the physiological abnormalities in chronic obstructive lung disease?**

1. Reduced total lung capacity (TLC)
2. Increased functional residual capacity
3. Increased residual volume (RV)
4. Increased RV/TLC ratio

Select the correct answer using the code given below:

(a) 1 and 2 only (b) 2, 3 and 4 (c) 1, 3 and 4 (d) 3 and 4 only

EXPLANATION

Spirometry

- Total lung capacity (TLC) is the maximum volume of air present in the lungs at the end of maximum inspiration.
- **Functional Residual Capacity** (FRC) is the volume of air present in the lungs at the end of passive expiration. In emphysema, FRC is increased, because the lungs are more compliant and the equilibrium between the inward recoil of the lungs and outward recoil of the chest wall is disturbed.
- The **residual volume**, the **volume** of air left in the lungs following full expiration, is often **increased** in **COPD**, as is the total lung capacity, while the vital capacity remains relatively normal.

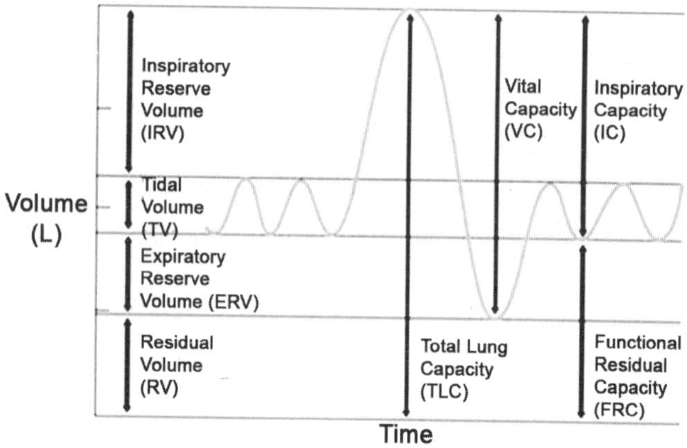

Ans. (B) i.e., 2, 3 and 4

32. **Consider the following statements:**

Acute respiratory distress syndrome characteristically occurs in

1. **Gram negative septicaemia**
2. **Gastric aspiration**
3. **Pancreatitis**
4. **Severe burns**
5. **Myocarditis**

Which of the statements given above are correct?

(a) 2, 3, 4 and 5 (b) 1, 3, 4 and 5

(c) 1, 2 and 5 (d) 1, 2, 3 and 4

EXPLANATION

Acute respiratory distress syndrome (ARDS) is a medical condition occurring in critically ill or critically wounded patients characterized by widespread inflamation in the lungs. Diffuse compromise of the pulmonary system resulting in ARDS generally occurs in the setting of critical illness. ARDS may be seen in the setting of severe pulmonary (pneumonia) or systemic infection (sepsis), following trauma, multiple blood transfusions (TRALI), severe burns, severe inflammation of the pancreas (pancreatitis), near drowning or other aspiration events, drug reactions, or inhalation injuries.

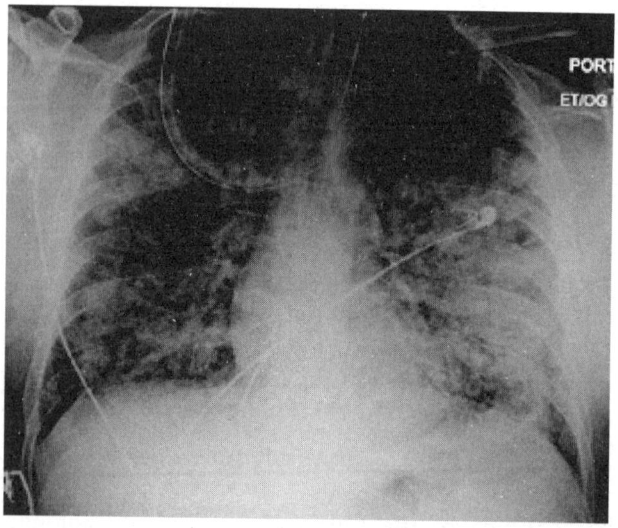

Ans. (D) i.e., 1, 2, 3 and 4

2016

33. **Botulism can have the following clinical features except:**

(a) Hyperpyrexia
(b) Sudden onset quadriplegia
(c) Cranial nerve deficits
(d) Respiratory failure

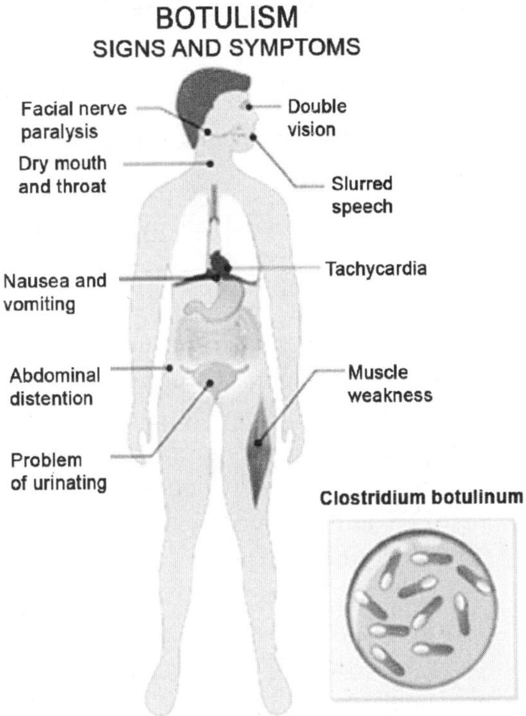

EXPLANATION

Botulism is a rare and potentially fatal illness caused by a toxin produced by the bacterium *Clostridium Botulinum*. The disease begins with weakness, blurred vision, feeling tired, and trouble speaking. This may then be followed by weakness of the arms, chest muscles, and legs. Vomiting, swelling of the abdomen, and diarrhea may also occur. The disease does not usually affect consciousness or cause a fever.

Ans. (A) i.e., Hyperpyrexia

34. **A 55-year old man, non smoker presents with sudden onset of shortness of breath. On examination, pulse rate is 110/minute and B.P. 180/110mmHg. Patient is restless and anxious. Examination of chest shows bilateral rhonchi and crepitation. S3 gallop is heard on auscultation of precordium. There is no history of chronic bronchitis. The most likely diagnosis is:**

(a) Bronchial asthma
(b) Acute LVF
(c) Pneumothorax
(d) Acute exacerbation of COPD

EXPLANATION

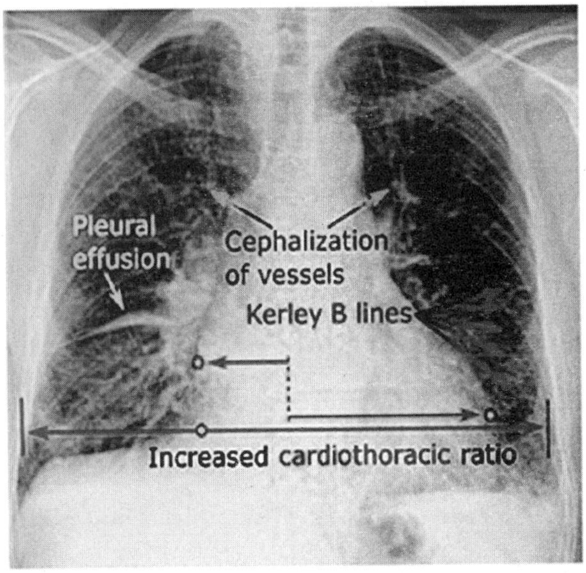

Features of left ventricular failure

- Increased rate of breathing (tachypnea) and increased *work* of breathing (non specific signs of respiratory distress).
- Rales or crackles or crepitations, heard initially in the lung bases, and when severe, throughout the lung fields suggest the development of pulmonary edema (fluid in the alveoli).
- Cyanosis which suggests severe low blood oxygen, is a late sign of extremely severe pulmonary edema.
- Laterally displaced apex beat (which occurs if the heart is enlarged) and
- A gallop rhythm (additional heart sounds) may be heard as a marker of increased blood flow or increased intracardiac pressure.

Ans. (B) i.e., Acute LVF

35. Consider the following statements:

Small cell carcinoma of lung is commonly associated with following paraneoplastic syndromes:

1. Ectopic ACTH production
2. Lambert Eaton syndrome
3. Syndrome of inappropriate ADH (SIADH)
4. Addison's disease

Which of the statements given above are correct?

(a) 1, 2 and 3 (b) 2, 3 and 4
(c) 1, 3 and 4 (d) 1, 2 and 4

EXPLANATION

Due to its high grade neuroendocrine nature, small cell carcinomas can produce ectopic hormones, including adrenocorticotropic hormone (ACTH) and anti diuretic hormone (ADH). Ectopic production of large amounts of ADH leads to syndrome of inappropriate antidiuretic hormone hypersecretion (SIADH). Lambert Eaton myasthenic syndrome (LEMS) is a well known paraneoplastic condition linked to small cell carcinoma.

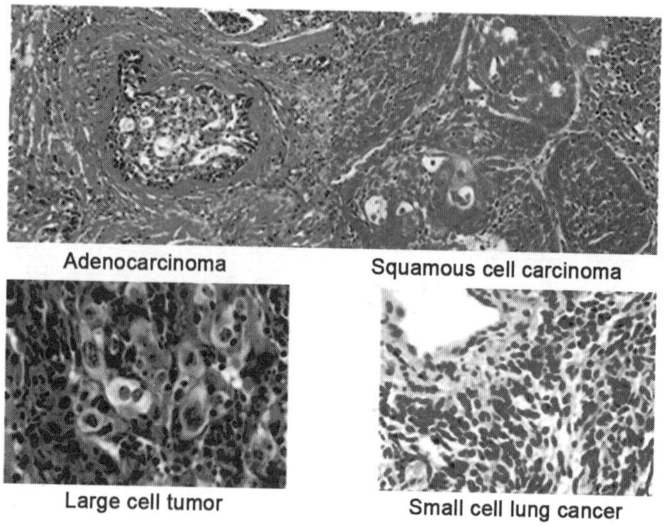

Ans. (A) i.e., 1, 2 and 3

36. On abdominal percussion, liver dullness may be obliterated in the following except:

(a) Fatty liver (b) Emphysema (c) Perforated viscus (d) Fulminant hepatitis

EXPLANATION

Liver dullness is obliterated in following conditions

- Severe emphysema
- Right pneumothorax
- Gas under the diaphragm (perforation of a viscus)
- Shrunken liver: Massive hepatic necrosis in fulminant hepatocellular failure, Advanced cirrhosis of liver.

Ans. (A) i.e., Fatty liver

37. Consider the following statements regarding *Helicobacter pylori*:

1. It is a gram negative bacterium
2. It invades the epithelium
3. It produces urease
4. It produces chronic gastritis

Which of the statements given above are correct?

(a) 1, 2 and 4
(b) 1 and 3 only
(c) 2 and 4 only
(d) 1, 3 and 4

EXPLANATION

Helicobacter pylori, previously known as *Campylobacter pylori*, is a gram negative, microaerophilic bacterium usually found in the stomach. It was identified in 1982 by Australian scientists Barry Marshall and Robin Warren, who found that it was present in a person with chronic gastritis and gastric ulcers, conditions not previously believed to have a microbial cause. It is also linked to the development of duodenal ulcers and stomach carcinoma. However, over 80% of individuals infected with the bacterium are asymptomatic, and it may play an important role in the natural stomach ecology. It produces oxidase, catalase, and urease.

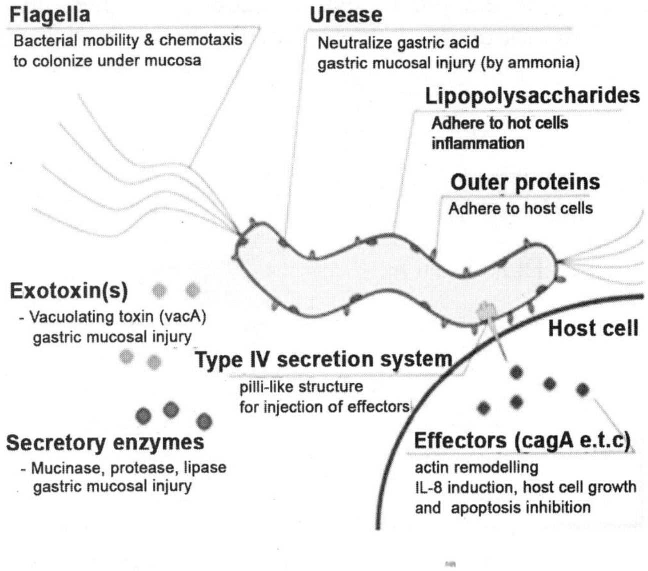

Ans. (D) i.e., 1, 3 and 4

38. **Consider the following conditions:**

1. **Steroid therapy**
2. **Hypertriglyceridaemia**
3. **Hypercalcaemia**
4. **Azathioprine therapy**

Acute pancreatitis may occur in which of the above conditions?

(a) 1, 2 and 3 only
(b) 2 and 4 only
(c) 1, 3 and 4 only
(d) 1, 2, 3 and 4

EXPLANATION

Common causes of acute pancreatitis

- Biliary Pancreatitis due to gallstones, constriction of ampulla of Vater in 40% of cases
- Alcohol in 30% of cases
- Idiopathic in 15–25% of cases
- Metabolic disorders: hereditary pancreatitis, hypercalcemia, elevated triglycerides, malnutrition
- Post ERCP
- Abdominal trauma
- Penetrating ulcers
- Carcinoma of the head of pancreas, and other cancer
- Drugs: diuretics (e.g., thiazides, furosemide), gliptins (e.g., vildagliptin, sitagliptin, saxagliptin, linagliptin), tetracycline, sulfonamides, estrogen, azathioprine and mercaptopurine, pentamidine, salicylates, steroids etc.

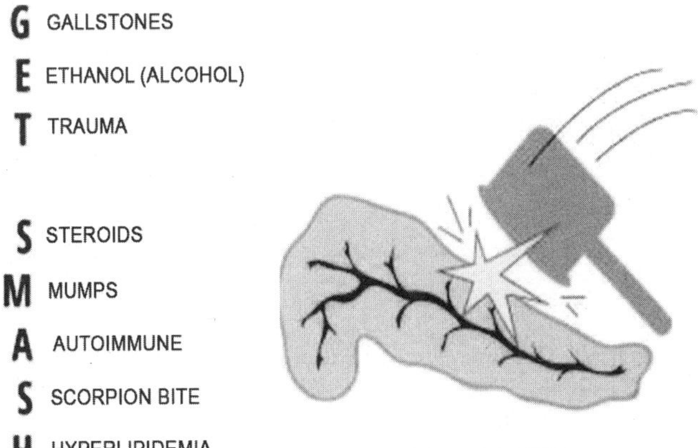

ACUTE PANCREATITIS MNEMONIC

Ans. (D) i.e., 1, 2, 3 and 4

39. **A 60-year old patient presents with gradually increasing dysphagia to solids for 3 months with significant loss of weight. The most probable diagnosis is:**

(a) Stricture oesophagus
(b) Carcinoma oesophagus
(c) Reflux oesophagitis
(d) Neurogenic oesophagus

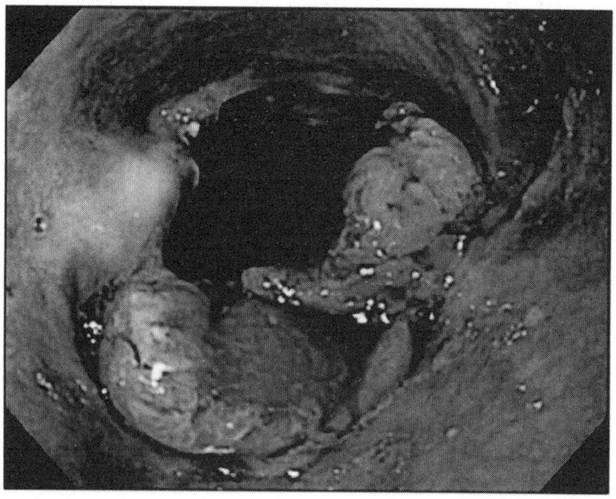

EXPLANATION

The first and the most common symptom is usually difficulty in swallowing, which is often experienced first with solid foods and later with softer foods and liquids. Pain while swallowing is less usual at first. Weight loss is often an initial symptom in cases of squamous cell carcinoma, though not usually in cases of adenocarcinoma. Eventual weight loss due to reduced appetite and undernutrition is common.

Ans. (B) i.e., Carcinoma oesophagus

40. **Consider the following statements:**

1. **Gentamicin should be added to empirical regime for acute meningitis for patients aged more than 55 years.**
2. **Ampicillin covers listeria monocytogenes.**

Which of the statements given above is/are correct?

(a) 1 only
(b) 2 only
(c) Both 1 and 2
(d) Neither 1 nor 2

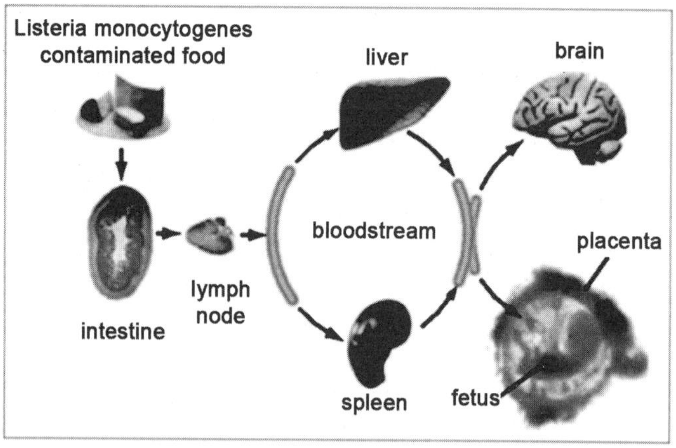

EXPLANATION

Ampicillin in combination with an aminoglycoside such as **gentamicin** is the therapy of choice for listerial infections. **Listeria** is not susceptible to cephalosporins of any generation.

Ans. (B) i.e., 2 only

41. **Which one of the following gases is used for sterilization of pharmaceutical products?**

(a) Ethylene oxide
(b) Ammonia
(c) Halothane
(d) Nitrous oxide

EXPLANATION

Ethylene Oxide (EtO) sterilization is mainly used to sterilize medical and pharmaceutical products that cannot support conventional high temperature steam sterilization—such as devices that incorporate electronic components, plastic packaging or plastic containers.

Ans. (A) i.e., Ethylene oxide

2016

42. The following statements about peptic ulcer are true except:

(a) Eradication of *H. pylori* is a part of medical management.

(b) Duodenal ulcer invariably changes into malignant.

(c) Complications are indication for surgery.

(d) Zollinger Ellison syndrome is associated with intractable peptic ulceration.

EXPLANATION

Malignant degeneration is the most serious complication of gastric ulcer. Its recognition is difficult both in the early stage and in advanced cases in which only the evidence of a previous ulcer cavity, and the radiating folds of the mucous membrane indicate progressive development of carcinoma from an original ulcer. It is impossible to say how often gastric ulcer becomes malignant; one can only state the frequency of ulcer carcinoma, found in gastric resections.

Ans. (B) i.e., Duodenal ulcer invariably changes into malignant.

43. In a patient with lacerated injury foot who is not actively immunised against tetanus, which one of the following is indicated for tetanus prophylaxis?

(a) Penicillin
(b) Tetanus toxoid
(c) Tetanus immunoglobulin
(d) Triple vaccine

EXPLANATION

Antitetanus immunoglobulin, also known as **tetanus immune globulin** (TIG) and **tetanus antitoxin**, is made up of antibodies against the tetanus toxin. It is used to prevent tetanus in those who have a wound that is at high risk and have not been fully vaccinated with tetanus toxoid. It is also used to treat tetanus along with antibiotics and muscle relaxants.

Ans. (C) i.e., Tetanus immunoglobulin

2016

44. Which one of the following neoplasms can lead to 'water intoxication'?

(a) Oat cell carcinoma of bronchus
(b) Hepatocarcinoma
(c) Testicular tumours
(d) Rhabdomyosarcoma

EXPLANATION

Syndrome of inappropriate antidiuretic hormone secretion(SIADH) is characterized by excessive unsuppressible release of antidiuretic hormone (ADH) either from the posterior pituitary gland, or an abnormal non pituitary source. Unsuppressed ADH causes an unrelenting increase in solute free water being returned by the tubules of the kidney to the venous circulation. SIADH was originally described in 1957 in two people with small cell carcinoma of the lung.

Ans. (A) i.e., Oat cell carcinoma of bronchus

45. The Swan Ganz catheter is used to measure:

(a) Peripheral arterial blood pressure

(b) Portal venous pressure

(c) Pulmonary wedge pressure

(d) Intracranial pressure monitoring

EXPLANATION

Pulmonary Artery Catheterization (PAC) is the insertion of a catheter into a pulmonary artery. Its purpose is diagnostic; it is used to detect heart failure or sepsis, monitor therapy, and evaluate the effects of drugs. The pulmonary artery catheter allows direct, simultaneous measurement of pressures in the right atrium, right ventricle, pulmonary artery, and the filling pressure ("wedge" pressure) of the left atrium. The pulmonary artery catheter is frequently referred to as a **Swan Ganz catheter**, in honor of its inventors Jeremy Swan and William Ganz, from Cedars Sinai Medical Center.

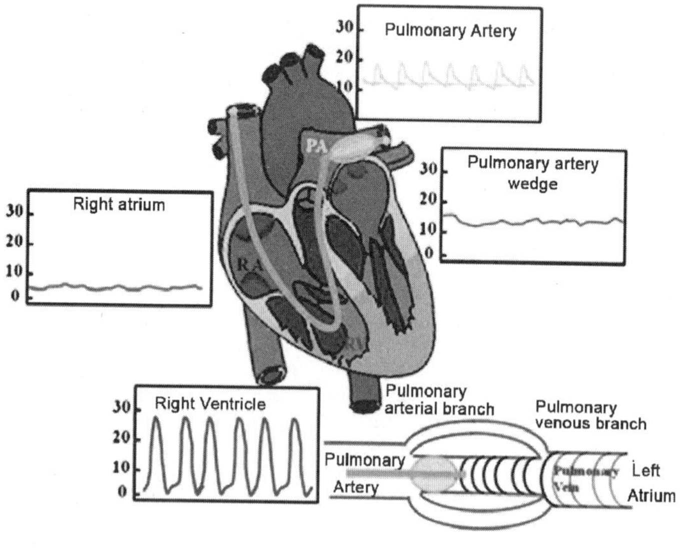

Ans. (C) i.e., Pulmonary wedge pressure

46. **Delirium is usually seen in:**

(a) Acetaminophen toxicity

(b) Atropine toxicity

(c) Kerosene poisoning

(d) Digitalis toxicity

EXPLANATION

Adverse reactions to atropine include ventricular fibrillation, supraventricular or ventricular tachycardia, dizziness, nausea, blurred vision, loss of balance, dilated pupils, photophobia, dry mouth and potentially extreme confusion, deliriant hallucinations, and excitation especially among the elderly. A common mneomonic used to describe the physiologic manifestations of atropine overdose is: "hot as a hare, blind as a bat, dry as a bone, red as a beet, and mad as a hatter".

Ans. (B) i.e., Atropine toxicity

47. **The following statements regarding Hodgkin's disease are true except:**

(a) It usually presents as painless lymph-adenopathy.

(b) The Pel Ebstein fever is a characteristic feature.

(c) Stage III disease is confined to one side of the diaphragm.

(d) Reed Sternberg cells are a diagnostic feature.

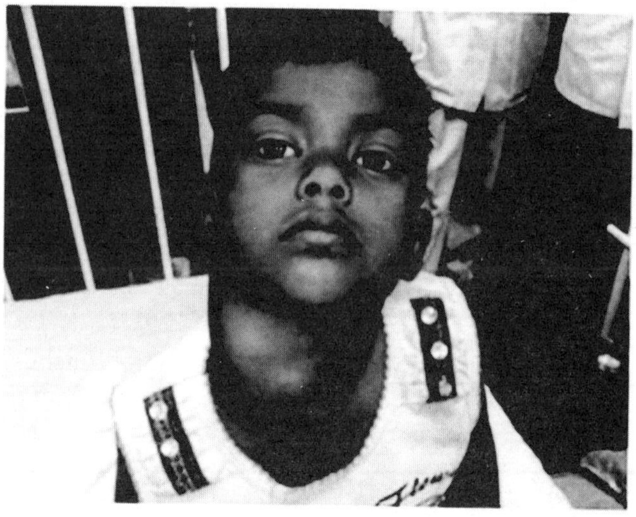

EXPLANATION

Stage III Hodgkin disease is involvement of lymph node regions on both sides of the diaphragm, which may include the spleen (IIIs) or limited contiguous extralymphatic organ or site (IIIe, IIIes)

Ans. (C) i.e., Stage III disease is confined to one side of the diaphragm.

48. **Following are causes of bleeding except:**

(a) Heparin induced thrombocytopenia
(b) Dengue fever
(c) ITP
(d) Aspirin

EXPLANATION

Heparin induced thrombocytopenia (HIT) is the development of thrombocytopenia (a low platelet count), due to the administration of various forms of heparin, an anticoagulant. HIT predisposes to thrombosis (the abnormal formation of blood clots inside a blood vessel) because platelets release microparticles that activate thrombin, thereby leading to thrombosis. When thrombosis is identified the condition is called **heparin induced thrombocytopenia and thrombosis** (HITT).

Ans. (A) i.e., Heparin induced thrombocytopenia

49. **The combination of cyanosis with clubbing can be seen in the following conditions except:**

(a) Eisenmenger syndrome
(b) Lung abscess
(c) Chronic bronchitis
(d) Pulmonary AV fistula

Finger clubbing

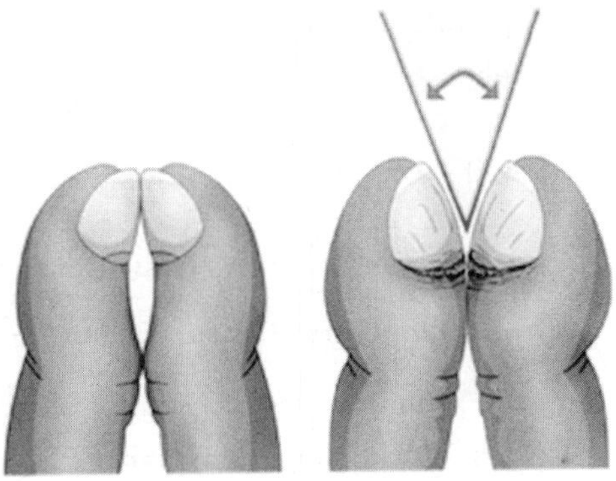

EXPLANATION

Fingernail clubbing is not specific to COPD and should prompt investigations for an underlying lung cancer or other heart/lung conditions.

Ans. (C) i.e., Chronic bronchitis

50. **Diagnosis and grading of multi-organ failure is based on all the following criteria except:**

(a) Serum bilirubin
(b) Serum albumin
(c) Serum creatinine
(d) PaO2/FiO2 ratio

EXPLANATION

Multiple organ dysfunction syndrome (MODS), **also known as** multiple organ failure (MOF), total organ failure (TOF) **or** multisystem organ failure (MSOF), **is altered organ function in an acutely ill patient requiring medical intervention to achieve homeostasis. Evaluation of systems is done by:**

(a) the respiratory system (PaO2/FiO2 ratio);
(b) the renal system (serum creatinine concentration);
(c) the hepatic system (serum bilirubin concentration);
(d) the hematologic system (platelet count); and
(e) the central nervous system (Glasgow Coma Scale).

Ans. (B) i.e., Serum albumin

51. **A 16-year old boy presents with exertional dyspnea, haemoptysis and occasionally paroxysmal nocturnal dyspnea. There was history of joint pains five years back. The most probable diagnosis is:**

(a) Aortic regurgitation
(b) Mitral stenosis
(c) Tricuspid stenosis
(d) Aortic stenosis

EXPLANATION

Signs and symptoms of mitral stenosis:

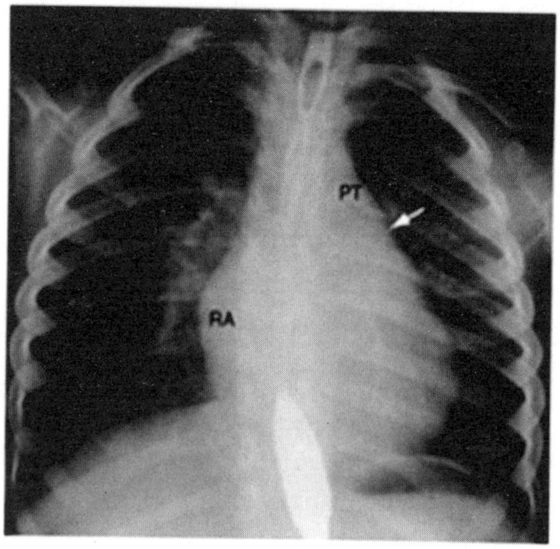

- Heart failure symptoms, such as dyspnea on exertion, orthopnea and paroxysmal nocturnal dyspnea (PND)
- Palpitations
- Chest pain
- Hemoptysis
- Thromboembolism in later stages when the left atrial volume is increased (i.e., dilation). The latter leads to increase risk of atrial fibrillation, which increases the risk of blood stasis (motionless). This increases the risk of coagulation.
- History of joint pains five years back suggests the episode of acute rheumatic fever (migrating polyarthritis).

Ans. (B) i.e., Mitral stenosis

52. **Consider the following statements:**

The Adrenocortical insufficiency may result in:

1. Hyponatremia **2. Hypokalemia** **3. Acidosis** **4. Hyperglycemia**

Which of the statements given above is/are correct?

(a) 1 only (b) 1 and 3 (c) 2 and 4 only (d) 2, 3 and 4

EXPLANATION

Routine laboratory investigations in Addison's disease

- Hypoglycemia, low blood sugar (worse in children due to loss of glucocorticoid's glucogenic effects)
- Hyponatremia (low blood sodium levels), due to loss of production of the hormone aldosterone, to the kidney's inability to excrete free water in the absence of sufficient cortisol, and also the effect of corticotropin releasing hormone to stimulate secretion of ADH.
- Hyperkalemia (raised blood potassium levels), due to loss of production of the hormone aldosterone.
- Eosinophilia and lymphocytosis (increased number of eosinophils or lymphocytes, two types of white blood cells).
- Metabolic acidosis (increased blood acidity), also is due to loss of the hormone aldosterone because sodium reabsorption in the distal tubule is linked with acid/hydrogen ion (H^+) secretion. Absent or insufficient levels of aldosterone stimulation of the renal distal tubule leads to sodium wasting in the urine and H^+ retention in the serum.

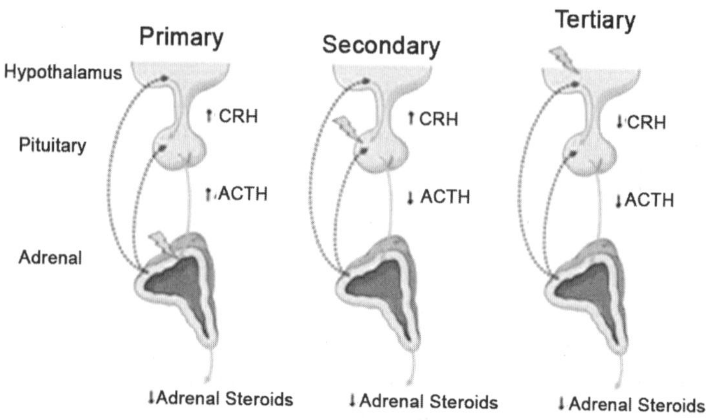

Ans. (B) i.e., 1 and 3

53. Consider the following statements:

Life threatening pneumococcal infection is a complication seen in:

1. Idiopathic thrombocytpaenic purpura
2. Sickle cell disease
3. Thalassemia minor
4. Nephrotic syndrome

Which of the statements given above is/are correct?

(a) 1 only (b) 1 and 3 (c) 2 and 4 only (d) 2, 3 and 4

EXPLANATION

Pneumococcal infections

- The risk of pneumococcal infection is much increased in persons with impaired IgG synthesis, impaired phagocytosis, or defective clearance of pneumococci. In particular, the absence of a functional spleen, through congenital asplenia, surgical removal of spleen, or sickle cell anemia predisposes one to a more severe course of infection (overwhelming post splenectomy infections).
- Children with idiopathic ***nephrotic syndrome*** are at risk of potentially severe ***pneumococcal infections***, such as pneumonia, meningitis and peritonitis. This susceptibility is due to losses of immunoglobulin and complement system components.

Ans. (C) i.e., 2 and 4 only

54. The following are true regarding Zollinger Ellison syndrome except:

(a) Common age group is 30 to 50 years

(b) Gastrin level is usually high

(c) Diarrhea can be an associated feature

(d) It occurs in association with MEN-2 syndrome

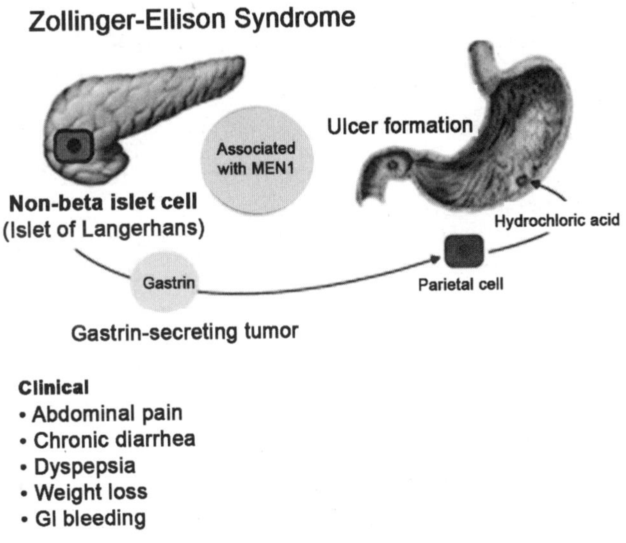

EXPLANATION

ZES may occur on its own or as part of an autosomal dominant syndrome called multiple endocrinal neoplasia 1 (MEN 1). The primary tumor is usually located in the pancreas, duodenum or abdominal lymph nodes, but ectopic locations (e.g., heart, ovary, gallbladder, liver, and kidney) have also been described.

Ans. (D) i.e., It occurs in association with MEN-2 syndrome

55. The following may be seen in a patient with chronic liver disease except:

(a) Prolonged PT (b) Prolonged PTT

(c) Thrombocytopenia (d) Decreased factor VIII

EXPLANATION

Factor VIII is produced in liver sinusoidal cells and endothelial cells outside the liver throughout the body.

Ans. (D) i.e., Decreased factor VIII

56. **Pseudo membranous colitis is caused by which of the following organisms?**

(a) *Shigella* (b) *Clostridium difficile*

(c) *E.coli* (d) *Clostridium perfringens*

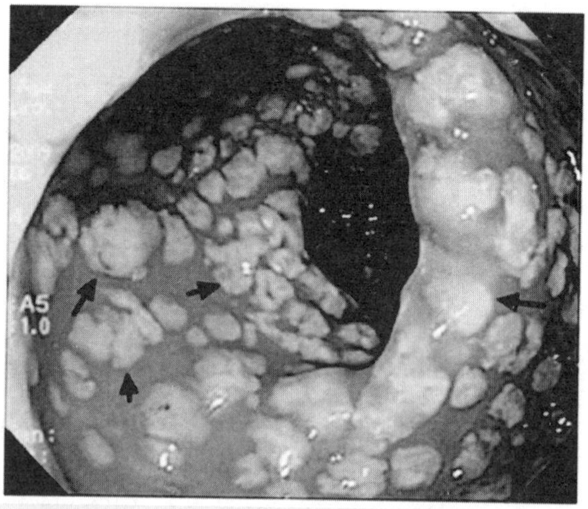

EXPLANATION

Clostridium difficile infection (CDI or C-dif) is a symptomatic infection due to the spore forming bacterium, Clostridium difficile. Symptoms include watery diarhhea, fever, nausea, and abdominal pain. It makes up about 20% of cases of antibiotic associated diarrhea. Complications may include pseudomembranous colitis, toxic megacolon, perforation of the colon, and sepsis.

Ans. (B) i.e., *Clostridium difficile*

57. **A patient presents with breathlessness and occasional dry cough. On physical examination, he is found to have bilateral basal crepitations. His pulmonary function tests reveal a decrease in total lung capacity and vital capacity (VC), with normal FEV1/FVC ratio. He is most likely suffering from:**

(a) Chronic bronchitis (b) Idiopathic pulmonary fibrosis

(c) Cystic fibrosis (d) Allergic bronchopulmonary aspergillosis

EXPLANATION

Most common clinical features of IPF:

- Age over 50 years
- Dry, non productive cough on exertion
- Progressive exertional dyspnea (shortness of breath with exercise)
- Dry, inspiratory bibasilar "velcro like" crackles on auscultation (a crackling sound in the lungs during inhalation similar to Velcro being torn apart slowly, heard with a stethoscope).
- Clubbing of the digits, a disfigurement of the finger tips or toes.
- Abnormal pulmonary function test results, with evidence of restriction and impaired gas exchange. Spirometry classically reveals a reduction in the vital capacity (VC) with either a proportionate reduction in airflows, or increased airflows for the observed vital capacity. The latter finding reflects the increased lung stiffness (reduced lung compliance) associated with pulmonary fibrosis, which leads to increased lung elastic recoil.

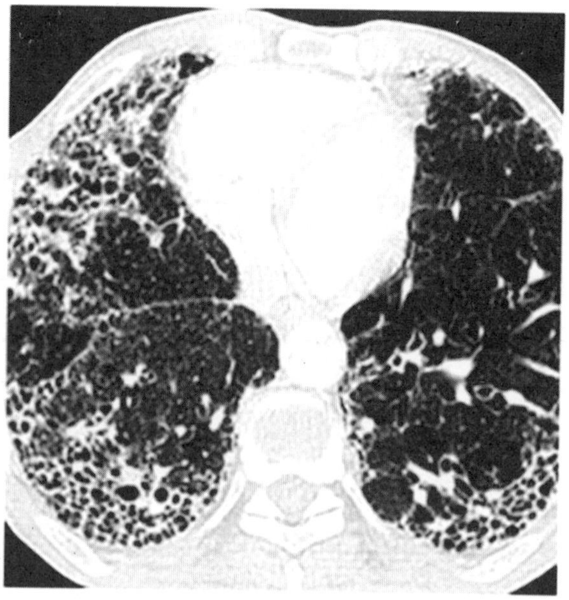

Ans. (B) i.e., Idiopathic pulmonary fibrosis

58. **A 45-year old hypertensive male patient presented to the casualty with 3 hour history of sudden onset severe headache associated with nausea and vomiting. On clinical examination, patient had right sided ptosis and neck stiffness. Rest of the neurological examination was normal. The most likely diagnosis in this case is:**

(a) Hypertensive brain damage
(b) Migraine
(c) Aneurysmal subarachnoid bleed
(d) Acute pyogenic meningitis

EXPLANATION

Subarachnoid hemorrhage (SAH) is bleeding into the subarachnoid space—the area between the arachnoid membrane and the pia mater surrounding the brain. Symptoms may include a severe headache of rapid onset, vomiting, decreased level of consciousness, fever, and sometimes seizures. Neck stiffness or neck pain are also relatively common. In about a quarter of people a small bleed with resolving symptoms occurs within a month of a larger bleed. SAH may occur as a result of a head injury or spontaneously, usually from a ruptured cerebral aneurysm.

Ans. (C) i.e., Aneurysmal subarachnoid bleed

59. Which one of the following is *not* a treatment of hepatic encephalopathy?

(a) Lactulose
(b) Rifaximin
(c) TIPS
(d) Electrolyte supplementation

EXPLANATION

Transjugular intrahepatic portosystemic shunt (TIPS or TIPSS) is an artificial channel within the liver that establishes communication between the inflow portal vein and the outflow hepatic vein. It is used to treat portal hypertension (which is often due to liver cirrhosis) which frequently leads to intestinal bleeding, life threatening esophageal bleeding (esophageal varices) and the buildup of fluid within the abdomen (ascites).

Ans. (C) i.e., TIPS

2016

60. Features of intravascular haemolysis are the following except:

(a) Increased LDH
(b) Haemoglobinuria
(c) Increased serum indirect bilirubin
(d) Increased serum haptoglobin

EXPLANATION

In clinical settings, the haptoglobulin assay is used to screen for and monitor intravascular haemolytic anemia. In intravascular hemolysis, free hemoglobin will be released into circulation and hence haptoglobin will bind the hemoglobin. This causes a decline in haptoglobin levels.

Tests for intra- and extravascular haemolysis

Test	Intravascular haemolysis	Extravascular haemolysis
Serum haptoglobin	↓	↓
Plasma Hb	Present	Absent
Haemoglobinuria	Present	Absent
Haemosiderinuria	Present	Absent
Serum lactate dehydrogenase	↑	↑
Serum unconjugated bilirubin	Normal	↑

Ans. (D) i.e., Increased serum haptoglobin

61. Consider the following statements:

1. Hypertrophic cardiomyopathy can lead to sudden cardiac death.
2. Dressler's syndrome is an early complication of acute myocardial infarction.

Which of the statements given above is/are correct?

(a) 1 only (b) 2 only (c) Both 1 and 2 (d) Neither 1 nor 2

EXPLANATION

Hypertrophic cardiomyopathy (HCM) is a condition in which a portion of the heart becomes thickened without an obvious cause. This results in the heart being less able to pump blood effectively. Symptoms vary from none to feeling tired, leg swelling, and shortness of breath. It may also result in chest pain or fainting. Complications include heart failure, an irregular heartbeat, and sudden cardiac death.

Ans. (A) i.e., 1 only

62. **The common sites of hypertensive bleed are the following except:**

(a) Basal ganglion (b) Pons

(c) Cerebellum (d) Frontal cortex

EXPLANATION

When due to raised blood pressure, intracerebral hemorrhages typically occur in the putamen (50%) or thalamus (15%), cerebrum (10–20%), cerebellum (10–13%), pons (7–15%), or elsewhere in the brainstem (1–6%).

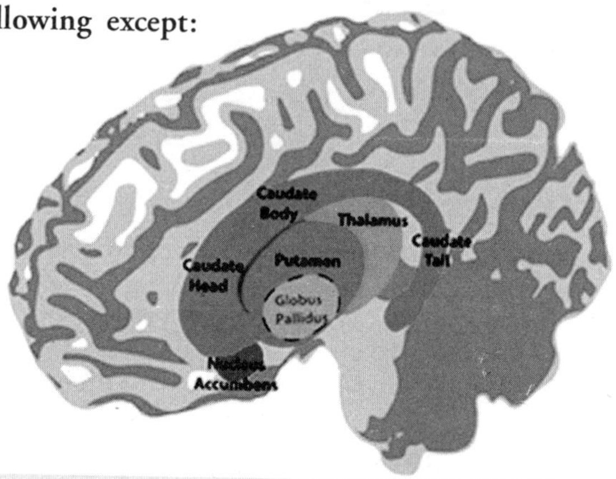

Ans. (D) i.e., Frontal cortex

63. **Hypoglycaemia as an adverse side effect is most commonly seen during the treatment with:**

(a) Dipeptyl peptidase IV inhibitors (b) Metformin

(c) a glucosidase inhibitors (d) Sulfonylureas

EXPLANATION

Sulfonylureas, as opposed to metformin, the thiazolidindiones, exenatide, pramlintide and other newer treatment agents may induce hypoglycemia as a result of excesses in insulin production and release. This typically occurs if the dose is too high, and the patient is fasting.

Ans. (D) i.e., Sulfonylureas

64. **Which of the following statements is/are correct regarding Gilbert's syndrome?**

1. **Inheritance of the disease is autosomal dominant.**
2. **Jaundice becomes very severe with time.**
3. **Fasting leads to increased bilirubin levels.**

Select the correct answer using the code given below:

(a) 1 and 3 only (b) 1 only (c) 2 and 3 only (d) 1, 2 and 3

EXPLANATION

Gilbert's syndrome

- Gilbert's syndrome is due to a mutation in the UGT1A1 gene which results in decreased activity of the bilirubin uridine diphosphate glucuronyl transferase enzyme. It is typically inherited in an autosomal recessive pattern and occasionally in an autosomal dominant pattern depending on the type of mutation.
- Episodes of jaundice may be triggered by stress such as exercise, menstruation, or not eating.

Ans. (A) i.e., 1 and 3 only

65. **The following are causes of secondary hypertension except:**

(a) Conn's syndrome
(b) Carcinoid syndrome
(c) Cushing's syndrome
(d) Pheochromocytoma

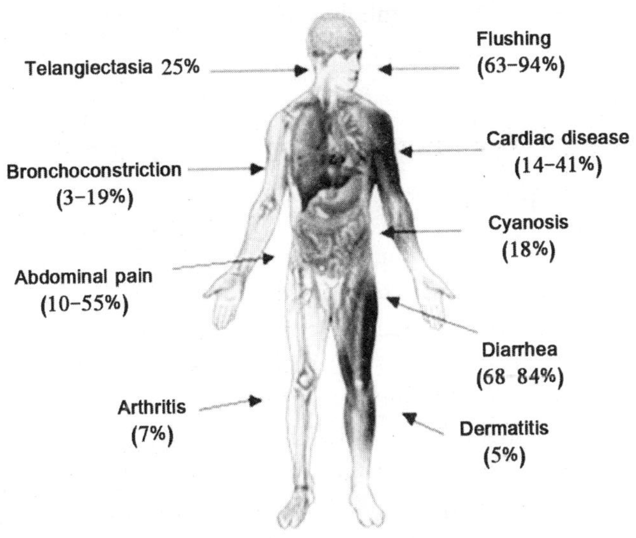

EXPLANATION

Carcinoid syndrome is a paraneoplastic syndrome comprising the signs and symptoms that occur secondary to carcinoid tumours. The syndrome includes flushing and diarrhoea, and less frequently, heartfailure, emesis and bronchoconstriction. It is caused by endogenous secretion of mainly serotonin and kallikrein.

Ans. (B) i.e., Carcinoid syndrome

66. **Tetrology of Fallot (Fallot's tetrology) is characterised by the following except:**

(a) Ventricular septal defect
(b) Overriding aorta
(c) Pulmonary hypertension
(d) Right ventricular hypertrophy

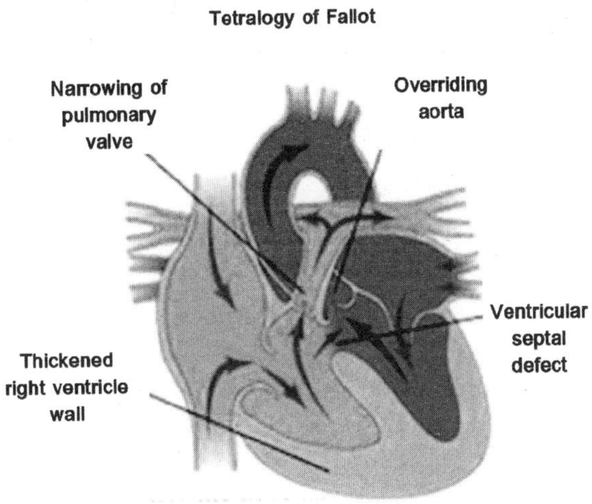

EXPLANATION

Classical four defects of TOF:

- Pulmonary stenosis, narrowing of the exit from the right ventricle
- A ventricular septal defect, a hole between the two ventricles
- Right ventricular hypertrophy, thickening of the right ventricular muscle
- An overriding aorta, which allows blood from both ventricles to enter the aorta.

Ans. (C) i.e., Pulmonary hypertension

67. **Regarding high altitude pulmonary oedema, the following statements are true except:**

(a) It can be caused by physical exertion at high altitude
(b) It does not occur in a physically fit person
(c) It occurs due to leak in the alveolar capillary membrane
(d) Portable hyperbaric chamber may be used for the treatment instead of descent to a lower altitude

EXPLANATION

High altitude pulmonary edema (HAPE) is a life threatening form of non cardiogenic pulmonary edema (fluid accumulation in the lungs) that occurs in otherwise healthy mountaineers at altitudes typically above 2,500 meters (8,200 ft).

Ans. (B) i.e., It does not occur in a physically fit person

2016

68. **Complications of myocardial infarction are all except:**

(a) Systemic embolisation
(b) Rupture of interventricular septum
(c) Dissection of aorta
(d) Ventricular fibrillation

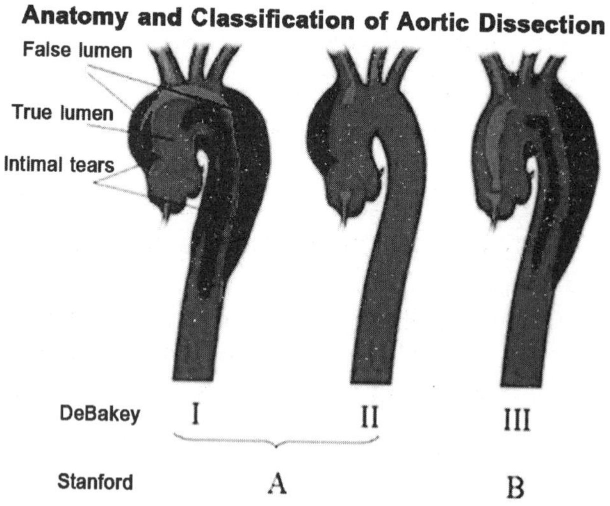

EXPLANATION

Aortic dissection is more common in those with a history of raised blood pressure, a number of connective tissue disorders that affect blood vessel wall strength such as Marfan syndrome, a bicuspid aortic valve, and previous heart surgery. Major trauma, smoking, cocaine use, pregnancy, a thoracic artery aneurysm, inflammation of the arteries, and abnormal lipid levels are also associated with an increased risk.

Ans. (C) i.e., Dissection of aorta

69. **Philadelphia chromosome can be detected by which of the following techniques?**

1. FISH 2. PCR 3. Cytogenetics

Select the correct answer using the code given below:

(a) 1 only (b) 1 and 3 only
(c) 2 and 3 only (d) 1, 2 and 3

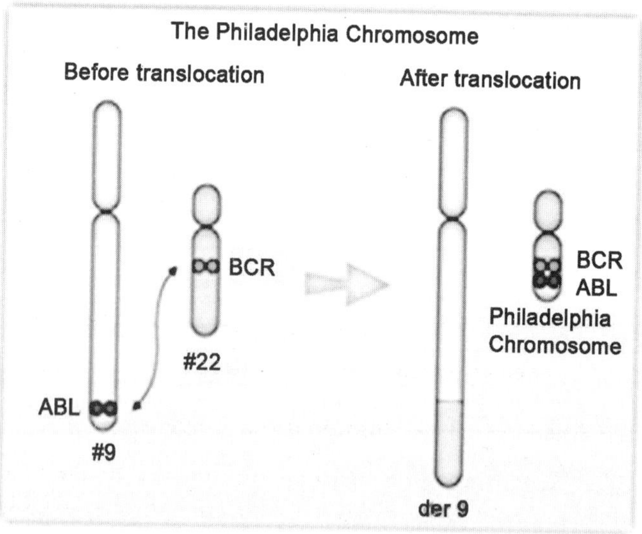

EXPLANATION

The chromosomal defect in the Philadelphia chromosome is a translocation, in which parts of two chromosomes, 9 and 22, swap places. The result is that a fusion gene is created by juxtaposing the ABL1 gene on chromosome 9 (region q34) to a part of the BCR (breakpoint cluster region) gene on chromosome 22 (region q11). This is a reciprocal translocation, creating an elongated chromosome 9 (termed a derivative chromosome, or *der 9*), and a truncated chromosome 22 (*the Philadelphia chromosome, 22q-).*

Ans. (D) i.e., 1, 2 and 3

70. **The following statements regarding celiac disease are correct except:**

(a) Absence of gastrointestinal symptoms rules out celiac disease
(b) Malabsorption syndrome may be a presenting feature
(c) Duodenal biopsy shows increased intraepithelial lymphocytes
(d) Steroid therapy may induce remission

2016

EXPLANATION

Coeliac disease is a long term autoimmune disorder that primarily affects the small intestine. Classic symptoms include gastrointestinal problems such as chronic diarrhoea, abdominal distension, malabsorption, loss of appetite and among children failure to grow normally. This often begins between six months and two years of age. There may be mild or absent gastrointestinal symptoms, a wide number of symptoms involving any other part of body or no obvious symptoms.

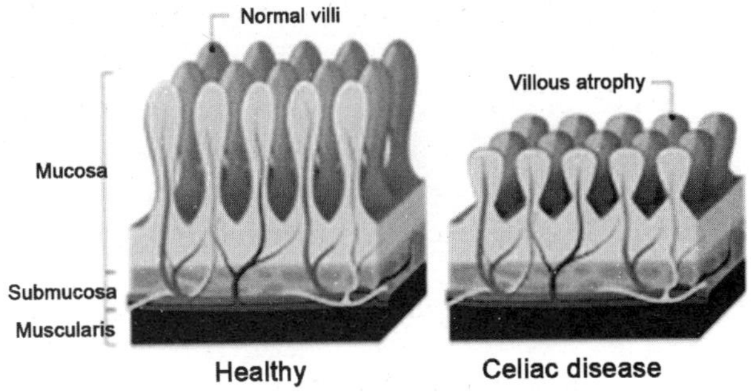

Ans. (A) i.e., Absence of gastrointestinal symptoms rules out celiac disease

71. **A 6-year old child presents with oliguria, haematuria, puffiness of face, convulsions, B.P. of 200/100mm Hg and blood urea 80mg%. What is the most likely diagnosis?**
   - (a) Haemolytic uraemic syndrome
   - (b) Nephrotic syndrome
   - (c) Acute glomerulonephritis with hypertensive encephalopathy
   - (d) Obstructive uropathy

EXPLANATION

Hypertensive encephalopathy (HE) is general brain dysfunction due to significantly high blood pressure. Symptoms may include headache, vomiting, trouble with balance, and confusion. In hypertensive encephalopathy, generally the blood pressure is greater than 200/130 mmHg. Hypertensive encephalopathy is caused by an increase in blood pressure. Several conditions may evoke blood pressure elevation: acute nephritis, eclampsia, crises in chronic essential hypertension, sudden withdrawal of antihypertensive treatment.

Ans. (C) i.e., Acute glomerulonephritis with hypertensive encephalopathy

2016

72. **A 3-year old child is brought for sudden inability to walk following fever of two days duration. On clinical examination, sensorium is normal, both the lower limbs are hypotonic with the right limb more affected than the left. Plantar reflex is equivocal and deep tendon reflexes are not elicitable in the lower limbs on both sides. The most probable diagnosis is:**
   - (a) Acute poliomyelitis
   - (b) Acute rheumatic fever
   - (c) Acute transverse myelitis
   - (d) Acute infective polyneuritis

THE TYPICAL CONTRACTURES OF POLIO

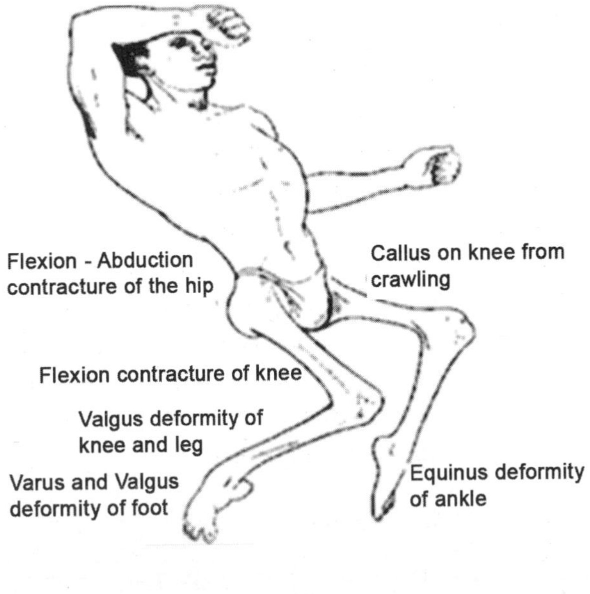

EXPLANATION

Poliomyelitis, often called **polio** or **infantile paralysis**, is an infectious disease caused by the poliovirus. In about 0.5 percent of cases there is muscle weakness resulting in an inability to move. This can occur over a few hours to a few days. The weakness most often involves the legs but may less commonly involve the muscles of the head, neck and diaphragm. Many people fully recover. In those with muscle weakness about 2 to 5 percent of children and 15 to 30 percent of adults die. Another 25 percent of people have minor symptoms such as fever and a sore throat and up to 5 percent have headache, neck stiffness and pains in the arms and legs. These people are usually back to normal within one or two weeks. In up to 70 percent of infections there are no symptoms. Years after recovery post polio syndrome may occur, with a slow development of muscle weakness similar to that which the person had during the initial infection.

Ans. (A) i.e., Acute poliomyelitis

73. X-ray of the skull in an infant shows periventricular calcification in:

(a) Tuberculous meningitis
(b) Cytomegalovirus infection
(c) Japanese B encephalitis
(d) Congenital syphilis

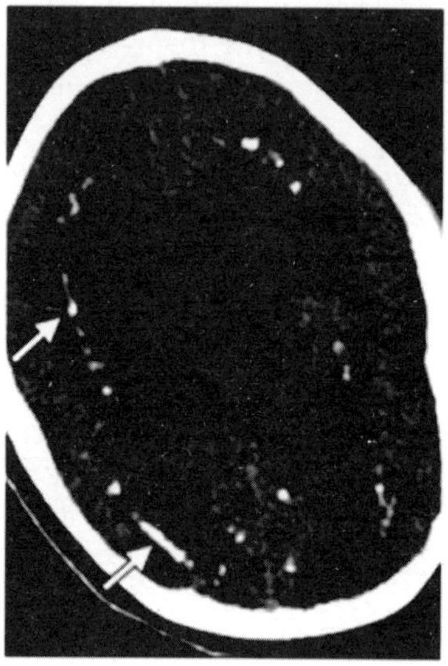

EXPLANATION

CT brain findings in congenital CMV infection

- Intracranial calcifications: Particularly thick and chunky in germinal matrix and periventricular regions with faint and punctate basal ganglia calcifications.
- White matter low density regions.
- Ventriculomegaly/cerebral atrophy/destructive encephalopathy.
- Neuronal migration disorders.

Ans. (B) i.e., Cytomegalovirus infection

74. A 4 year old boy diagnosed as a case of sickle cell disease presents with pain and swelling of bones, marked in small bones of hand and feet along with severe pain in abdomen. Investigation reveals necrosis of femoral head and upper third of tibia. The symptoms have resolved after one week. The possible explanation is:

(a) Aplastic crisis
(b) Sequestration crisis
(c) Vasoocclusive crisis
(d) Hemolytic crisis

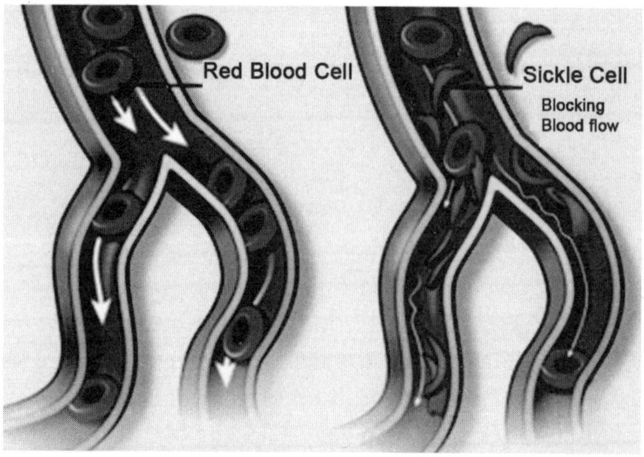

EXPLANATION

Sickle cell disease (SCD) usually manifests early in childhood. For the first 6 months of life, infants are protected largely by elevated levels of Hb F; soon thereafter, the condition becomes evident. The most common clinical manifestation of SCD is vasoocclusive crisis. A vasoocclusive crisis occurs when the microcirculation is obstructed by sickled RBCs, causing ischemic injury to the organ supplied and resultant pain.

Ans. (C) i.e., Vasoocclusive crisis

75. **Match *List I* with *List II* and select the correct answer using the code given below the lists:**

List I (Genetic disorder)	*List II* (Genotype)
A. Down Syndrome	1. 47, XY, +21
B. Turner Syndrome	2. 46, XY
C. Noonan Syndrome	3. 46, XX, 5p -
D. Cri-du-chat Syndrome	4. 45, XO
	5. 47, XXY

Code: A B C D

(a) 1 4 2 3 (b) 1 4 5 3 (c) 3 1 2 4 (d) 3 1 5 4

EXPLANATION

Genetic conditions and genotype

- **Down syndrome** (DS or DNS), also known as **trisomy 21**, is a genetic disorder caused by the presence of all or part of a third copy of chromosome 21. Trisomy 21 (also known by the karyotype 47, XX, +21 for females and 47, XY, +21 for males) is caused by a failure of the 21st chromosome to separate during egg or sperm development.
- **Turner syndrome** (TS), also known as 45, X or 45, X0, is a condition in which a female is partly or completely missing an X chromosome.
- **Noonan syndrome** (NS) is a relatively common autosomal dominant congenital disorder and is named after Jacqueine Noonan, a pediatric cardiologist. It used to be referred to as a male version of Turner's syndrome. NS is a RASopathy, and is one of several disorders that are caused by a disruption of RAS MAPK signaling pathway.

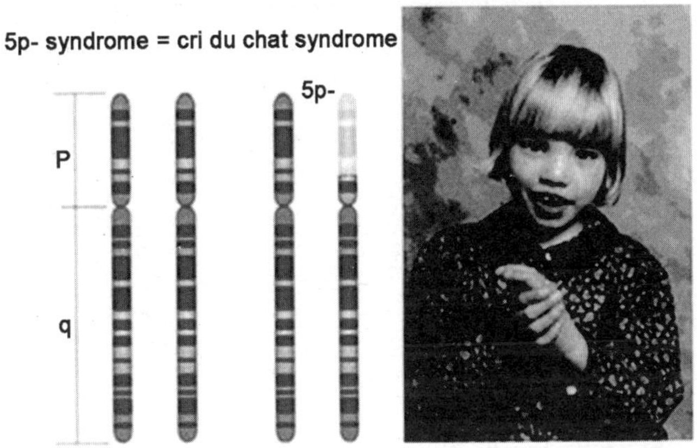

- **Cri du chat syndrome**, also known as **chromosome 5p deletion syndrome, 5p" syndrome** (pronounced "five P minus") or **Lejeune's syndrome**, is a rare genetic disorder due to chromosome deletion on chromosome 5. Its name is a french term ("cat cry" or "call of the cat") referring to the characteristic cat like cry of affected children.

Ans. (A) i.e., 1 4 2 3

76. **With reference to Paediatrics, the following are true of breath holding spells except:**

(a) They occur during inspiration (b) They are involuntary
(c) Cyanosis may not occur (d) Bradycardia may occur

EXPLANATION

Breath holding spells (BHS) are the occurrence of episodic apnea in children, possibly associated with loss of consciousness, and changes in postural tone. The most common is termed *simple breath holding spell*, in which the manifestation is the holding of breath in and expiration. The usual precipitating event is a frustration or injury leading to the temporary cessation of breathing in and expiration. There is no major alteration of circulation or oxygenation and the recovery is spontaneous.

Ans. (A) i.e., They occur during inspiration

77. **Match *List I* with *List II* and select the correct answer using the code given below the lists:**

List I (Drugs for epilepsy)	*List II* (Side effects dose dependent)
A. Sodium volproate	1. Raised liver enzymes
B. Carbamazepine	2. Hirsutism
C. Phenytoin	3. Hyperactivity
D. Phenobarbitone	4. Drowsiness

Code: A B C D

(a) 1 4 2 3 (b) 1 4 3 2 (c) 4 1 2 3 (d) 4 1 3 2

EXPLANATION

Anti epileptic drugs and side effects

- Common side effects of valproate include nausea, vomiting, sleepiness, and a dry mouth. Serious side effects can include liver problems and regular monitoring of liver function tests is therefore recommended.
- Common side effects of carbamazepine include nausea and drowsiness. Serious side effects may include skin rashes, decreased bone marrow function, suicidal thoughts, or confusion.
- Common side effects of phenytoin include nausea, stomach pain, loss of appetite, poor coordination, increased hair growths, and enlargement of the gums. Potentially serious side effects include sleepiness, self harm, liver problems, bone marrow suppression, low blood pressure, and toxic epidermal necrolysis.
- Sedation and hypnosis are the principal side effects (occasionally, they are also the intended effects) of phenobarbital. Central nervous system effects, such as dizziness, nystagmus and ataxia, are also common. In elderly patients, it may cause excitement and confusion, while in children, it may result in paradoxical hyperactivity. Another very rare side effect is amelogenesis imperfecta.

Ans. (A) i.e., 1 4 2 3

2016

78. **The confirmatory diagnostic test for thalassemia carrier status is:**

(a) Low haemoglobin level (b) Haemoglobin A2 more than 3.5%

(c) Foetal haemoglobin more than 10% (d) Positive osmotic fragility test

EXPLANATION

Sometimes, people with only one *HBB* gene mutation in each cell (carriers) do have mild anemia. These people are said to have 'beta thalassemia minor' or 'beta thalassemia trait. The normal Hb A2 level in an adult is less than 3.5% and it is elevated (>4%) in beta thalassaemia trait.

Type of Hb	Levels	Indication
Hemoglobin A1	12.1 – 16.3g/dL, 90% of total hemoglobin	Low levels indicate anemia or blood loss.
Hemoglobin A2	1.5% – 3.5% of total hemoglobin	High levels may indicate thalassemia.
Hemoglobin F	50 – 90% in neonates, 0% – 1% of total hemoglobin in adults	Normally high in neonates, long-term elevations may indicate a thalassemia.
Hemoglobin S	Presence is abnormal	Indicative of sickle cell disease

Ans. (B) i.e., Haemoglobin A2 more than 3.5%

79. **A three year old male child has a poor stream of urine and strains at micturition. After voiding, the bladder is still palpable. The patient should be advised**

(a) Abdomen X-ray (b) Urine examination (c) Circumcision (d) Excretory urogram

EXPLANATION

Presentation of a boy with posterior urethral valve will depend on the severity of obstruction. The boy may present at birth or as late as 3–4 years. The symptoms are the same difficulty in passing urine, straining to pass urine, dribbling of urine, poor stream of urine. There may be distension of the lower abdomen caused by a stretched out filled up bladder. The common mistake that can be made is to diagnose this condition as phimosis and then get a circumcision done. Investigations are done to look for the complications associated with this entity like electrolyte imbalances and infection of urine and also in the blood stream by sending both blood and urine for Culture studies and treating the infection first before specific therapy for the PUV.

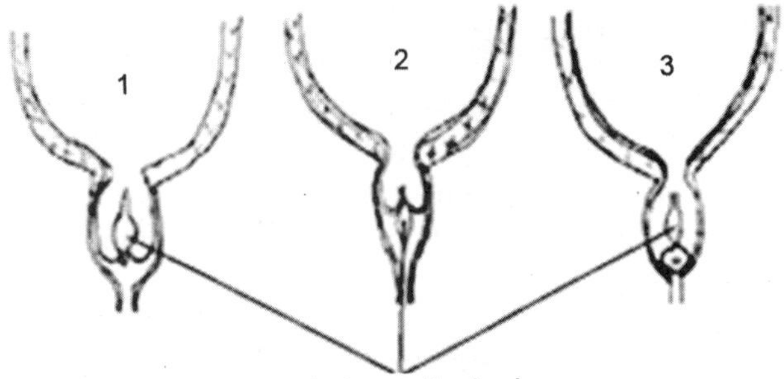

Posterior urethral valves

Ans. (B) i.e., Urine examination

80. A two year old child has weight less than 3 SD (less than 3 Z score) as per WHO growth chart and mid upper arm circumference (MUAC) less than 11 cm. What is the correct diagnosis for this child?

(a) Acute malnutrition
(b) Chronic malnutrition
(c) Severe acute malnutrition
(d) Moderate acute malnutrition

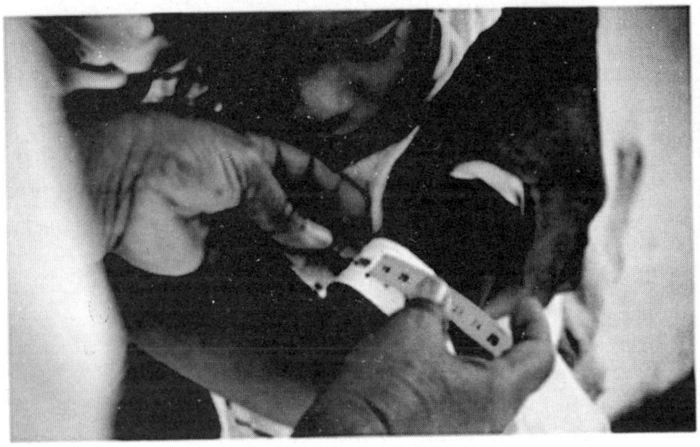

EXPLANATION

Indicators of Severe Acute malnutrition/SAM

- SAM is defined as a weight to height ratio less than -3 Standard Deviations on the Z score for the reference population.
- MUAC < 110mm with or without Oedema corresponds to SAM.

Ans. (C) i.e., Severe acute malnutrition

81. For a three year old male child, the height for age is 82% of the expected for that age and weight for height is 65% of the expected value. The child is labelled as:

(a) Normal (b) Wasted (c) Stunted (d) Wasted and stunted

EXPLANATION

Anthropometric indices of malnutrition

- Low *weight for height*: ***Wasting*** or thinness indicates in most cases a recent and severe process of ***weight*** loss, which is often associated with acute starvation and/or severe disease. However, ***wasting*** may also be the result of a chronic unfavourable condition.
- The definition of stunting according to the WHO is for the "height for age" value to be less than two standard deviations of the WHO Child Growth Standards median.

Ans. (D) i.e., Wasted and stunted

82. For an early infant diagnosis of HIV infection, which of the following tests is used as per national programme?

(a) ELISA (IgG antibody test)
(b) DNA PCR test
(c) p24 antigen test
(d) CD4 count

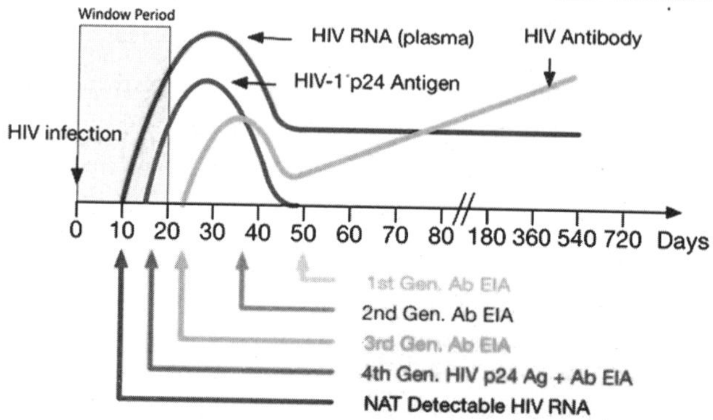

EXPLANATION

HIV DNA PCR is a sensitive technique used to detect intracellular *HIV* viral *DNA* in peripheral blood mononuclear cells. The specificity of the *HIV DNA PCR* is 99.8% at birth and 100% at ages 1, 3, and 6 months.

Ans. (B) i.e., DNA PCR test

83. A normal three year old baby should be able to do the following tasks except:

(a) Using hands and feet simultaneously
(b) Riding tricycle
(c) Copying a square
(d) Using pair of scissors

EXPLANATION

A 4 year old child can draw circles, squares or crosses.

Ans. (C) i.e., Copying a square

84. A seven year old child presents with intermittent claudication, pain and weakness of legs and dyspnea on running. Examination shows delayed and weak femorals compared to brachial arteries. The heart size is normal with a left ventricular forcible apex. The most probable diagnosis is:

(a) Ventricular septal defect
(b) Patent ductus arteriosus
(c) Atrial septal defect
(d) Coarctation of aorta

EXPLANATION

Features of Coarctation of aorta

- Patients have cold legs and feet or have pain in their legs with exercise (intermittent claudication).
- Patients may experience dizziness or shortness of breath, fainting or near fainting episodes, chest pain, abnormal tiredness or fatigue, headaches, or nose bleeds.
- Arterial hypertension in the arms with low blood pressure in the lower extremities is classic.
- In the lower extremities, weak pulses in the femoral arteries and arteries of the feet are found.

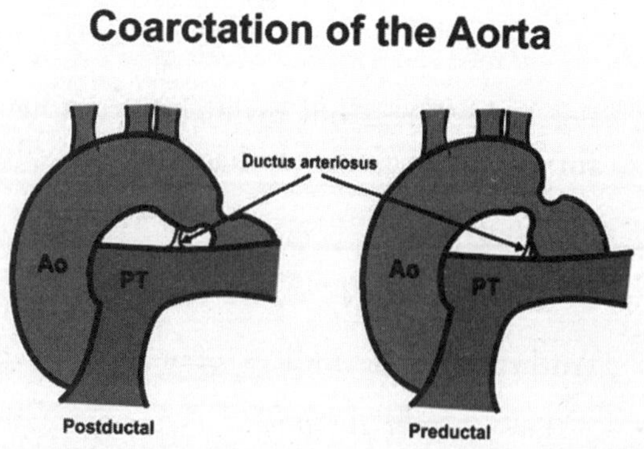

Ans. (D) i.e., Coarctation of aorta

85. A seven day old baby presents with complaints of vomiting and diarrhoea. Examination reveals cataract in both the eyes and jaundice. What is the most probable diagnosis?

(a) Rh incompatibility
(b) Galactosemia
(c) Congenital rubella syndrome
(d) Congenital syphilis

EXPLANATION

Galactosemia

- Infants affected by galactosemia typically present with symptoms of lethargy, vomiting, diarrhea, failure to thrive, and jaundice.
- The presence of presenile cataract, noticeable in galactosemic infants as young as a few days old, is highly associated with two distinct types of galactosemia: GALT deficiency and to a greater extent, GALK deficiency.

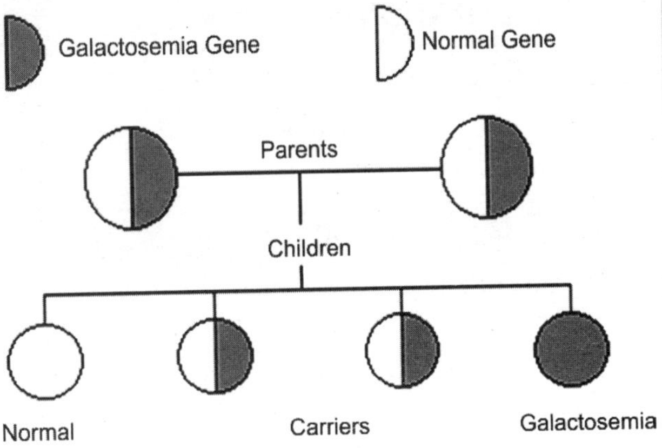

Ans. (B) i.e., Galactosemia

86. **The treatment of choice for Guillain Barre syndrome/GBS is:**

(a) Corticosteroids
(b) Intravenous immunoglobulins
(c) Cyclosporins
(d) ACTH

EXPLANATION

Plasmapheresis and intravenous immunoglobulins (IVIG) are the two main immunotherapy treatments for GBS. Plasmapheresis attempts to reduce the body's attack on the nervous system by filtering antibodies out of the bloodstream. Similarly, administration of IVIG neutralizes harmful antibodies and inflammation.

Diagnostic Criteria for GB Syndrome

Required
1. Progressive weakness of 2 or more limbs due to neuropathy*
2. Areflexia
3. Disease course < 4 weeks
4. Exclusion of other causes (e.g., vasculitis, toxins, botulism, diphtheria, prophyria, localized spinal cord or cauda equina syndrome)
Supportive
1. Relatively symmetrical weakness
2. Mild sensory involvement
3. Facial or other cranial nerve involvement
4. Absence of fever
5. Typical CSF profile (cytoalbumin dissociation)
6. Electrophysiologic evidence of demyelination

Ans. (B) i.e., Intravenous immunoglobulins

87. **A two years old child is admitted with history of fever for two weeks and convulsions for the last one day. CSF examination shows CSF pressure elevated to 30–40 cm H_2O, clear CSF, lymphocytic pleocytosis (250 cells/mm3), elevated protein and low chloride levels. What is the most probable diagnosis?**

(a) Pyogenic meningitis
(b) Tubercular meningitis
(c) Acute encephalitis
(d) Sabacute sclerosing panencephalitis (SSPE)

EXPLANATION

TBM

- Fever and headache are the cardinal features; confusion is a late feature and coma bears a poor prognosis. Meningism is absent in a fifth of patients with TB meningitis. Patients may also have focal neurological deficits.
- The CSF in TBM usually has a high protein, low glucose and a raised number of lymphocytes. Acid fast bacilli are sometimes seen on a CSF smear, but more commonly, *M. tuberculosis* is grown in culture. A spiderweb clot in the collected CSF is characteristic of TB meningitis, but is a rare finding.

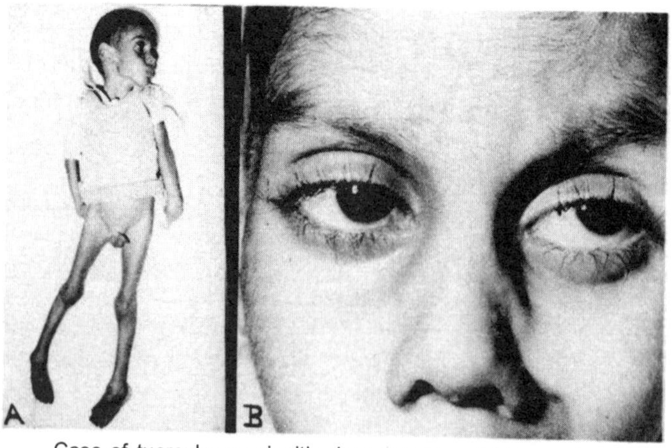

Case of tuercular meningitis demonstrating (A) Decerebrate rigidity (B) With conjugate deviation of eyes to the left.

Ans. (B) i.e., Tubercular meningitis

88. **Features of Turner syndrome in childhood include the following except:**

(a) Webbed neck
(b) Cubitus valgus
(c) Shield chest with widely spaced nipples
(d) Polydactyly

EXPLANATION

Features of Turner syndrome

- Short stature
- Lymphedema (swelling) of the hands and feet of a newborn
- Broad chest (shield chest) and widely spaced nipples
- Low posterior hairline
- Low set ears
- Reproductive sterility
- Rudimentary ovaries gonadal streak (underdeveloped gonadal structures that later become fibrotic)
- Amenorrhoea, the absence of a menstrual period
- Increased weight, obesity
- Shortened fourth metacarpal
- Small fingernails
- Characteristic facial features
- Webbed neck from cystic hydroma in infancy
- Aortic valve stenosis
- Coarctation of aorta
- Bicuspid aortic valve (most common cardiac problem)
- Horse shoe kidney

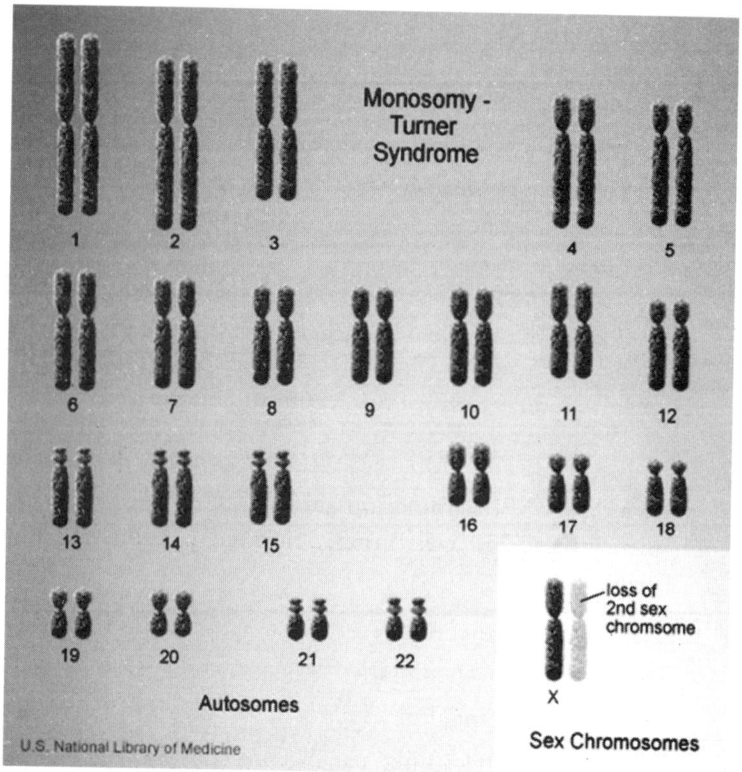

- Visual impairments—Sclera, cornea, glaucoma, etc.
- Ear infections and hearing loss
- High waist to hip ratio (the hips are not much bigger than the waist)
- Attention deficit hyperactivity disorder (problems with concentration, memory, attention with hyperactivity seen mostly in childhood and adolescence)
- Nonverbal learning disability (problems with maths, social skills, and spatial relations).

Ans. (D) i.e., Polydactyly

89. The following drugs can be used as steroid sparing agents in the treatment of nephrotic syndrome in children except:

(a) Levamisole
(b) Aspirin
(c) Cyclophosphamide
(d) Mycophenolate mofetil

EXPLANATION

Steroid sparing drugs

- Frequent relapses of nephrotic syndrome (after prednisone therapy) are treated by: cyclophosphamide or nitrogen mustard or cyclosporin or levamisole.
- Mycophenolate mofetil is an immunosuppressant that has decreased the incidence of acute rejection in solid transplant recipients. Mycophenolate is increasingly utilized as a steroid sparing treatment in auto immune diseases and similar immune mediated disorders including Behcet's disease, pemphigus vulgaris, refractory incomplete systemic lupus erythematosus, immunoglobulin A nephropathy, small vessel vasculitides, and psoriasis.

Ans. (B) i.e., Aspirin

2016

90. In childhood acute lymphoblastic leukemia, the following are good prognostic factors except:

(a) Age between 1 and 9 years
(b) Female sex
(c) Leukocyte count less than 50,000/mm3
(d) Hypodiploidy

EXPLANATION

Prognosis of ALL based on bone marrow cytogenetics	
Prognosis	**Cytogenetic findings**
Favorable	Hyperdiploidy > 50; t (12;21)
Intermediate	Hyperdiploidy 47–50; Normal (diploidy); del (6q); Rearrangements of 8q24
Unfavorable	Hypodiploidy–near haploidy; Near tetraploidy; del (17p); t (9;22); t (11q23)

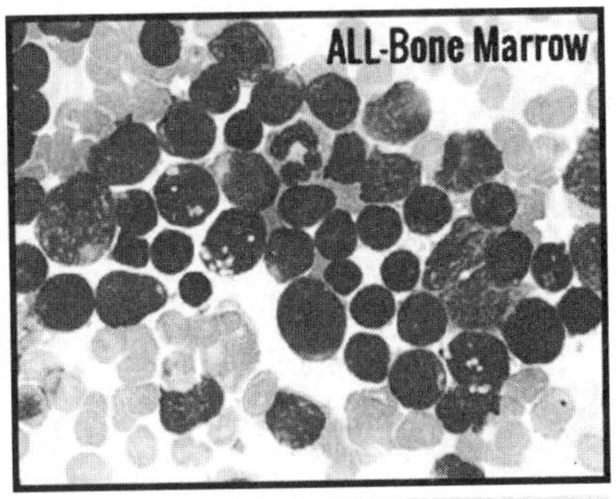

Ans. (D) i.e., Hypodiploidy

91. Consider the following statements:

1. Biodiversity is normally greater in the lower latitudes as compared to the higher latitudes.
2. Along the mountain gradients, biodiversity is normally greater in the lower altitudes as compared to the higher altitudes.

Which of the statements given above is/are correct?

(a) 1 only
(b) 2 only
(c) Both 1 and 2
(d) Neither 1 nor 2

EXPLANATION

Biodiversity

- Generally, there is an increase in biodiversity from the poles to the tropics. Thus localities at lower latitudes have more species than localities at higher latitudes. This is often referred to as the latitudinal gradient in species diversity.
- Higher you go = colder atmosphere = less biodiversity

Ans. (C) i.e., Both 1 and 2

92. There is a growing concern about the melting of Arctic permafrost. Why?

(a) It will result in the increase of methane concentration in atmosphere.
(b) All the countries surrounding North Pole will be permanently submerged.
(c) The temperature of ocean currents will be drastically altered.
(d) The pH of the ocean water will be drastically changed.

EXPLANATION

Sea ice loss is correlated with warming of Northern latitudes. This has melting effects on permafrost, both in the sea, and on land. Lawrence et al. suggest that current rapid melting of the sea ice may induce a rapid melting of arctic permafrost. This has consequential effects on methane release, and wildlife. Some studies imply a direct link, as they predict cold air passing over ice is replaced by warm air passing over the sea. This warm air carries heat to the permafrost around the Arctic, and melts it. This permafrost then releases huge quantities of methane.

Ans. (A) i.e., It will result in the increase of methane concentration in atmosphere.

2016

93. With reference to Pre Conception and Pre Natal Diagnostics Techniques (Prohibition of Sex Selection) Act, 1994, which of the following statements is/are correct?

1. Every offence under this Act is cognizable non bailable.
2. For the first offence, the penalty for the doctor is 'upto 7 years of imprisonment with a fine up to ₹ 1,00,000.'

Select the correct answer using the code given below:

(a) 1 only (b) 2 only (c) Both 1 and 2 (d) Neither 1 nor 2

EXPLANATION

PCPNDT Act

- The offence being cognizable, non bailable and non compoundable, they put up a criminal case.
- Any medical geneticist, gynecologist, registered medical practitioner or any person who owns a Genetic Counseling Centre, a Genetic Laboratory or a Genetic Clinic or is employed in such a Centre, Laboratory or Clinic and renders his professional or technical services to or at such a Centre, Laboratory or Clinic, whether on an honorary basis or otherwise, and who contravenes any of the provisions of this Act or rules made thereunder shall be punishable with imprisonment for a term which may extend to three years and with fine which may extend to ten thousand rupees and on any subsequent conviction, with imprisonment which may extend to five years and with fine which may extend to fifty thousand rupees.

Ans. (A) i.e., 1 only

94. 'Nagoya Protocol', sometimes seen in news refers to:

(a) Convention on International Trade in Endangered Species of Wild Fauna and Flora
(b) Convention on the Conservation of Migratory Species of Wild Animals

(c) Convention on Biological Diversity

(d) Convention on Wetlands of International Importance especially as Waterfowl Habitat

EXPLANATION

The Nagoya Protocol on Access to Genetic Resources and the Fair and Equitable Sharing of Benefits Arising from their Utilization to the Convention on Biological Diversity, also known as the **Nagoya Protocol on Access and Benefit Sharing** (ABS) is a 2010 supplementary agreement to the 1992 Convention on Biological Diversity (CBD). Its aim is the implementation of one of the three objectives of the CBD: the fair and equitable sharing of benefits arising out of the utilization of genetic resources, thereby contributing to the conservation and sustainable use of biodiversity.

Ans. (C) i.e., Convention on Biological Diversity

95. Some substances known as 'Short Lived Climate Forcers' (SLCF) assume importance in the context of climate change. Which of the following is/are SLCF?

1. Black carbon
2. Carbon dioxide
3. Hydrofluorocarbons
4. Methane

Select the correct answer using the code given below:

(a) 1 and 2 only (b) 1, 3 and 4 only (c) 3 and 4 only (d) 1, 2, 3 and 4

EXPLANATION

The main ***short lived climate*** pollutants are black carbon, methane, tropospheric ozone, and fluorinated gases. Currently, fluorinated gases (HFCs, perfluorocarbons (PFCs), SF6, and NF3) account for 3 percent of domestic greenhouse gas emissions in terms of carbon dioxide equivalency.

Ans. (B) i.e., 1, 3 and 4 only

2016

96. Consider the following statements:

1. **Production of cement blended with fly ash or slag (blended cement) is less energy efficient compared to the production of ordinary portland cement.**
2. **'Electricity and heat production' together constitute the single largest contributor of greenhouse gases in India.**

Which of the statements given above is/are correct?

(a) 1 only (b) 2 only (c) Both 1 and 2 (d) Neither 1 nor 2

EXPLANATION

Electricity and Heat Production

- 25% of 2010 global greenhouse gas emissions
- The burning of coal, natural gas, and oil for electricity and heat is the largest single source of global greenhouse gas emissions.

Ans. (B) i.e., 2 only

97. What is the present share of agriculture and allied sectors in the Gross Domestic Product of India?

(a) Less than 20%
(b) Between 20% and 30%
(c) Between 31% and 35%
(d) Above 35%

EXPLANATION

Agriculture and Allied Sector includes forestry and fishing also. This sector is also known as the **primary sector of the economy**. At the time of Indian independence this sector had biggest share in the Gross Domestic Product of India. But year by year its contribution goes on declining and currently it contributes only 17% of Indian GDP at current prices.

Ans. (A) i.e., Less than 20%

98. The global warming potential is highest among which of the following greenhouse gases?

(a) CO_2 (b) CH_4 (c) N_2O (d) SF_6

EXPLANATION

Sulfur hexafluoride (SF_6) is an inorganic, colorless, odorless, non flammable, extremely potent greenhouse gas, and an excellent electrical stimulator.

Ans. (D) i.e., SF_6

99. Which of the following is/are included in Kyoto Protocol?

1. Brominated flame retardants

2. Methyl alcohol

3. Hydrofluorocarbons

Select the correct answer using the code given below:

(a) 1 and 2 (b) 2 and 3 (c) 3 only (d) 1 only

EXPLANATION

The **Kyoto Protocol** is an international treaty which extends the 1992 United Nations Framework Convention on Climate Change (UNFCCC) that commits state parties to reduce greenhouse gas emissions, based on the scientific consensus that (part one) global warming is occurring and (part two) it is extremely likely that human made CO_2 emissions have predominantly caused it.

Ans. (C) i.e., 3 only

2016

100. In the context of food processing, the addition of sulfites (sulphites) to fruits and vegetables has which of the following effects?

1. Prevention of browning **2. Increase in sour taste**

3. Destruction of thiamine **4. Preservation of thiamine**

Select the correct answer using the code given below:

(a) 1 and 3 only (b) 2 and 3 only (c) 2 and 4 (d) 1, 2 and 3

EXPLANATION

Sulfite in food processing

- The main reason why ***sulfites*** are able to inhibit a wide range of ***browning*** reactions is the nucleophilic reactivity of ***sulfite*** ion.
- ***Vitamin B1*** is extremely sensitive to alcohol and ***sulfites*** and in the presence of either it is ***destroyed.***

Ans. (A) i.e., 1 and 3 only

101. Which of the following has/have antioxidant properties?

1. Ascorbic acid **2. Butylated hydroxyanisole** **3. Stannous chloride** **4. Tocopherol**

Select the correct answer using the code given below:

(a) 1, 2 and 3 only (b) 2, 3 and 4 only (c) 1 and 4 only (d) 1, 2, 3 and 4

EXPLANATION

Antioxidants

- Oxidation is a chemical reaction that can produce free radicals, thereby leading to chain reactions that may damage the cells of organisms.
- Antioxidants such as thiols or ascorbic acid (vitamin C) terminate these chain reactions.
- **Butylated hydroxyanisole** (BHA) is an antioxidant consisting of a mixture of two ismoeric organic compounds, 2-*tert*-butyl-4-hydroxyanisole and 3-*tert*-butyl-4-hydroxyanisole.
- Stannous chloride is added as a food additive with E number **E512** to some canned and bottled foods, where it serves as a color retention agent and antioxidant.
- Tocopherols and tocotrienols are fat soluble antioxidant but also seem to have many other functions in the body.

Ans. (D) i.e., 1, 2, 3 and 4

102. In food processing, which of the following is/are used as emulsifiers?

1. Carboxymethyl cellulose
2. Ethylene diamine tetra acetate
3. Propylene glycol

Select the correct answer using the code given below:

(a) 1 only (b) 2 and 3 only (c) 1 and 3 only (d) 1, 2 and 3

EXPLANATION

Emulsifiers

- **Emulsifying agents** are substances that are soluble in both fat and water and enable fat to be uniformly dispersed in water as an emulsion.
- Carboxymethyl cellulose/CMC is used in food under the E number E466 as a viscosity modifier or thickener, and to stabilize emulsions in various products including ice cream.
- Propylene glycol is an emulsifying agent.

Ans. (C) i.e., 1 and 3 only

103. To test the adulteration of milk, 3 ml of milk is boiled, then cooled to room temperature; and two or three drops of iodine solution is added. The milk turned blue. This indicates that the milk is adulterated with:

(a) Sodium bicarbonate (b) Glucose

(c) Starch (d) Urea

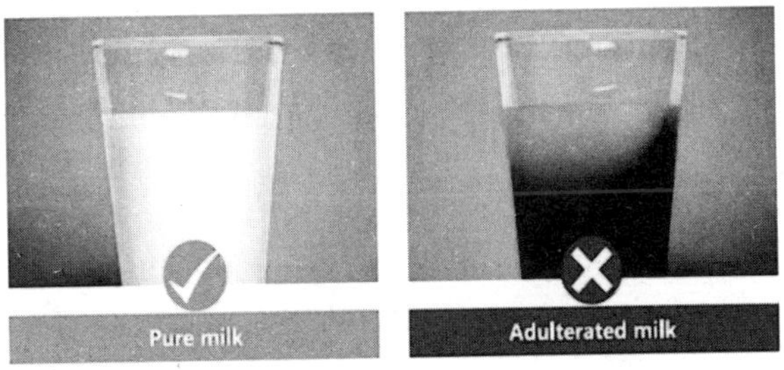

EXPLANATION

TEST 3 : **Detection of starch in milk and milk products (khoya, chenna, paneer)**

Testing method:

1. Boil 2–3 ml of sample with 5ml of water.
2. Cool and add 2–3 drops of tincture of iodine.
3. Formation of blue colour indicates the presence of starch. (In the case of milk, addition of water and boiling is not required)

Ans. (C) i.e., Starch

104. With reference to food preservation, which of the following statements is/are correct?

1. Pasteurization means the heating of a food product to a sufficiently high temperature to kill all the microorganisms present in it.
2. In the case of food preservation by sterilization by heat, foods high in acid are very easily sterilized as compared to those low in acid.

Select the correct answer using the code given below:

(a) 1 only (b) 2 only (c) Both 1 and 2 (d) Neither 1 nor 2

EXPLANATION

In the case of foods with high acidity, i.e. pH 4.6 or lower, it is much easier to obtain commercial sterility, because the lower pH value decreases the heat resistance of bacteria and their destruction can be effected in a relatively short time and at a temperature much lower than that needed for low-acid foods.

Ans. (B) i.e., 2 only

105. Consider the following statements:

1. Pasteurization by heat is used in the processing of fruit juices.
2. Water glass is used in the preservation of eggs.

Which of the statements given above is/are correct?

(a) 1 only (b) 2 only (c) Both 1 and 2 (d) Neither 1 nor 2

EXPLANATION

Preservation of food stuffs

- **Heat** treatment plays an essential role in securing product quality and shelf life. It has long been thought that much of the vitamin C content in orange **juice** is destroyed during the **pasteurization** process.
- Water glass, a bacteria-**resistant** solution of **sodium silicate**, discouraged the entrance of spoilage organisms and evaporation of water from eggs. It didn't penetrate the eggshell, imparted no odor or taste to the eggs and was considered to have somewhat antiseptic properties.

Ans. (C) i.e., Both 1 and 2

2016

106. With reference to irradiation for food processing, which of the following statements is/are correct?

1. Cobalt 60 produces ionizing radiation, therefore it is used in the process of irradiation of food.
2. Ultra violet rays are the only ionizing radiation used for irradiation of food.

Select the correct answer using the code given below:

(a) 1 only (b) 2 only (c) Both 1 and 2 (d) Neither 1 nor 2

EXPLANATION

Cobalt 60 is the most common source of gamma rays for food irradiation in commercial scale facilities as it is water insoluble and hence has little risk of environmental contamination by leakage into the water systems.

Ans. (A) i.e., 1 only

107. Among the following pairs of States, in India, major deposits of bauxite are concentrated in:

(a) Jharkhand and Odisha
(b) Assam and West Bengal
(c) Bihar and Haryana
(d) Punjab and Rajasthan

EXPLANATION

More than half of India's bauxite reserves are in Orissa and Andhra Pradesh states. Recently extensive deposits of bauxite have been discovered in the Jammu and Poonch areas of the Jammu and Kashmir state. The other states which have rich reserves of bauxite are Jharkhand, Madhya Pradesh, Gujarat, Maharashtra, Karnataka, Tamil Nadu, Kerala, Goa and Uttar Pradesh.

Ans. (A) i.e., Jharkhand and Odisha

108. Doha Development Agenda, sometimes seen in news, refers to the affairs of:

(a) UNFCCC (b) UNCTAD (c) UNDP (d) WTO

EXPLANATION

The **Doha Development Round** or **Doha Development Agenda** (DDA) is the trade negotiation round of the World Trade Organization (WTO) which commenced in November 2001 under then director general Mike Moore. It's objective was to lower trade barriers around the world, and thus facilitate increased global trade.

Ans. (D) i.e., WTO

109. With reference to 'monosodium glutamate' (MSG) used in processed foods, which of the following statements is/are correct?

1. MSG is not a naturally occurring substance.

2. MSG is a neurotransmitter.

Select the correct answer using the code given below:

(a) 1 only (b) 2 only (c) Both 1 and 2 (d) Neither 1 nor 2

2016

EXPLANATION

MSG

- To verify that ionized glutamate was responsible for *umami*, Ikeda studied the taste properties of glutamate salts: calcium, potassium, ammonium, and magnesium glutamate. All these salts elicited *umami* and a metallic taste due to the other minerals. Of them, sodium glutamate was the most soluble, most palatable, and easiest to crystallize. Ikeda called his product "monosodium glutamate", and submitted a patent to produce MSG; the Suzuki brothers began commercial production of MSG in 1909 as *Aji-no-moto* ("essence of taste").
- Glutamate, the main component of ***MSG***, is the primary excitatory ***neurotransmitter*** in the brain.

Ans. (C) i.e., Both 1 and 2

110. In the parliamentary form of government, the

(a) Executive is responsible to the legislature (b) Legislature is responsible to the executive

(c) Judiciary is responsible to the executive (d) Legislature is responsible to the judiciary

EXPLANATION

In a **Parliamentary form of Government**, real **executive** power lies with the Council of Ministers headed by the Prime Minister which is **responsible to the legislature**. In other words, they hold office only if the majority in Lok Sabha supports them and must resign if they loose confidence.

Ans. (A) i.e., Executive is responsible to the legislature

111. The term 'Ramsar Convention', sometimes seen in news, refers to:

(a) conservation of forests
(b) conservation of wetlands
(c) reduction of greenhouse gas emissions
(d) controlling wildlife trafficking

EXPLANATION

The **Ramsar Convention on Wetlands of International Importance especially as Waterfowl Habitat** is an international treaty for the conservation and sustainable use of wetlands. It is also known as the **Convention on Wetlands**. It is named after the city of Ramsar in Iran, where the Convention was signed in 1971.

Ans. (B) i.e., Conservation of wetlands

112. In India, who heads the National Disaster Management Authority?

(a) Prime Minister
(b) Union Minister for Home Affairs
(c) Cabinet Secretary
(d) Secretary, Union Ministry of Environment, Forests and Climate Change

EXPLANATION

National Disaster Management Authority, abbreviated as **NDMA** is an agency of the Ministry of Home Affairs whose primary purpose is to coordinate response to natural or manmade disasters and for capacity building in disaster resiliency and crisis response. NDMA was established through the Disaster management Act enacted by the Government of India in <ay 30 2005. The Prime minister is the exofficio chairperson of the same.

Ans. (A) i.e., Prime Minister

113. Natural gas is used for the production of which of the following?

1. **Detergents and soaps**
2. **Electricity**
3. **Fertilizers for crops**

Select the correct answer using the code given below:

(a) 1, 2 and 3
(b) 2 and 3 only
(c) 2 only
(d) 3 only

EXPLANATION

Natural gas

- It is a naturally occurring hydrocarbon gas mixture consisting primarily of methane, but commonly including varying amounts of other higher alkanes, and sometimes a small percentage of carbon dioxide, nitrogen, hydrogen sulfide, or helium.
- Natural gas is a major source of electricity generation through the use of cogeneration, gas turbines and steam turbines.
- Natural gas is a major feedstock for the production of ammonia, via the Haber process, for use in fertilizer production.

Ans. (B) i.e., 2 and 3 only

114. Which of the following parts of the human body can be used as a sample/samples for the presence of mercury?

1. **Blood**
2. **Hair**
3. **Nail**

Select the correct answer using the code given below:

(a) 1 only (b) 2 and 3 only (c) 3 only (d) 1, 2 and 3

EXPLANATION

Mercury poisoning

- Mercury is also eliminated in saliva, through the pancreas, through intestinal wall secretion, and through nails and hair.
- Both blood and hair are used to detect mercury toxicity. In the study by Marsh et al. (1974), hair levels generally correlated directly with blood levels. Absolute levels in the hair were about 300 times higher than in the blood. (Prasad 1976). Hair can also provide a chronological account of mercury excretion by measuring mercury content of different segments of a hair sample.

Ans. (D) i.e., 1, 2 and 3

115. Which of the following is/are known as 'ozone depleting substance(s)'?

1. Black carbon 2. Halons 3. Oxides of nitrogen

Select the correct answer using the code given below:

(a) 1 and 2 only (b) 2 only (c) 1 and 3 only (d) 1, 2 and 3

EXPLANATION

The main cause of ozone depletion and the ozone hole is manufactured chemicals, especially manufactured halocarbon refrigerants, solvents, propellants, and foam blowing agents (chlorofluoro carbons (CFCs), HCFCs, halons), referred to as **ozone depleting substances** (ODS).

Ans. (B) i.e., 2 only

2016

116. Consider the following statements:

1. All organochlorine pesticides (OCPs) enter the human bodies through food chain only.

2. Some of the OCPs are categorized as Persistent Organic Pollutants.

Which of the statements given above is/are correct?

(a) 1 only (b) 2 only (c) Both 1 and 2 (d) Neither 1 nor 2

EXPLANATION

Persistent organic pollutants (POPs) are organic compounds that are resistant to environmental degradation through chemical, biological, and photolytic processes. Because of their persistence, POPs bioaccumulate with potential adverse impacts on human health and the environment. Many POPs are currently or were in the past used as pesticides, solvents, pharmaceuticals, and industrial chemicals.

Ans. (B) i.e., 2 only

117. With reference to mercury pollution, which of the following statements are correct?

1. Once released into environment, mercury can turn into methyl mercury.

2. Mercury can enter the human body through inhalation.

3. As regards the entry and accumulation of mercury in humans, contaminated fish is an important source.

Select the correct answer using the code given below:

(a) 1 and 2 only (b) 2 and 3 only (c) 1 and 3 only (d) 1, 2 and 3

EXPLANATION

Mercury pollution

- Mercury occurs naturally in the earth's crust, but human activities, such as mining and fossil fuel combustion, have led to widespread global mercury pollution. Mercury emitted into the air eventually settles into water or onto land where it can be washed into water. Once deposited, certain microorganisms can change it into methylmercury, a highly toxic form that builds up in fish, shellfish and animals that eat fish.
- When metallic **mercury** vapors are **inhaled**, they readily **enter** the bloodstream and are carried **throughout** the **body** and **can** move into the brain. **Breathing in** or swallowing large amounts of methylmercury also results **in** some **of the mercury** moving into the brain and affecting the nervous system.

Ans. (D) i.e., 1, 2 and 3

118. Consider the following statements:

1. In India, the executive power of a State is vested in its Chief Minister.
2. Union Territories are administered by the President of India through an Administrator appointed by him.

Which of the statements given above is/are correct?

(a) 1 only (b) 2 only (c) Both 1 and 2 (d) Neither 1 nor 2

EXPLANATION

Administration of the Union Territories (Article 239)

- The **Union Territories are administered by the President through an administrator**, who is **appointed by him with** a suitable designation.
- This designation is called either Lieutenant Governor or Chief Commissioner or **Administrator.**

Ans. (B) i.e., 2 only

119. The quantity of water required to produce 1 kg of which of the following foods is largest?

(a) Barley (b) Mutton (c) Potato (d) Wheat

EXPLANATION

Typical values for the volume of water required to produce common foodstuffs

Foodstuff	Quantity	Water consumption, litres
Beef	**1 kg**	15,415
Sheep **Meat**	**1 kg**	10,412
Pork	**1 kg**	5,988
Butter	**1 kg**	5,553

Ans. (B) i.e., Mutton

120. What is 'CRISPR-Cas9' sometimes seen in the news?

(a) A targetted genome editing technique

(b) A cancer causing gene

(c) A robotic surgical procedure

(d) A technique of two dimensional electrophoresis

EXPLANATION

CRISPR is a family of DNA sequences in bacteria and archaea. The sequences contain snippets of DNA from viruses that have attacked the prokaryote. These snippets are used by the prokaryote to detect and destroy DNA from similar viruses during subsequent attacks. These sequences play a key role in a prokaryotic defense system, and form the basis of a technology known as **CRISPR/Cas9** that effectively and specifically changes genes within organisms.

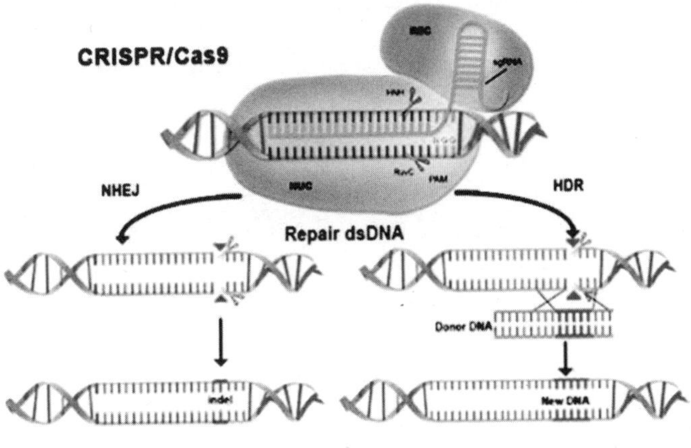

From Advanced Analytical.

Ans. (A) i.e., A targeted genome editing technique